Artificial Kidney,
Artificial Liver,
and Artificial Cells

Artificial Kidney, Artificial Liver, and Artificial Cells

Edited by
Thomas Ming Swi Chang, M.D., C.M., Ph.D., F. R.C. P. (C)

Professor of Physiology, Professor of Medicine
Associate, Medical Research Council of Canada
Director, Artificial Organs Research Unit
Faculty of Medicine, McGill University
Montreal, Quebec, Canada

Springer Science+Business Media, LLC

Library of Congress Cataloging in Publication Data

Main entry under title:

Artificial kidney, artificial liver, and artificial cells.
   Includes index.
   1. Hemodialysis—Congresses. 2. Artificial kidney—Congresses. 3. Artificial liver—
Congresses. I. Chang, Thomas Ming Swi. II. McGill University. Artificial Organs Re-
search Unit. [DNLM: 1. Perfusion—Congresses. 2. Kidney, Artificial—Congresses. 3.
Artificial organs—Congresses. 4. Liver—Congresses. 5. Membranes, Artificial—Con-
gresses. 6. Cells—Congresses. 7. Hemodialysis—Congresses. 8. Charcoal—Congresses.
WO665 A791 1977]

RC901.7.A7A74   617'.95   77-18738

ISBN 978-1-4684-2480-5   ISBN 978-1-4684-2478-2 (eBook)
DOI 10.1007/978-1-4684-2478-2

Proceedings of the McGill Artificial Organs Research Unit
International Symposium, McGill University, April 20, 1977

© 1978 Springer Science+Business Media New York
Originally published by Plenum Press, New York in 1978
Softcover reprint of the hardcover 1st edition 1978

A Division of Plenum Publishing Corporation
227 West 17th Street, New York, N.Y. 10011

Preface

There is a rapid increase in interest related to novel approaches in artificial kidneys, artificial liver, and detoxification. Recent research has included the successful clinical applications of the principle of artificial cells for adsorbent hemoperfusion. Since it is 20 years ago at McGill that the first report on "Artificial Cells" was presented, I thought it might be useful to get together a small group of speakers and participants for a day before the ASAIO meeting to discuss some recent advances in the area of the clinical applications of artificial kidney, artificial liver and artificial cells with emphasis on adsorbent hemoperfusion. However, the enthusiastic supports of distinguished speakers, session chairmen and participants were such that the original projection of 100 participants had expanded to a preregistration total of 250, from Australia, Canada, England, France, Germany, Israel, Italy, Japan, The Netherlands, Scotland, Sweden and U.S.A. The program also expanded to include a review section on hemodialysis, dialysate regeneration, hemofiltration, resin hemoperfusion and oxystarch given by their respective originators. The remaining of the symposium emphasizes the status of the art on different encapsulated adsorbent hemoperfusion approaches. I would like to apologize to those who we could not accommodate because of space limitations. It is hoped that this symposium volume may be useful for them and for others who are interested in this area.

Special thanks are due to Ms Joanne Toms for her excellent secretarial assistance for the conference and Mrs. Carol Fautrel for her help in the preparation of this volume; Dr. A. Chawla for organizing the audiovisual aspects; Professor F.C. MacIntosh for his suggestions in organizing the post conference special events; and the McGill Conferences and Special Events especially for organizing the reception and banquets. The members of the Artificial Organs Research Unit who have volunteered their help for this symposium included: M. Berman, Dr. A. Chawla, Dr. E. Chirito, G. Colantoni, Dr. J. Cousineau, Dr. J. Grunwald, C. Hayward, N. Kunterian, C. Lister, P. Nasielski, P. O'Keefe, Dr. B. Reiter, E. Resurreccion and J. Toms. Many thanks are due to my wife, Lancy, for preparing the index for this volume.

The research in this Unit has been enriched by past and present collaborators and members, especially: Dr. P. Barre, Mr. D. Cameron, Dr. J. Campbell, Dr. A. Chawla, Dr. E. Chirito, Dr. S. Chung, Dr. J. Coffey, Dr. C. Cole, Dr. J. Cousineau, Prof. J. Dirks, Mrs. P. Douglas, Dr. H. Duff, Mrs. C. Fautrel, Dr. A. Gonda, Dr. J. Grunwald, Dr. M. Habib, Mrs. C. Hayward, Mrs. M. Hewish, Mr. K. Holeczek, Mrs. L. Johnson, Mrs. N. Kunterian, Mrs. T. Lee-Burns, Mr. B. Lessor, Dr. M. Levy, Mr. C. Lister, Dr. K.S. Lo, Prof. F.C. MacIntosh, Mrs. N. Malave, Miss Celeste Malouf, Prof. S.G. Mason, Dr. M. McGoldrick, Miss M. Migchelsen, Mr. P. Nasielski, Dr. M. Poznansky, Dr. S. Prichard, Miss P. O'Keefe, Dr. B. Reiter, Mrs. E. Resurreccion, Dr. A. Rosenthal, Dr. J. Seely, Dr. E. Siu-Chong, Dr. A. Sniderman, Miss A. Stark, Miss J. Toms, Dr. P. Tung, Mrs. A. Versaza, Dr. B. Watson, and Miss W. Yensen. The support and encouragements in the past or at present in other ways by many others are also gratefully acknowledged, especially, Professor D. Bates, Professor J. Beck, Sir Arnold V.S. Bergen, Professor A. Burton, Professor R.F.P. Cronin, Professor O. Denstedt, Professor S. Freeman, Professor W. Kolff, Professor F.C. MacIntosh, Professor S.G. Mason, Professor G. Malcolm Brown, Professor M. McGregor, Professor R.J. Rossiter, Dr. P. Selkej and many others.

The collaboration of Plenum Publishing Corp. in agreeing to publish this symposium volume is appreciated.

The grant supports for this symposium from the following are gratefully acknowledged: Department of Physiology; McGill University Faculty of Medicine; McGill University Administration; Amicon Corp., U.S.A.; Becton & Dickenson Co., U.S.A.; Extracorporeal Medical Specialties Inc., U.S.A.; Gambro Dialysatoren GmH, Germany; and Warner Lambert Foundation, U.S.A.

The research of the Artificial Organs Research Unit is being supported by the Medical Research Council of Canada.

Thomas Ming Swi Chang

Contents

OTHER ADSORBENT HEMOPERFUSION APPROACHES

COMMUNICATIONS

ADDRESS OF WELCOME

L. Yaffe

Vice Principal, McGill University

Montreal, Quebec, Canada

I am very happy to welcome you here on behalf of Principal
Bell and the Board of Governors. McGill is extremely proud of its
Faculty of Medicine. McGill also prides itself on the fact that
it has a tradition of excellence. In these days of egalitarianism,
democratic society, etc., it is virtually considered elitist to be
excellent, but I think your presence here today at a conference
like this, shows that you yourselves are committed to this very
same principle of excellence. Without this, scholarship in any
discipline, especially in the sciences, could never survive. I
want to congratulate Professor Chang on attracting such a distinguished group of people but I also want to congratulate the audience
because when I took a look at the program and the length and content
of the program, I recognized that it would take a certain kind of
stamina to be able to endure this. I would be interested to see
what you look like at about 5:30 or 6:00 this afternoon. I know
you did not come here to hear me. You have a very long and a very
good program. May I wish you a great deal of success in this conference. Thank you very much.

INTRODUCTION

T.M.S. Chang

Artificial Organs Research Unit
McIntyre Medical Sciences Building
McGill University
Montreal, Quebec, Canada

HEMODIALYSIS

Introduction

In 1913, Abel et. al. demonstrated that using the principle of
hemodialysis, they were able to remove diffusible substances from
the circulating blood of rabbits. This principle of hemodialysis
remained as an experimental curiosity until about 30 years later
when Kolff successfully developed a hemodialyser that can be used
effectively for the treatment of patients with renal failure (Kolff,
1944, 1947, also in this volume). However, long-term maintenance
of patients was associated with the difficulty of repeated accesses
to the blood vessels. It took another 15 years for Scribner's group
(Quinton et. al., 1961) to develop the arteriovenous shunt which
makes it possible for long-term intermittant accesses to blood
vessels of patients. Since that time the use of hemodialysis for
the long-term maintenance of patients with chronic renal failure
has become an established procedure. At present there are many
patients who have been maintained alive for more than 10 years by
long-term hemodialysis. The standard hemodialysers are based on the
principle of, (1) dialysis for the removal of diffusible molecules
and (2) ultrafiltration for the removal of water and sodium chloride
(Fig. 1). Although hemodialysis has been conclusively demonstrated
to be effective for the maintenance of chronic renal failure patients
there are a number of problems related to its use. The major problems are related to the complexity and size of the machine and the
cost and time required for treatment (6–12 hours three times a week).

3

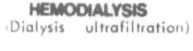

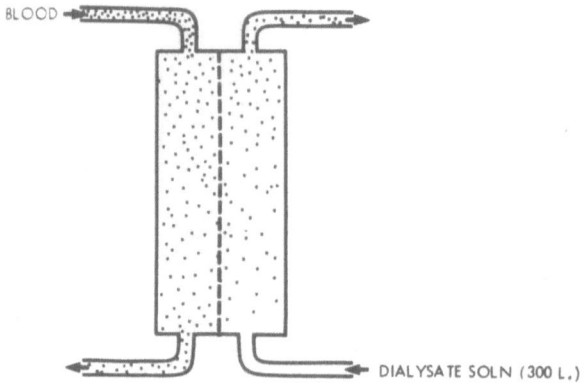

Figure 1

At present the exact type of toxic molecules that has to be removed
and the essential molecules which should not be removed still have
not been established. Hemodialysis though useful in treating some
form of drug intoxication (Maher and Schreiner, 1969) can be further
improved. The standard hemodialysers have not been demonstrated to
be effective for treating liver failure. A large amount of research
has therefore been carried out in the areas of artificial kidney,
artificial liver and detoxifiers. Most of the developments have
been related to the improvements, modificiations and extensions of
the principle of hemodialysis. Thus, the earlier developments involved the use of different membrane configurations in the form of
coils, plates, and capillaries. This has resulted in substantial
improvements in the membrane component of the hemodialysis machine.
A great deal of advance has also been made in the monitoring system.
The development of the internal AV fistula (Brescia et. al., 1966)
has overcome a number of the problems related to the external A-V
shunts. The single needle approach (Kopp et. al., 1972) has less-
ened problems related to needle puncture in internal AV fistula.

Dialysate Regeneration

One of the major problems of standard hemodialysis machine is

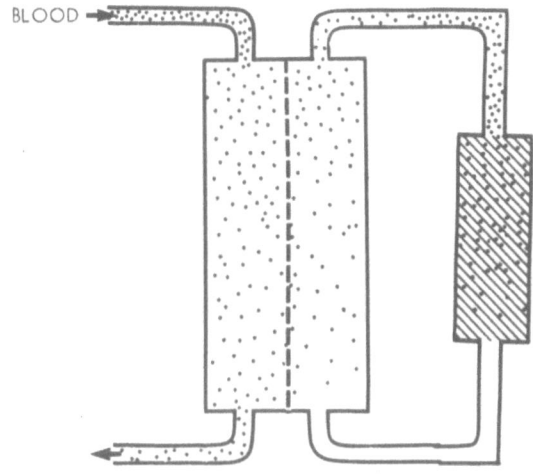

Figure 2

the dialysate required for removing uremic metabolites (Fig. 1).
Approximately 300 litres of fluid is required for each treatment.
This means that about 900 litres per week is required for the 3
times a week treatment. In addition to the very high cost of dialysate, there are other problems related to possible trace element
being absorbed by the patients from this large volume of fluid. The
principle of dialysate regeneration is a successful attempt to decrease the dialysate volume required by using sorbents in the dialysate fluid compartment to remove the uremic metabolites (Fig. 2)
(Gordon et. al., 1969, also in this volume). This principle has
been used for the construction of a "wearable artificial kidney"
(Kolff, in this volume).

Middle Molecules

The proposal that uremic toxins are molecules in the middle
molecular weight range(Babb et. al., 1972) has led to modifications
of hemodialysers. Thus the total membrane area has been increase to
facilitate the removal of these "middle molecules". Membranes with
high permeability to middle molecules (e.g. Rhone-Poulone) have
also been developed.

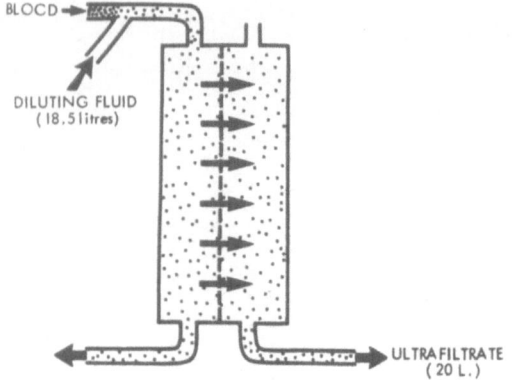

Figure 3

Hemofiltration

Another approach related to middle molecules is the use of the principle of hemofiltration whereby instead of using a combination of dialysis and ultrafiltration (Fig. 1) only ultrafiltration is used (Fig. 3) (Henderson et al., 1967; Henderson, in this volume). Hemofiltration (Fig. 3) is based on the principle that, unlike dialysis, permeant molecules of different molecular weight can move across a membrane at the same rate in ultrafiltration. This way, middle molecules can be removed as effectively as the smaller molecules. The ultrafiltrate removed has to be replaced very accurately with diluting solution in order not to deplete or overload the fluid volume of the patients.

Reviews

Some of these recent novel approaches related to new extension and modifications of hemodialysis will be reviewed by their originators.

ADSORBENTS

Many adsorbents like activated charcoal, oxystarch, ion-exchange resins, and others have been used. Activated charcoal is used in the dialysate regeneration system described above. It has also been used for hemoperfusion (Yatzidis, 1964) however, complications related to embolism and platelet depletion has prevented its clinical use as free granules for hemoperfusion. The use of oxystarch (Giordano, in this volume) and amberlite (Rosenbaum, in this volume) will be reviewed by their original proponents in this volume.

ARTIFICIAL CELLS

Introduction

With the thought that most of the novel approaches in artificial kidney have been extensions and modifications of hemodialysis;
and also with the thought that perhaps completely different approaches
may also contribute to the further development of artificial kidney,
artificial liver and detoxification, a new area of research was
started here. This involved investigations into the possible uses
of artificial cells (microencapsulation) as the basis for the construction of artificial liver, artificial kidney and detoxifier(Fig.4)
(Chang, 1964, 1966, 1972). The ultrathin membrane and the large
surface to volume relationship of artificial cells is such that a
very small volume of suspension allows for extremely high transport
rates of metabolites. Studies carried out to use enzyme systems in
the artificial cells for the removal and conversion of metabolites
have recently been reviewed in more detail elsewhere (Chang, 1977).

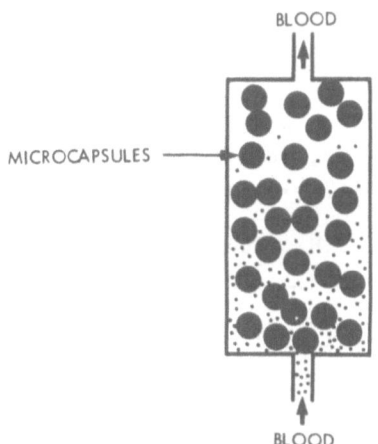

Figure 4

Microencapsulated Adsorbents

This volume reviews in some detail the use of artificial cells
or other extensions to encapsulate adsorbents for clinical applications as artificial kidneys, artificial livers, and detoxifiers.
Most centers working in this area at present have contributed to
this volume.

REFERENCES

Abel, J.J., Rowntree, L.G. and Turner, B.B. (1913). Trans. Assoc.
     Amer. Physicians, 28, 51.
Babb, A.L., Farrell, D.A., Uvelli, D.A. and Scribner, B.H. (1972).
     Trans. Amer. Soc. Artif. Intern. Organs, 13, 98.
Brescia, M.J., Crimino, J.E., Appel, K. and Hurwith, B.J. (1966).
     New England J. Med., 275, 1089.
Chang, T.M.S. (1964). Science, 146, 524.
Chang, T.M.S. (1966). Trans. Amer. Soc. Artif. Intern. Organs, 12,
     13.
Chang, T.M.S. (1972). Artificial Cells, Charles C. Thomas,
     Publisher, Springfield, Illinois.
Chang, T.M.S. (1977). Biomedical Application of Immobilized Enzymes
     and Proteins, Plenum Publishing Corp., New York. Volumes 1 & 2.
Giordano, C. In this volume.
Gordon, A., Greenbaum, M.A., Marantz, L.B., McArthur, M.H. and
     Maxwell, M.H. (1969). Trans. Amer. Soc. Artif. Intern. Organs,
     15, 347.
Gordon, A. In this volume.
Henderson, L.W., Besarab, A., Michaels, A.S. and Blume, L.W. (1967).
     Trans. Amer. Soc. Artif. Intern. Organs, 13, 216.
Henderson, L.W. In this volume.
Kolff, W.J. (1944). Acta. Med. Scand., 117, 121.
Kolff, W.J. (1947). "New Ways of Treating Uremia", J. & A. Churchill
     Ltd., London, U.K.
Kopp, K.F., Gutch, C.F. and Kolff, W.J. (1972). Trans. Amer. Soc.
     Artif. Intern. Organs, 18, 75.
Maher, J.E. and Schreiner, G.E. (1969). Trans. Amer. Soc. Artif.
     Intern. Organs, 15, 461.
Quinton, W.E., Dillard, D.H., Cole, J.J. and Scribner, B.H. (1961).
     Trans. Amer. Soc. Artif. Intern. Organs, 7, 60.
Rosenbaum, J. In this volume.
Yatzidis, D. (1964). Pro. Eur. Dial. Transpl. Assoc., 1, 83.

REVIEWS OF HEMODIALYSIS, DIALYSATE REGENERATION,

HEMOFILTRATION AND OXYSTARCH

THE PRESENT STATUS AND PERSPECTIVES OF HEMODIALYSIS

HONOURED GUEST LECTURE

W. J. Kolff, M.D., Ph.D.

Institute for Biomedical Engineering
University of Utah
Salt Lake City, Utah 84112, U.S.A.

     I accepted this invitation to speak to you only because I have
so much admiration for the work of Dr. Chang. Figure 1 shows the
City of Kampen in The Netherlands, which was about as large
(23,000 inhabitants) when I worked there during the war as it was on
the slide made from a gravure anno 1495. We did not go to the
movies for 5 years during the German occupation, so we had nothing
better to do than to make artificial kidneys. Here are some of these
artificial kidneys (Figure 2), wooden drums, because other material
could not be obtained. Later, after World War II one of these
kidneys was sent to the Royal Victoria Hospital in Montreal so that
les Canadiens and the Canadians would both be treated with hemodialysis. This rotating drum rotates slowly, and as a result, blood
in the cellophane tubing which is wrapped around the drum tends to
go down by gravity. As the drum turns, the blood will continuously
go down and run through the 20 metres of cellophane tubing from one
end of the drum to the other. The principle involved is that both
the dialyzing fluid which is in the tank, and the blood in the cellophane tubing are continuously moving. I feel that in some of the
sorption devices, if you would have a better movement of either the
dialysate or the blood through the sorbent, you would also get a
much higher yield. Maybe the Italian oxystarch would work a little
better if it were continuously moved and dispersed through the
material you want to purify.

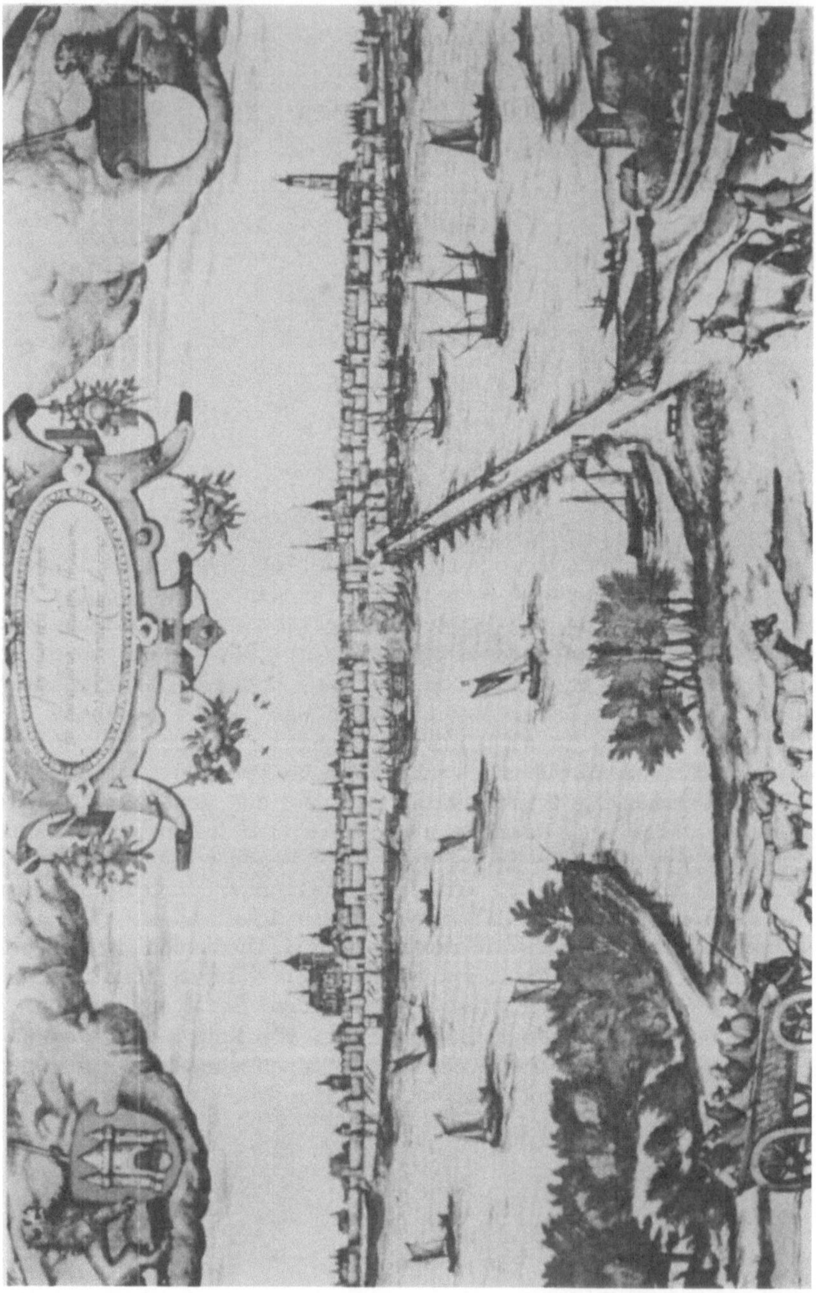

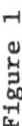

Figure 1

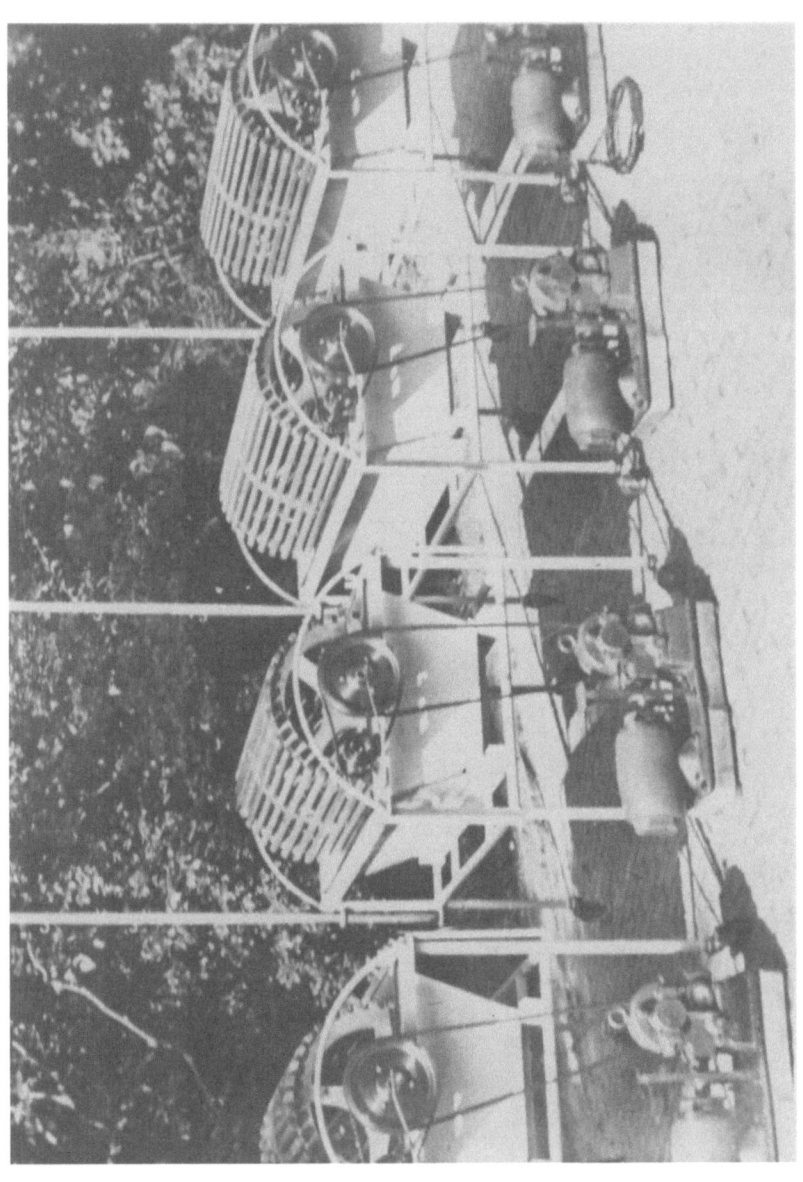

Figure 2

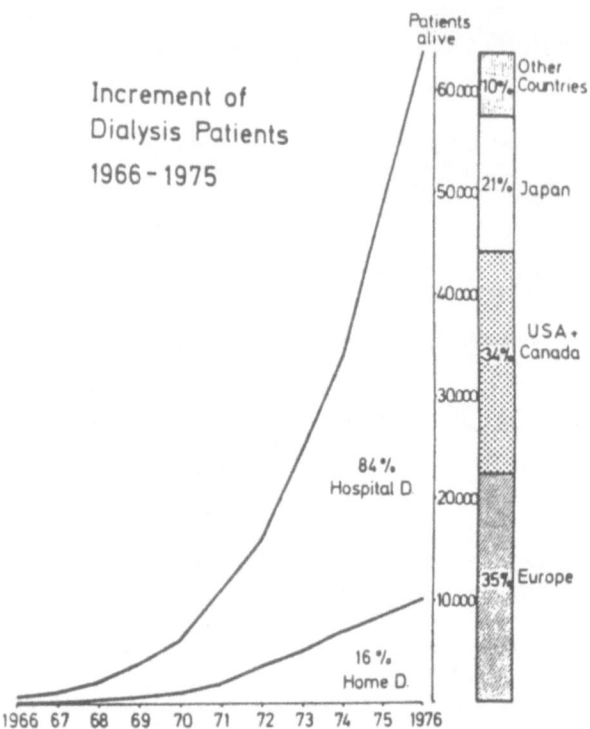

Figure 3

Figure 3 was received from Dr. Gurland; it is taken from EDTA 1976.
You see the exponential rise of the number of patients treated with
the artificial kidney, and the very slow rise and relative
decrease in the patients treated with home dialysis. I think this
is a great shame and that we should try to go back to more home
dialysis, not only to save costs, but also because it makes more
complete rehabilitation possible. (You can obviously not do home
dialysis if there is no home.) One of the means to promote home
dialysis is to make the machines more portable. Some years ago this
field was quite dead, but now it is very much alive. We are presently engaged in making:

A Wearable Artificial Kidney (WAK),

A Wearable Filtration Artificial Kidney (FAK),

A Wearable Peritoneal Artificial Kidney (PAK),

A Hemoperfusion Artificial Kidney (HAK).

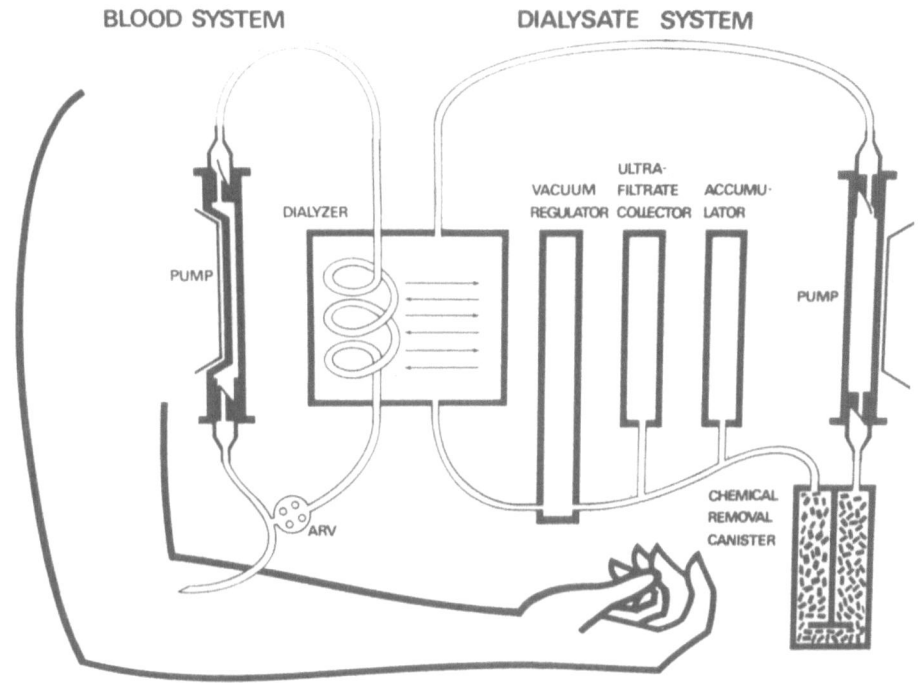

Figure 4

Here you see Figure 4, the diagram of the WAK, the Wearable
Artificial Kidney. I would like to point out that we have usually
championed a single needle dialysis where the blood goes in and out
through the same lumen. The only place where it goes back and forth
is in the needle. It is possible both in this country and in Germany
to buy needles that have a double lumen. In the WAK the blood compartment of the dialyser, and the dialyzing fluid circulates around
adsorbents. Since we do not have the ideal adsorbent for urea yet,
we also use a 20 litre tank. I think it's not that despicable. It
has some very good advantages. If there are minor changes in the
electrolyte content of the patient, the 20 litre tank will take care
of it. Also with a 20 litre tank, you do not have to go through
the cost of reverse osmosis equipment which is quite expensive. Unless you leave the sodium chloride completely out of the dialysate,
if you make errors in the composition of the solutes, with a 20 litre
tank it is not immediately deadly. I would like to stress that the

patient does not have to be connected with the 20 litre tank all the time - he can go for a walk for 15 minutes and provided that he hooks himself on again, there is no penalty in terms of a longer dialysis that day.

The REDY system guides the dialyzing fluid over a column with urease, zirconium compounds, and charcoal. I wonder about the wisdom of having phosphate binder in it. I think the sudden decrease in phosphate content of the blood tends to confuse the parathyroids and I think I would leave it out. The Wearable Artificial Kidney weighs about 6 to 8 pounds.

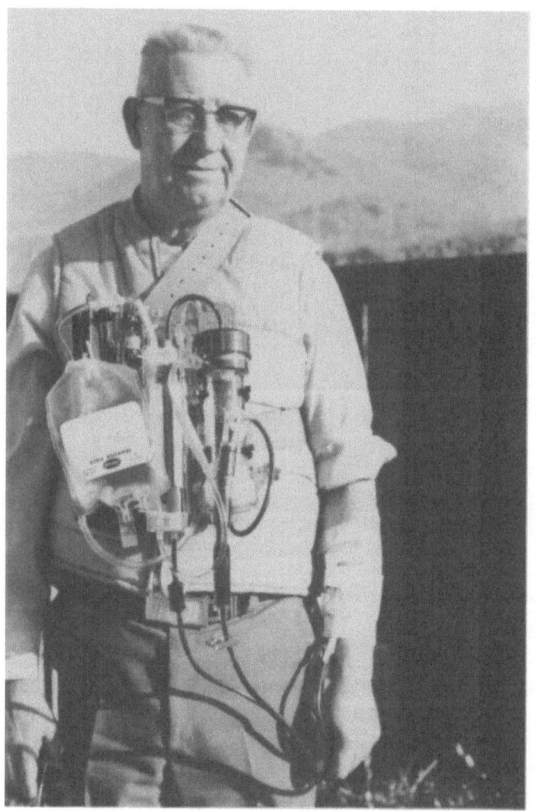

Figure 5

Figure 5 shows a patient wearing this Artificial Kidney. The Wearable Artificial Kidney can be put on top of a 20 litre tank. This has the advantage that the patient does not have to wear it when he sits at his desk or at the dinner table. But if the door bell rings

- all he has to do is disconnect the dialyzing fluid tubing from the
20 litre tank and then he can open the door, let in the dog, welcome
the children, etc.

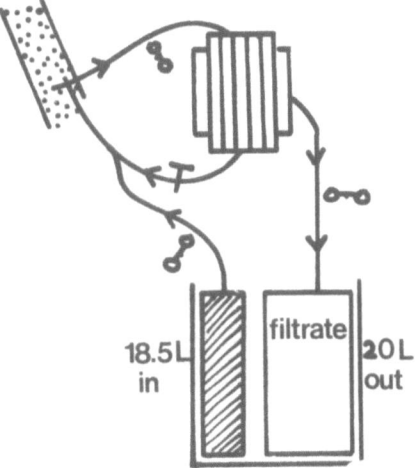

Figure No. 6.   FAK - 1977

Figure 6 is the FAK (Filtration Artificial Kidney.) You have
heard from Dr. Henderson that it removes the middle molecules at the
same clearance as the smaller molecules. You can put a screw clamp
on your blood lines to increase the pressure and you can also apply
suction on the dialysis fluid compartment so that you get a high
gradient. By the way, our WAK can do both, and the WAK can be used
for ultrafiltration.

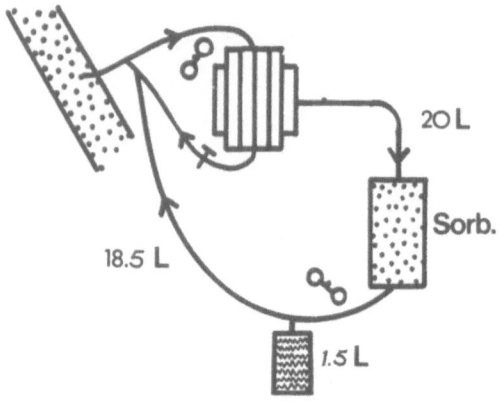

Figure 7. FAK - 1980

      The Germans have a 20 litre bath of infusion fluid roughly
equivalent to our usual dialyzing fluid and while the ultrafiltrate
accumulates on one side of a membranous septum, fluid is reinfused
into the patient. They also reinfuse only 18.5 litres and remove
20 litres. This 20 litre for the size of the tank is a magic figure.
I'm sure it was independently derived from the fact that 20 litres
also seems to be enough for our WAK. The Germans state that they
can remove ultrafiltrate from patients without causing shock and
also confirm that you can reduce blood pressure if it is too high.

      Figure 7 - is the FAK as I think it will be in 1980. In other
words, you should regenerate your ultrafiltrate over charcoal and
perhaps other substances, and if you remove 20 litres you will
reinfuse 18.5 litres into the patient.

      Figure 8 - brings me to the PAK. (Wearable Peritoneal Lavage
Kidney). We believe strongly that you should have a closed system
and I fully agree with Dr. Gordon that the future for wearable
systems should be a Wearable Peritoneal Dialysis System, but it
should be a closed system. You begin by putting 2 litres of fluid
in the abdominal cavity (which most people can take) and then you
exchange about 600 ml at a time, in and out of the body. To do that
practically, we have a "mouse."

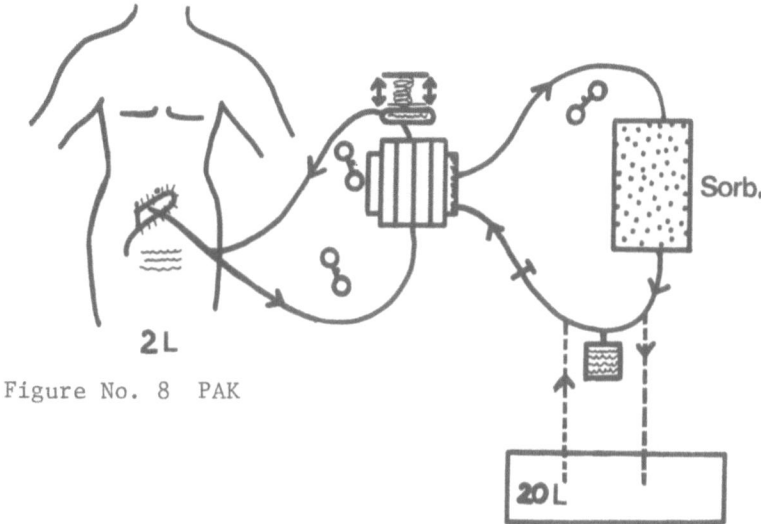

Figure No. 8 PAK

Figure 9 - A good "mouse" has a hairy body, is hollow, and it has
a tail which hangs in the peritoneal cavity so you can get access to
the peritoneal cavity by sticking the needle in the "mouse." You
take the needle out when you do not dialyze and the puncture will
reseal itself. The rest of the system is exactly the same as our
Wearable Artificial Kidney, and one could use the same pumps, etc.
Here too we have the 20 litre bath and a charcoal cannister. You
can disconnect the dialysate from the 20 litre tank and go for a
walk. This "mouse" has two tails. You can use it with two valves
in it so you have unidirectional flow, but in our later experience,
it seems that 1/2 of a "mouse" with only one tail is quite sufficient.
We have the same adsorbing systems as in the WAK.

Fig.10 is the HAK (Hemoperfusion Artificial Kidney) with the
charcoal hemoperfusion as we use it now. It can also be used with
a gel in series with the charcoal. This gel when started in a dry
form, could absorb about 1.5 litres of fluid, and of course, with
this 1.5 litres of fluid it would also absorb all the electrolytes
including sodium that are present in the 1.5 litre blood plasma
water. That is about as much as we remove otherwise by dialysis.

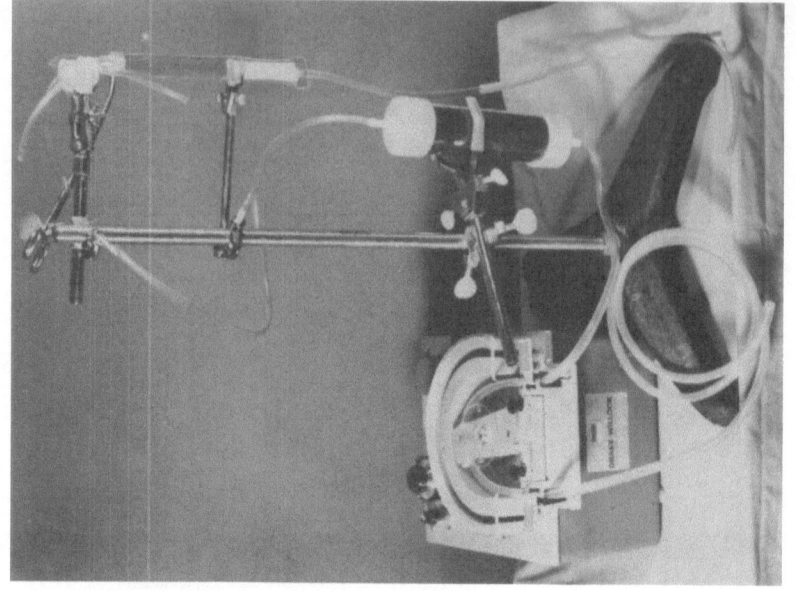

Figure No. 10

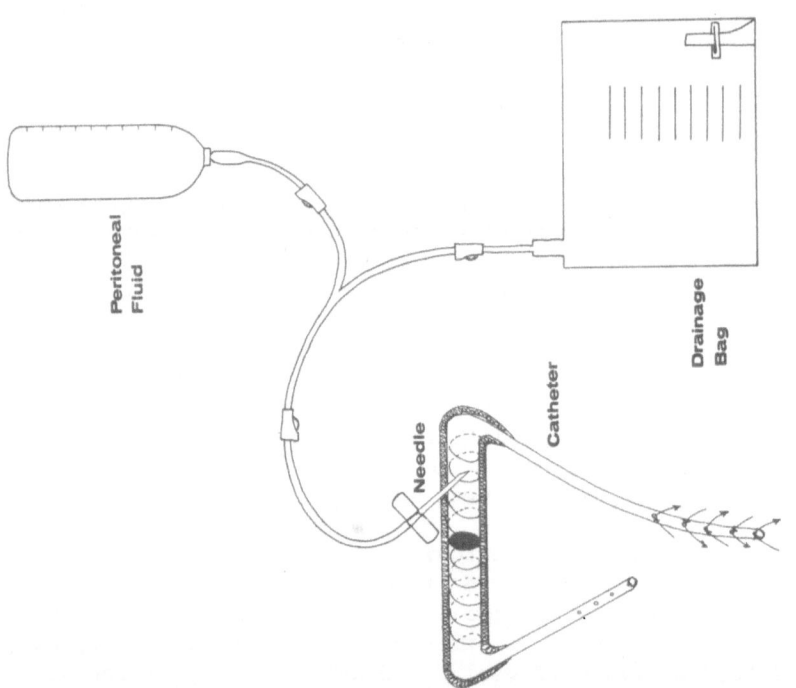

Figure No. 9

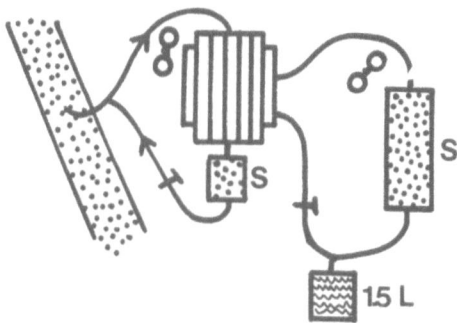

Figure 11:   WAK-HAK 1980

     Figure 11 is a combination of the WAK and the HAK. You have
·the regular volume of sorbents for the dialysing fluid in the WAK
and a much smaller volume for the HAK. The HAK part will adsorb
directly from the blood and will remove large and middle molecules.
Remember that their number is small. The WAK-HAK using ordinary
cellophane in the WAK part should be able to compete with the
Filtration Artificial Kidneys (FAK's) that use highly permeable
membranes such as Rhone Poulenc-6 which uses polyacrylonitrile.

     You recall the biblical story where Lot was allowed to leave
the doomed cities of Sodom and Gomorrah provided he would not look
back. His wife couldn't resist the temptation, looked back and was
changed into a column of urea. What we are really aiming for is the
kind of a system that you see here where the flamingos are standing
in a shallow pond, fertilizing it all the time. In the resulting
media a culture of bacteria converts urea to amino acid, and it is
very palatable, at least to the flamingos. This kind of system
still uses the kidneys of the flamingo; it is not quite perfect, so
we have a look at how the cow does it. It has a wonderful collection of bacteria and protozoa in its rumen which can take cellulose
and urea and build it up to very palatable amino acids and other
useful substances. We should adapt this kind of a system. Dr.
Bryant can do this. You could have your own grown yogurt like
bacterial culture that would adsorb the urea, send the amino acids
back, and what you don't need you could empty in the bathroom. 500 ml
of bacteria would be sufficient to remove 20 gm of urea per 24 hours.
If you don't like the idea of the cow, why not have the termites on
your side and do the same thing. There's only one thing wrong with
it, and that is termites eat wood and probably would eat through the
cellulose tubing. So, you should build a special house for the
termites.

CURRENT STATUS OF DIALYSATE REGENERATION FOR THE TREATMENT OF CHRONIC UREMIA

Arthur Gordon, M.D., Andrew J. Lewin, M.D., Morton H. Maxwell, M.D. and Martin Roberts, Ph.D.

Cedars-Sinai Medical Center
8700 Beverly Blvd., Los Angeles, California 90048

The removal of uremic solutes from dialysate by chemical compounds with adsorptive capacity provides a methodology for achieving a major reduction in the volume of dialysate necessary for conducting effective dialysis. Sorbent regeneration of dialysate permits a system with a small volume of recirculating dialysate to maintain maximal blood to dialysate concentration gradients and to potentially achieve mass transfer efficiency equal to that of a large volume recirculating or single pass dialysate flow system. Activated carbon, by virtue of its ability to adsorb organic nitrogenous compounds has served as the basic component of virtually all sorbent systems applied to the treatment of uremia. Yatzidis(1) demonstrated that activated carbon could adsorb creatinine, uric acid, phenols, indolic compounds, guanidines and organic acids. The adsorption of endogenous uremic metabolites of middle molecular weight configuration has also been demonstrated and there is presumptive clinical evidence derived from patients treated with sorbent systems that activated carbon probably adsorbs all organic uremic metabolites, known or as yet unidentified, which are of toxic significance(2-4). Unfortunately, there is one exception to this remarkable affinity of carbon for nitrogenous uremic metabolites. Urea proves to be a relatively unreactive molecule and at physiologic ranges of pH and temperature is only poorly adsorbed by activated carbon. Although direct evidence for urea toxicity may be limited, there are few who deny the need for any system of end stage renal disease to provide for a rate of urea removal approximating or exceeding its generation rate.

Table 1 lists the various investigators who have clinically or experimentally evaluated various systems for dialysate regeneration. All are based primarily on the use of activated carbon to remove

23

dialyzed uremic metabolites from dialysate. They vary, however,
in the approaches used to achieve adequate urea removal.

TABLE I

METHODS FOR UREA REMOVAL IN SORBENT BASED
DIALYSATE REGENERATION SYSTEMS

1. Dialysis
   Sparks, Blaney and Lindan
   Kolobow and Dedrick
   Twiss and Paulssen
   Jutzler, et al
   Maeda, et al
   Malchesky, Surovy and Nosé
   Kolff, et al

2. Cold charcoal adsorption
   Giordano, Esposito and Bello

3. Oxycellulose adsorption
   Giordano, et al

4. Sulfonated polystyrene adsorption
   Hydén

5. Urease hydrolysis
   Gordon, et al

The early attempts at augmentation of dialysate by activated carbon
recognized the potential for sorbent regeneration to reduce dialysate
volumes to quantities capable of functioning as a wearable system
but were thwarted by the inability to adsorb urea(5-9). Maeda, et
al, utilizing a system of 500 gms of activated charcoal and 200 gms
of alumina (to provide for phosphate adsorption), effect urea removal by using dialysate volumes of 30 liters or 10 liters(10).
Although urea removal is reduced in comparison to standard dialysis
systems, clinical results have been satisfactory and, for reasons
not yet clearly defined, predialysis BUN gradually decreased over a
period of months to mean pre-dialysis levels of 60-70 mg per cent.
A similar system termed the charcoal-coil has received preliminary
in vitro evaluation by Malchesky et al(11). Efficiency for creatinine, uric acid and phosphate were comparable to standard coil dialyses but urea removal was less efficient and related to the dialysate volume used and its relationship to the initial urea body pool
volume. Kolff and his associates(12) have developed, described and
clinically used a wearable artificial kidney (WAK) utilizing charcoal regeneration of dialysate. This device is cleverly designed so

that a single battery operated pump propels both blood and dialysate
and a special system of valves permits unidirectional flow and ultrafiltration. Unfortunately, the need to remove urea and potassium
and maintain fluid and electrolyte balance requires the use of a 20
liter dialysate tank in conjunction with this system. When this
dialysate is changed midway through a dialyses of 4 to 5 hours duration, biochemical and clinical results are comparable to those
obtained with standard dialyses methods of equal duration. Total
urea removal of 28-38 grams can be achieved in this manner. The
need for the 20 liter dialysate reservoir prevents this system from
being truly wearable. However, it does demonstrate that mechanically
a wearable artificial kidney configuration is attainable.

Giordano, et al(13), taking note of the fact that urea adsorption by carbon is a physical type of binding and, therefore, subject
to being altered by thermal changes, have demonstrated that urea
adsorption on charcoal, maximally 4 gms/kg charcoal at 37^oC, could
be increased to 15 gms/kg charcoal at 1^oC and potentially to a maximum capacity of 33.8 gms/kg charcoal at BUN concentrations of 140
mg%, and using multiple charcoal minicartridges. They have confirmed these considerations with in vitro studies using a cold charcoal depurator system in which adsorption on charcoal takes place
at $0-1^oC$ and dialysate is then rewarmed to $37-40^oC$ as it returns to
the dialysis compartment. In addition they have demonstrated that
urea can be desorbed from charcoal at a temperature of 85^oC and pos-
tulate the potential development of a "cold trap-warm release" adsorption process which would have the advantage of functioning with
relatively small amounts of charcoal. Clinical testing of these
systems and concepts have not yet been reported.

Giordano, et al(14), having previously demonstrated the capacity of oxystarch to adsorb urea and ammonia, have developed an
insoluble form by treatment with periodic acid to produce oxycellulose. Insoluble oxycellulose also binds urea and ammonia and its
potential for dialysate regeneration has been studied. Affinity
for urea adsorption can be enhanced by simple water pretreatment,
further enhanced by pretreatment with alkali and maximally enhanced
by heating to 60^oC. As much as 16 gms of urea/kg oxycellulose
could be adsorbed in simulated dialysis experiments. This system
too has not yet received clinical trial.

Most recently, Hydén(15) has reported on a highly crosslinked
sulfonated polystyrene compound in hydrogen form, 200 gms of which
have the capacity to adsorb more than 40 gms of urea. This resin,
in combination with activated charcoal, is currently being subjected
to initial clinical trial as a means for regenerating dialysate.

The largest clinical experience to date with a sorbent system
for dialysate regeneration has been achieved with the REDY Ⓡ

system which achieves urea removal by enzymatic hydrolyses with
urease. The ammonium ion derived from this reaction is adsorbed
by zirconium phosphate, a cation exchange resin, which also adsorbs
potassium and divalent cations in exchange for hydrogen and sodium
ions. The hydrogen ion combines with carbonate derived from the
urea to form bicarbonate. Modification of the initial dialysate
sodium concentration permits adaptation for the sodium added to the
dialysate. Hydrated zirconium oxide, an anion exchange resin provides for phosphate adsorption in exchange for either chloride or
acetate, depending upon preparation and pretreatment of the zirconium oxide. Activated carbon completes the sorbent components of the
system. An infusion system is required to reconstitute the calcium
and magnesium composition of the dialysate and to maintain dialysate
potassium levels at prescribed levels. Infusion of these cations
as acetate salts provides additional buffering capacity. Although
this system has functioned with total dialysate volumes as low as
one to 1.5 liters, as currently designed it utilizes 5.5 liters of
dialysate to permit its use with all types of dialyzers. This
larger dialysate volume also provides more buffer and greater capacity to accept the sodium ions derived from the zirconium phosphate. The dialysate is maintained free of all uremic nitrogenous
waste products, including urea and ammonium. Each sorbent cartridge
has the capacity to adsorb the ammonium derived from 48 grams of
urea. Clinical experience with the REDY(R) system has shown clinical and biochemical results closely paralleling those of conventional dialyses methods(16). The use of dialysate flow rates of
200 ml/min reduces the efficiency of mass transfer of low molecular
weight solutes by 10-15 per cent and in any given patient may account for pre-dialysis urea and creatinine levels correspondingly
higher than seen with standard systems using dialysate flow rates
of 500 ml/min or more. Similarly, the rate of acetate transfer
into the patient is reduced and in certain patients this may contribute to mild to moderate pre-dialysis acidosis. This has been
largely overcome by changing the zirconium oxide from the chloride
to the acetated form, thereby providing higher dialysate acetate
concentrations. Similar results have been obtained when standard
dialyses systems are operated at dialysate flow rates of 200 ml/min
(17,18). Despite this reduced efficiency of low molecular weight
solute transfer, the suggestion has been made that a dialysate flow
rate of 200 ml/min is not only acceptable but perhaps preferable.
Recent clinical studies indicate that dialysate flow rates of the
REDY(R) system can be raised to 300 ml/min with further augmentation in capacity to correct acidosis. With the REDY(R) system,
less acetate influx is required for acidosis correction since less
bicarbonate is dialyzed from the patient because dialysate bicarbonate concentrations of 10-20 meq/L are maintained in the dialysate.
Recent evidence that bicarbonate as a buffer is preferable to
acetate has led to preliminary studies for using the REDY with bicarbonate rather than acetate as the principle buffer. This is
possible since the high dialysate pCO_2 of the REDY(R) system permits

TABLE II

COMPARISON OF PREDIALYSIS PATIENT CHEMISTRIES WITH REDY^(R) AND SINGLE PASS (SP) DIALYSIS

Serum Urea Nitrogen mg%

    REDY   84 $\pm$ 20
    SP   84 $\pm$ 19

Creatinine mg%

    REDY   11.8 $\pm$ 3.1
    SP   14.4 $\pm$ 4.0

Hematocrit vol%
    REDY   24.6 $\pm$ 5.0
    SP   23.4 $\pm$ 6.7

Sodium mEq/L
    REDY   141 $\pm$ 3.1
    SP   141 $\pm$ 3.7

Potassium mEq/L
    REDY   4.9 $\pm$ 0.5
    SP   5.2 $\pm$ 0.6

Calcium mg%
    REDY   9.2 $\pm$ 1.2
    SP   9.1 $\pm$ 0.9

Magnesium mEq/L
    REDY   2.3 $\pm$ 0.5
    SP   2.7 $\pm$ 0.8

Chloride mEq/L
    REDY   102 $\pm$ 5.9
    SP   103 $\pm$ 4.8

Phosphorous mg%
    REDY   5.2 $\pm$ 1.5
    SP   5.2 $\pm$ 1.1

Bicarbonate mEq/L
    REDY   17.8 $\pm$ 3.7
    SP   19.8 $\pm$ 1.8

carbonate and bicarbonate salts to remain in solution. Although
some adsorption of bicarbonate by zirconium oxide occurs, significant dialysate concentrations of bicarbonate result and bicarbonate
loss by the patient can be minimized and in certain instances bicarbonate is dialyzed into the patient(19).

Since uremic toxins remain undefined and the possibility
exists that unknown or undetectable uremic toxins may escape adsorption, since the REDY(R) system represents such a major depart-
ure from conventional techniques and since there is the possibility
that toxic contaminants might derive from the sorbents (the sorbents
themselves are insoluble) or from sorbent-solute interactions, the
ultimate test of the REDY(R) system must lie in the clinical results
obtained with long term use. Of 45 patients dialyzed with the REDY
for a period of one to $3\frac{1}{2}$ years, seven have died for an overall
mortality of 15 per cent and yearly mortalities ranging from 5 to
14 per cent. All deaths were due to cardiovascular disease and
occurred in patients ranging in age from 55 to 72 years with the
exception of one diabetic, aged 40. These mortality rates are comparable to those reported for standard dialysis methods. Twenty-
one patients have now been dialyzed with the REDY for periods of
two to four years. Table II compares the predialysis chemistries
of these patients with a matched group of patients on standard single
pass dialysis. There are no significant differences except for the
lower bicoarbonate concentrations in the REDY patients. This difference, however, has been minimized since a change to the acetated
form of zirconium oxide which has resulted in an average predialysis
bicarbonate concentration of 18.5 meq/L. No unusual clinical syn-
dromes or evidence of toxicity has been noted. One patient did
develop an apparent dialysis dementia syndrome.

These successful clinical results with the REDY(R) system
validate the concept of sorbent regeneration of dialysate and demonstrate that the requirements of such a system as listed on
Table III are capable of being met. In its present state the system offers the advantages of portability, independence from fixed
sources of large volumes of water requiring treatment for purification and the ability to accurately and continuously monitor the
rate and volume of ultrafiltrate removal. Unfortunately, the quantities of sorbent required and the need for reinfusion of divalent
cations obviates the use of the REDY sorbents in a simple wearable
hemodialysis system. Although Kolff, et al(12) have demonstrated
that a wearable artificial kidney is potentially achievable, the
need for repeated access to the circulation, for extracorporeal
circulation and for anticoagulation makes ambulatory hemodialysis
a complex undertaking.

Such restraints do not exist for peritoneal dialysis and
accordingly we have evaluated the potential for development of an
ambulatory peritoneal dialyses system utilizing regeneration by the

sorbents of the REDY (R) system to reduce dialysate volumes to wearable quantities(16). Sterilization of the system has been achieved
with gamma radiation and a system of filters has been shown to be
capable of maintaining the dialysate free of significant particulate
matter contamination. The adsorption of glucose by the activated
carbon is limited, allowing maintenance of desired peritoneal dialysate glucose concentrations. Furthermore, glucose adsorption
does not impair adsorption of other solutes. As with the hemodialyses system, the sorbents maintain the dialysate free of dialyzed
uremic solutes and biochemical efficiency equivalent to that achieved
with conventional peritoneal dialyses has been obtained in clinical
peritoneal dialyses with dialysate volumes as low as four liters.
Efficiency of dialysis can be augmented by increasing recirculating
dialysate flow rates(20-22). Unfortunately, large scale clinical
testing of this system has been hampered to date by the occurrence
of reversible sterile and bacterial peritonitis. If this problem
can be overcome, an ambulatory peritoneal dialysis system based on
sorbent dialysate regeneration seems a realistic goal, especially
if the technique for equilibrium peritoneal dialysis requiring an
exchange of only ten to twelve liters of peritoneal dialysate daily
proposed by Popovich, et al(23) is validated.

TABLE III

REQUIREMENTS OF A DIALYSATE REGENERATION SYSTEM

1. Removal of all uremic solutes of
   potential toxic significance

2. Provide for correction of fluid and
   electrolyte abnormalities

3. Provide for correction of acid-base
   abnormalities

4. Removal of dialysate contaminants

5. Add no toxic contaminants to dialysate

6. Offer significant advantages

The methodology for sorbent regeneration of peritoneal dialysate, especially those aspects relating to sterility and exclusion
of particulate matter are also potentially applicable to regeneration of the large volumes of ultrafiltrate derived by the various
methods of diafiltration. This technique is receiving increasing
attention and it is readily apparent that it can be simplified
appreciably and the large volumes of reconstituting fluid virtually
eliminated by sorbent regeneration of the ultrafiltrate. No studies
have yet been reported of sorbent regeneration of diafiltrate.

Current techniques of dialysate regeneration have permitted
the development of truly portable dialysis systems and have laid
the foundation for the potential future development of wearable
artificial kidney systems. They have the capacity to enhance the
efficiency of peritoneal dialysis and simplify the methodology for
diafiltration. The need to utilize indirect methods for urea removal limit the simplicity and flexibility of regeneration systems but
it is to be hoped that increasing interest in sorbent applications
to uremia therapy will soon result in the development of new sorbent
agents and technology.

BIBLIOGRAPHY

1. Yatzidis, H. A convenient hemoperfusion microapparatus over
    charcoal for the treatment of endogenous and exogenous intoxi-
    cation. Its use as an effective artificial kidney. Proc Eur
    Dial Transpl Assoc 1,83,1964

2. Chang, T.M.S., Migchelsen, M., Coffey, J.F. and Stark, R.
    Serum middle molecule levels in uremia during long-term inter-
    mittent hemoperfusion with the ACAC (coated charcoal) micro-
    capsule artificial kidney. Trans Amer Soc Artif Int Organs
    20-A,364,1974

3. Gordon, A., Lewin, A., Rosenfeld, J., et al. Adsorption of
    uremic toxins. Proc. 6th Int. Congr. Nephrol., Florence, 1975,
    pp. 612-7, (Karger,Basel,1976)

4. Yatzidis, H., Psimenos, G. and Mayopoulou-Symvolidis, D. Non-
    dialysable toxic factor in uremic blood effectively removed by
    the activated charcoal. Experientia 25,1144,1969

5. Sparks, R.E., Blaney, J.L. and Lindan, O. Adsorption of nitro-
    genous waste metabolites from artificial kidney dialyzing
    fluids. Chem Engr Prog Symp Series 62,2,1966

6. Blaney, J.L., Lindan, O. and Sparks, R.E. Adsorption - a step
    toward a wearable artificial kidney. Trans Amer Soc Artif Int
    Organs 12,7,1966

7. Kolobow, J. and Dedrick, R.L. Dialysate capacity augmentation
    at ultra-low flow rates with activated carbon slurry. Trans
    Amer Soc Artif Int Organs 12,1,1966

8. Twiss, E.E. and Paulssen, M.M.P. Dialysis system incorporating
    the use of activated charcoal. Proc Eur Dial Transpl Assoc
    3,262,1966

9. Jutzler, G.A., Keller, H.E., Klein, J., et al. Physico-
    chemical investigations in regeneration of dialyzing fluid
    Proc Eur Dial Transpl Assoc 3,265,1966

10. Maeda, K., Ohta, K., Manji, T., et al. Dialysate regeneration:
    30 liter dialysate supply system with sorbents. Kidney Int 10
    (Suppl.7),S-289,1976

11. Malchesky, P.S., Surovy, R.M. and Nosé, Y. The charcoal coil:
    A dialysis-dialysate regeneration system. Kidney Int 10 (Suppl.
    7),S-296,1976

12. Kolff, W.J., Jacobsen, S., Stephen, R.L. and Rose, D. Towards
    a wearable artificial kidney. Kidney Int 10, (Suppl.7),S-300,
    1976

13. Giordano, C., Esposito, R. and Bello, P. A cold charcoal
    depurator for the adsorption of high quantities of urea.
    Kidney Int 10 (Suppl.7),S-284,1976

14. Giordano, C., Esposito, R., Pluvio, M. and Gonzalez, F. Oxy-
    celluloses: A group of sorbents to remove extracorporeal urea.
    Kidney Int (Suppl.7),S-348,1976

15. Hydén, H. Compact low volume self-regenerating artificial
    kidney. Presented at 10th Annual Contractor's Conf. NIAMDD.
    Jan. 17-19,1977,Bethesda, Md.

16. Gordon, A., Lewin, A., Marantz, L.B. and Maxwell, M.H. Sorbent
    regeneration of dialysate. Kidney Int 10, (Suppl.7)S-277,1976

17. Christopher, T.G., Cambi, V., Harker, L.A., et al. A study
    of hemodialysis with lowered dialysate flow rate. Trans Amer
    Soc Artif Int Organs 17,92,1971

18. Wathen, R.L., Shapiro, F.L., Comty, C.M. and Keshaviah, P.
    Low flow dialysate study. Presented at 10th Annual Contractor's
    Conf. NIAMDD. Jan. 17-19,1977,Bethesda, Md.

19. Gentile, D. Use of bicarbonate in dialysate of the sorbent
    delivery system. Abstract submitted to Amer. Soc. Artif. Int.
    Organs,1977

20. Raja, R.M., Kramer, M.S. and Rosenbaum, J.L. Recirculation
    peritoneal dialysis with sorbent REDY cartridge. Nephron 16,
    134,1976

21. Gordon, A., Lewin, A.J., Maxwell, M.H. and Morales, N.D.
    Augmentation of efficiency by continuous flow sorbent regenera-
    tion peritoneal dialysis. Trans Amer Soc Artif Int Organs

22,599,1976

22.   Stephen, R.L., Atkin-Thor, E. and Kolff, W.J.   Recirculating
      peritoneal dialysis with subcutaneous catheter.   Trans Amer
      Soc Artif Int Organs 22,575,1976

23.   Popovich, R.P., Moncrief, J.W., Decherd, J.F., et al.   Clinical
      development of the low dialyses clearance hypothesis via equi-
      librium peritoneal dialyses.   Presented at 10th Annual Con-
      tractor's Conf., NIAMDD. Jan. 17-19,1977,Bethesda, Md.

DEVISING A PRACTICAL SUITCASE HEMODIALYZER

Eli A. Friedman, James T. Hutchisson, Robert S.
Galonsky and Richard L. Hessert

Department of Medicine, Downstate Medical Center
450 Clarkson Avenue, Brooklyn, New York 11203

Following Kolff's invention of a practical hemodialysis system
in 1943 (1) and Scribner's demonstration in 1960 that repetitive
hemodialyses could extend the life of uremic patients indefinitely
(2), the long-term approach to uremia was altered dramatically.
In the United States in mid 1977 more than 36,000 patients are sustained by regular hemodialyses at a cost in excess of $650,000,000.
per year. For those patients who lack a donor or are either unsuitable or undesirous of a renal transplant, intermittent use of
a hemodialyzer is a necessary and limiting fact of life.

An important aspect of rehabilitation during maintenance hemodialysis is a resumption of preuremia life patterns including travel
as indicated by employment obligations or while on vacation. Con-
temporary dialysis systems are bulky and heavy, preempting their use
for treatments on location in a hotel room or at a camping site.
Several groups have addressed the task of reducing the mass and
weight of dialyzers and dialysate supply systems. Gordon and co-
workers (3,4) employed the principle of sorbent dialysate regeneration using zirconium phosphate, zirconium oxide, activated charcoal
and urease to fabricate the Redy Dialysate Delivery System which is
portable and requires only 1.5L of dialysate. Kolff's team has over
the past five years been trying to develop a wearable artificial
kidney relying on the reduction of dialysate volume permitted by dialysate regeneration over activated charcoal (5,6).

We approached the problem of mobilizing hemodialysis by mini-
aturizing components of the monitoring, blood and dialysate supply
system. Central to the compact design are new small, high speed
peristaltic blood and dialysate pumps. Pump heads are 2" in diameter and have triple rollers which compress a 6" segment of silastic

33

tubing of inner diameter 2/18" (7). A solid state motor speed control varies the blood pump speed from 0 to 270 RPM; 240 RPM results
in a blood flow rate of 200 ml/min. Dialysate flow is fixed at 500
ml/min.

Transmembrane negative pressure is adjustable for control of
the rate of ultrafiltration which can be as high as 600 ml/hr.
Housed in a 2" X 5" nylon block the dialysate manifold incorporates
a thermo-control system, conductivity cell, blood leak detector and
temperature monitoring thermistor. Dialysate temperature is maintained within $\pm0.5^{\circ}F$ by a 288 watt somox insulated flexible heating
strip. All sensors yield visual and audible alarms through the
electronics module. The dialysate delivery and monitoring systems
are contained in an aluminum case 21"X13"X6" weighing 22 lbs.

A separate 21L collapsible plastic bag is used to hold pre-
warmed dialysate which is mixed by the addition of premeasured dialysate powders (or liquid concentrate) to hotel sink water which
has been passed through a small deionizer (Figures 1,2).

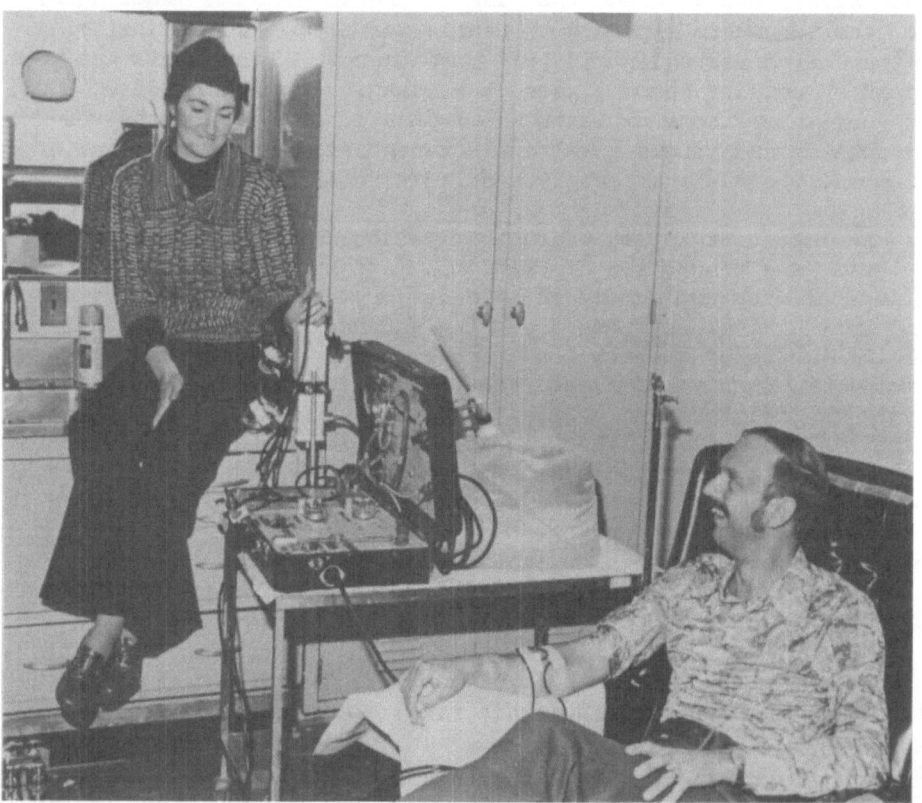

Figure 1. Patient and Wife Training to Use Suitcase Dialyzer
on Vacation.

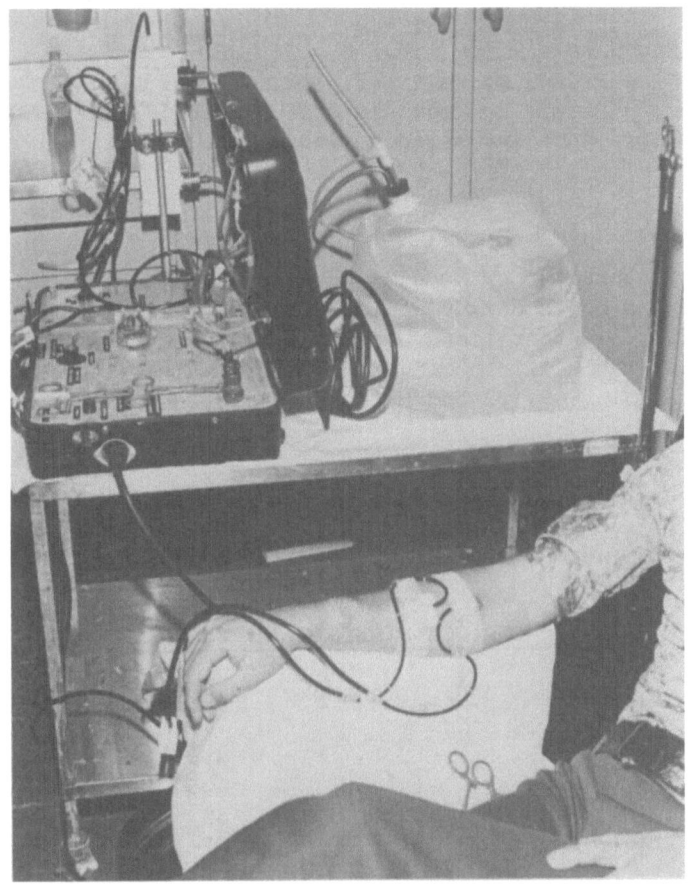

Figure 2.   Closeup View of Suitcase Dialyzer and 21L Dialysate Tank

In Vitro Testing

In vitro testing, utilizing expired whole blood was performed
in order to compare the high RPM blood pump with that of a conventional DeBakey type blood pump. A silastic tubing segment with
polyethylene adaptor was inserted in the blood tubing in place of
the PVC blood pump header. A unit of whole blood was recirculated
at a flow rate of 200 ml/min. After 120 minutes a 'c' clamp was
placed on the effluent tubing to create a 200 mmHg pressure. Samples for plasma hemoglobin were taken at 30 minute intervals for the
180 minute comparison runs. The mean plasma hemoglobin results of
3 runs (Table I) show that there is little difference in the acute
hemolytic effect caused by either pump.

TABLE I

IN VITRO BLOOD PUMP HEMOLYSIS COMPARISON (200 ml/min.)

Sample Time (min.)	0	30	60	90	120	150*	180
New Pump - Plasma Hgb mg%	15.5	16.3	16.9	18.0	19.0	22.3	25.7
DeBakey Pump - Plasma Hgb mg%	14.3	15.3	16.0	17.7	18.6	22.0	25.2

*Note: Back pressure increased to 200 mmHg after 120 min. samples

Two bilaterally nephrectomized dogs were dialyzed for 3 hrs. using a Cordis Dow Model IV Hollow Fiber Dialyzer. Dialysate was changed after 1-1/2 hrs. and was recirculated. Mean pre and post chemistries (Table II) showed adequate dialysis with mean percentage reductions of 69, 52 and 65 for urea, creatinine and phosphorous respectively.

TABLE II

THREE HOUR DOG DIALYSIS (2) SUMMARY

	UREA NITROGEN	CREATININE	PHOSPHOROUS
Pre (mg%)	59	3.9	6.3
Post (mg%)	19	1.9	2.2
% Reduction	69	52	65
Dialysance* (ml/min.)	127	97	69

*Mean BFR = 200 ml/min

Plasma hemoglobin levels in both artery and vein of one of the dogs (Table III) showed no essential hemolysis occurred during the dialysis.

TABLE III

DOG DIALYSIS - HEMOLYSIS STUDY

Sample Time (min.)	0	30	60	90	120	150	180
Plasma Hgb mg% Arterial	16	16	14	14	14	16	14
Plasma Hgb mg% Venous		14	16	14	14	14	16

Human Trials

Clinical trials on uremic patients were then begun with informed consent. The first volunteer ran for 3 hours with a bath change after 1-1/2 hours. Results of this dialysis (Table IV) show reductions of 54% for urea and 46% for creatinine with a mean blood flow rate of 178 ml/min.

TABLE IV

FIRST PATIENT DIALYSIS

	UREA NITROGEN	CREATININE	PHOSPHOROUS	URIC ACID
Pre (mg%)	63	9.5	4.8	6.9
Post (mg%)	29	5.1	4.0	3.0
% Reduction	54	46	20	57
Dialysance* (ml/min)	155	118	94	122

*Mean (4) BFR = 178 ml/min.

Further studies performed on six patients in 30 dialyses have shown that while dialysance remains relatively constant for creatinine (104±5 ml/min) and urea (148±10 ml/min), the clearances fell by 50% after 1-1/2 hours using one 21L bath. We currently prescribe a 5 hour dialysis during which the dialysate bath is changed twice, first at 1-1/2 hours and then at 3 hours with a mean blood flow rate of 187±12 ml/min. Using this protocol the mean reduction in serum levels were: Urea, 58±11%; creatinine 49±5%; phosphorous 35±9%; and uric acid 55±7%. Pre and post plasma hemoglobin, serum haptoglobin and methemalbumin assayed on 4 patients indicate no hemolysis.

Field Travel

In collaboration with Drs. John F. Sullivan at New York Hospital and Christopher R. Blagg of the Seattle Artificial Kidney Center we loaned suitcase kidney prototype systems for vacation travel by trained self dialysis patients (8). Seventeen patients performed 113 dialyses on 21 trips with only one patient having a system failure due to a burned out transformer. The 16 patients dialyzed without major incidents in hotels, motels, and at homes of friends and relatives. None of these patients visited a hospital during their trips and they had no subsequent after effects.

The suitcase kidney system offers a successful means of performing travel dialysis which should improve overall patient rehabilitation by permitting a more usual approximation of pre-illness patterns. Plans have been completed for nationwide testing of the system. It may be anticipated that the introduction of freedom to travel as a feature of the self dialysis regimen will serve as a stimulus to attract patients from center to home dialysis with substantial savings to the Federal government.

Acknowledgments

This work was supported in part by Contract No. NOl-AM-6-2203 from the NIAMDD. We are warmly appreciative of the volunteer services of Josephine Berman who served as a cheerful and willing guinea pig.

REFERENCES

1. Kolff WJ: New Ways of Treating Uremia. London, J.A. Churchill, 1947.

2. Quinton WE, Dillard DH, Cole JJ, Scribner BH: Eight months experience with silastic-teflon bypass cannulas. Trans Amer Soc Artif Int Organs 8:236-243, 1962.

3. Gordon A, Greenbaum MA, Marantz LB, McArthur MJ, and Maxwell MH: A sorbent based low volume recirculating dialysate system. Trans. Amer. Soc. Artif. Int. Organs, 15:347, 1969.

4. Gordon A, Better DS, Greenbaum MA, Marantz LB, Gral T, and Maxwell MH: Clinical maintenance hemodialysis with a sorbent-based low volume dialysate regeneration system. Trans. Amer. Soc. Artif. Int. Organs, 17:253, 1971.

5. Dharnidharka SG, Kirkham R, and Kolff WJ: Toward a wearable artificial kidney using ultrafiltrate as dialysate. Trans. Amer. Soc. Artif. Int. Organs, 19:92, 1973.

6. Porter L: How wearable artificial kidney has changed my life. National Association of Patients on Hemodialysis and Transplantation, August, 1975, p 8.

7. Briefel GR, Hutchisson JT, Galonsky RS, Hessert RL, and Friedman EA: Compact, travel hemodialysis system. Proc. Dialysis Transplant Forum, 1975, p 61.

8. Briefel GR, Galonsky RS, Hutchisson JT, Hessert RL and Friedman EA: Field trial of compact travel dialysis system. Journal of Dialysis, 1:57, 1976.

PRESENT STATUS OF HEMOFILTRATION*

Lee W. Henderson

Supported by the Medical Research Service of the
Veterans Administration and the University of
California, Division of Nephrology, San Diego,
California, U.S.A.

Introduction

Hemofiltration began in 1967 when serious attention was given
to the design of equipment for ultrafiltering whole blood on line
with maintenance of total blood volume within precise limits in a
manner analogous to the human kidney glomerulus and tubule (1).
Hemofiltration is defined as an extracorporeal process in which
uremic whole blood is cleansed by a combination of ultrafiltration
with convective solute loss and dilution with a physiologic saline
solution. Dilution may occur either before or after the ultrafiltration. I will spend no time on the rationale for this work,
but rather will address the present technical and clinical status
of hemofiltration. It should be appreciated that until recently
this technique for treating uremia was purely a laboratory endeavor.
Hence, the magnitude of the clinical experience is small. In the
present reporting, I have added my own speculation rather freely.

Technical

Membranes. At present, there are only two ultrafiltration
membranes that have been used clinically for hemofiltration and are
commercially available. Table 1 shows the format and properties of
these membranes. The RM-50 membrane was designed for the purpose

---

*Various terms have been used to describe this procedure, i.e.,
hemodiafiltration, hemoultrafiltration, diafiltration. Hemofiltration
was agreed upon as the best term by the workers in the field at a
meeting in Gstaad (Feb. 1977) and will be used throughout this
manuscript. Work was performed under NIH Contract #G-9091.

TABLE 1

Properties of Commercially Available Hemofiltration Membranes

Membrane	Manufacturer	Format	Transport Area M^2	Ultrafiltrate Flow Rate* cm^3/min	$cc/min\text{-}cm^2$	Sieving Coefficient for inulin (5200 daltons)
PM-50	Amicon polysulfone	200μ hollow fiber 4000 fibers 8 cm long	0.21	53	.025	1.0
PM-50	Amicon polysulfone	200μ hollow fiber 5000 fibers 16.5 cm long	0.54	76	.014	1.0
PM-50	Amicon polysulfone	200μ hollow fiber 12000 fibers 20 cm long	1.53	104	.007	1.0
RP-6	Rhone-Poulenc polyachriloni-trile	Sheet membrane 16 plates	1.2	70	.006	.77▲

*Flow rates are those that pertain to clinical operation with whole blood flow rates of 225 $cm^3/$min operated in the post dilution mode.

▲Data from Green et al (2).

of hemofiltration whereas the RP-6 membrane was designed as a dialyzer and found by Dr. Quellhorst and others to be useful as a
hemofilter. To date most experience has been had with the RP-6
membrane in that it has been widely available for clinical use as a
dialyzer whereas the PM-50 membrane has only recently been commercially available. The ultrafiltration rates of the RP-6 membrane
operated with whole blood (Table 1) is similar to that for the
1.53 m^2 PM-50 membrane. One may note for the PM-50 unit a fall in
ultrafiltration rate as overall membrane areas increases from 0.2
to 1.53 m^2. This fall in efficiency for water removal for a given
bloo flow rate agrees with previously advanced theory (3,4) which
correlates water removal rate (Q_f) for hollow fiber units with the
area (A), fiber diameter (d), ratio and blood flow rate at the
inlet (Q_{Bi}), i.e.,

$$Q_f \; \alpha \; \left(\frac{A}{d} \right) \; 2/3 \; \left(Q_{Bi} \right) \; 1/3$$

For the PM-50 devices the curve of ultrafiltration rate vs. transmembrane pressure shows a plateau above 250 mm Hg, i.e., for
increments of transmembrane pressure above 250 mm Hg there is little
or no concomitant increase in water flux. This is the result of
protein concentration polarization (5). There is no similar data
for the RP-6 sheet/plate device.

One may reasonably project an expanded use of PM-50 membrane
now that it is commercially available as it carries a sieving
coefficient for inulin that is equivalent to human glomerular basement membrane. Further, it is logical to expect polyacrylonitrile
membrane to be marketed in hollow fiber format in the not too
distant future. Other membranes such as that experimented with by
Quellhorst from Sartorius will undoubtedly find their way into
clinical use (6). It is my speculation that hollow fiber format
will win out as the most desirable in that a small (100-200 micron
height or diameter) dimensionally stable flow path is exceedingly
important in order to maintain the high shear rates (velocity
profile at the wall) necessary to reduce concentration polarization
and maximize water flux rate. Such a flow path is harder to
achieve in sheet plate format and still not "blind out" transporting
area at the 300-400 mm Hg transmembrane pressure required for hemofiltration.

Fluid cyclers. As of the present writing, there are very few
machines available to automate the task of balancing the flow rates
of ultrafiltrate and replacement or diluting fluid. Two principles
of operation have been used with the machines presently available.
The first is a volumetric matching of flow rates using a closely
matched pair of pumps. We have been largely responsible for
designing, building, and testing this kind of equipment. Details

of its operation are reported elsewhere and I will confine my
comments to critical comparison of this equipment with that using
a gravimetric principal for matching of flows (1,7-11). In our
volumetric equipment the pump delivering diluting fluid works
against a positive head of pressure (100 to 300 mm Hg) whereas that
casting ultrafiltrate away must operate against a vacuum (-300 to
-500 mm Hg). The flow rate in these pumps must be matched to within less than 1% for the flow rate (200 cc/min) and volume (40-60 L)
used each treatment to be within clinically acceptable limits of
error in overall fluid balance. We have encountered trouble with
this system as ultrafiltrate tends to "degas" in the outflow pump
and the microbubbles so generated make for errors in the volumetri-
cally matched flows. Redesign of this equipment so that ultrafiltrate flow rate was not governed by negative pressure fluctuations
would obviate this problem (e.g., develop transmembrane pressure by
pumping against a clamp on the blood return line rather than with
vacuum outside the fiber). Gravametric monitoring where net weight
of two receptacles one for ultrafiltrate and the other for diluting
fluid is held constant by adjusting the diluting fluid flow rate
insures fluid balance and obviates the problems of solution degassing.
Both systems may be programmed for net fluid removal with time. The
gravametric system (short of weighin the patient) does not lend itself easily to compact on line preparation and delivery of diluting
fluid while maintaining overall fluid balance. The ideal system
would involve flow probes of such sensitivity (< 1% at 2-300 cc/min)
that precise net fluid balance could be insured by using their
signaled difference to drive the diluting fluid pump.

At present, there are only 3-4 prototype fluid cycling units
that have been produced commercially for trial. There will undoubtedly be a period of trial and comparison with only 2 or 3 machines
that prove out to be satisfactory in terms of reliable performance
maintenance free.

Diluting fluid. Solutions designed to be comparable in composition of electrolyte to dialysis fluid have so far been used. We
have recently used a solution somewhat higher in sodium (140 meq/L
rather than the 130-135 meq/L commonly used) and containing glucose
at 100 mg%. Obviously, there is no need for a concentration gradient to remove sodium from the sodium/volume overloaded patient and
it is my speculation that patients will profit from a sodium and
glucose concentration in the plasma water that is held normal. It
is clear that formal studies of acid-base balance, Ca++ concentration, etc., will need to be done before establishing what composition is ideal.

The major cost difference between hemodialysis and hemofiltration lies with the need for sterile pyrogen-free diluting fluid in
large quantitiys. Until this can be made "on line" in a manner

analagous to dialysis fluid, there will remain a major cost disadvantage to hemofiltration.

Pre vs. post dilution. No studies are in hand as yet to permit a rational choice between these methods. Our laboratory began
using the predilution mode in order to achieve an arbitrarily set
goal of 100 ml/min clearance for inulin. If a physiologic filtration fraction (ultrafiltration rate/plasma flow rate) is maintained
(.25) and blood flow rate from the fistulas available to us averages
200-250 cc/min, then as previously detailed, (12) the predilution
mode is required to achieve the 100 cm^3/min goal clearance for
inulin and all smaller solutes.

Clinical Studies

At present there are some 50 patients who have been treated
or are now being treated with maintenance hemofiltration. Our
group in the United States comprises a total of 11 patients. Dr.
Quellhorst in Germany reports 13 patients (13). New groups using
hemofiltration are cropping up primarily in Germany and France
where the RP-6 dialyzer is widely marketed. I would expect to see
a logarythmic growth phase over the next 3-5 years as hemofiltration
establishes itself as a competitive, and for some, a more desirable
form of treatment than hemodialysis. The reason for this is the
promising initial findings so far reported clinically and detailed
below.

Symptoms. The observation that removal of excess total body
water and salt by hemofiltration produces far fewer symptoms in a
given patient than does hemodialysis is of high interest. We
observed this first with predilution, but others using post dilution
format also have found fewer symptoms. All patients studied by us
noted markedly fewer cramps and malaise with hemofiltration than
during bracketing control periods on hemodialysis. Similarly,
reports from Drs. Quellhorst, Funck-Brentano and others using post
dilution mode make this point (13,14,15). There is considerable
speculation, but little or no hard data on why this should be. Dr.
Quellhorst has noted that the pattern of serum osmolality change
with time for the two techniques is different, i.e., the fall in
serum osmolality during hemodialysis. As the pathophysiologic
mechanism for muscle cramps remains obscure, it is not clear whether
these events are related. It remains an important benefit for the
patient.

Thirst and attendant weight gain between treatments has been
more prominent in the group of eleven patients treated with predilution than has been reported from the European workers using post
dilution mode. This is a statistically significant observation when

interfiltration weight gains are compared with bracketing control
periods on hemodialysis. The fact that this is not seen with post
dilution suggests that this is more than just the impact of drinking
habits on patient awareness that large sodium/volume excesses may be
asymptomatically repaired.

Hypertension. Only 3 patients of 26 reported at the Gstaad
Conference (16) who had hypertension and were treated for 3 months
or more with hemofiltration failed to show either return to normal
or significant amelioration of hypertension. As reported elsewhere,
our studies point away from simple improvement in sodium/volume
status and toward the correction of an autonomic neuropathy that a
significant subset of the uremic hypertensive population manifests
(17,18). Further studies now under way here and in Europe will be
required to establish the incidence of responders and both the
mechanisms of response and failure to respond.

Triglycerides. Quellhorst has shown a significant fall in
plasma triglyceride levels in patients moving from maintenance hemodialysis to hemofiltration (19). Schneider et al (20) has seen this
in 2 out of 2 patients with high triglycerides on hemodialysis.
Further stidues with close attention to diet and other parameters
of lipid handling will be needed to establish the incidence and
mechanism of response.

Electroencephalogram. In 3 of four patients we have so far
studied, examination of the power spectrum of the compressed spectral
array has shown return to normal. As previously reported (12), this
has occurred with concurrent measurements of BUN, creatinine and
uric acid showing higher pretreatment values than in bracketing
control periods on conventional hemodialysis. This is of high
interest in the context of work from Vanderbilt showing improvement,
but not return to full normality of this parameter with conventional
dialysis and further improvement to normal on successful renal transplantation (21,22).

Hormones. Using the post dilution mode (Kramer et al (23), has
shown no major perturbations in measured circulating levels of HGH,
TSH, testosterone, cortisone, gastrin, GIP, insulin and glucagon.
However, somatomedin concentrations showed a fall.

Other clinical applications. In addition to hemofiltration,
ultrafiltration has also been applied in other clinical applications
(24-28).

This brief review of the preliminary clinical experiments with
hemofiltration in the treatment of chronic renal failure is offered
with the hope of stimulating further questions and pointing up the
need for further studies.

References

1. HENDERSON, L.W., BESARAB, A., MICHAELS, A. and BLUEMLE, L.W.,
    JR.: Blood purification by ultrafiltration and fluid replace-
    ment (diafiltration). Trans. Amer. Soc. Artif. Organs 13:216,
    1967.

2. GREEN, D.M., ANTWILER, G.D., MONCRIEF, J.W., DECHERD, J.F.,
    POPOVICH, R.P.: Measurement of the transmitance coefficient
    spectrum of cuprophan and RP 69 membranes: Applications to
    middle molecule removal via ultrafiltration. Trans. Amer.
    Soc. Artif. Int. Organs 22:627, 1976.

3. COLTON, C.K., HENDERSON, L.W., FORD, C.A. and LYSAGHT, M.H.:
    Kinetics of hemodiafiltration. I. In vitro transport charac-
    teristics of a hollow fiber blood ultrafilter. J. Lab. Clin.
    Med. 85:355, 1975.

4. HENDERSON, L.W., COLTON, C.K. and FORD, C.: Kinetics of Hemo-
    diafiltration. II. Clinical characterization of a new blood
    modality. J. Lab. Clin. Med. 85:372-391, 1975.

5. BLATT, W.F., DRAVID, A., MICHAELS, A.S., NELSEN, L.: Solute
    polarization and cake formation in membrane ultrafiltration:
    Causes, consequences and control techniques; in Flinn Membrane
    Science and Technology, p. 47, (Plenum, New York).

6. REIGER, J., QUELLHORST, E., LOWITZ, H.D., KONG, R.G., SCHELER,
    G.: Ultrafiltration for middle molecules in uraemia. Proc.
    EDTA 11:158, 1974.

7. HENDERSON, L.W., FORD, C., COLTON, C.K., BLUEMLE, L.W., JR.
    and BIXLER, H.J.: Uremic blood cleansing by diafiltration
    using a hollow fiber ultrafilter. Trans. Amer. Soc. Artif.
    Int. Organs 16:107, 1970.

8. HAMILTON, R., FORD, C., COLTON, C., CROSS, R., STEINMULLER, S.
    and HENDERSON, L.W.: Blood cleansing by diafiltration in
    uremic dog and man. Trans. Amer. Soc. Artif. Int. Organs 17:
    259, 1971.

9. HENDERSON, L.W., LIVOTI, L., FORD, C., KELLY, A., and LYSAGHT,
    M.: Clinical experience with intermittent hemodiafiltration.
    Trans. Amer. Soc. Artif. Int. Organs 19:119, 1973.

10. SILVERSTEIN, M.E., FORD, C.A., LYSAGHT, M.J. and HENDERSON,
    L.W.: Response to rapid removal of intermediate molecular
    weight solutes in uremic man. Trans. Amer. Soc. Artif. Int.
    Organs 20:614, 1974.

11. HENDERSON, L.W., SILVERSTEIN, M.E., FORD, C.A. and LYSAGHT,
    M.J.: Clinical response to maintenance hemodiafiltration.
    Kidney International Suppl. 2:S-58, 1975.

12. HENDERSON, L.W.: Development of a Convective Blood Cleansing
    Technique NIH, 10th Annual Contractors' Conference, January
    1977, Bethesda, Maryland. (in press).

13. QUELLHORST, E., SCHUENEMANN, B., RIEGER, H.: Treatment of
    severe hypertension in chronic renal insufficiency by hemo-
    filtration. Abstract 14th Congress EDTA 1977.

14. MAN, N.K., FUNCK-BRENTANO, J.L.: Hemofiltration an alternative method for treatment of end stage renal failure. Advances in Nephrology Year Book Med. Publishers 1977 (in press).
15. SCHÄFER, K.: Unpublished presentation. Conference on Hemo-filtration, Gstaad, Switzerland, March 1977.
16. Conference on Hemofiltration, Gstaad, Switzerland, March 1977.
17. LILLEY, J.J., GOLDEN, J., STONE, R.A.: Adrenergic regulation of blood in chronic renal failure. J. Clin. Invest. 57:1190, 1976.
18. LEVY, S.B., STONE, R.A., FORD, C.A., BEANS, E. and HENDERSON, L.W.: The influence of hemodiafiltration on blood pressure regulation. Trans. ASAIO 1977 (in press).
19. QUELLHORST, E., RIEGER, J., DOHT, B., BECKMANN, H., JACOB, I., KRAFT, B., MIETZCH, G., SCHELER, F.: Treatment of chronic uraemia by an ultrafiltration artificial kidney - First clinical experience. Proc. European Dial. and Trans. Assoc. p.134, 1976.
20. SCHNEIDER, H., STREICHER, E., HACHMANN, H., CHMIEL, H., MYLIUS, H.: Clinical experience with hemodiafiltration. Abstract 14th Congress EDTA 1977.
21. TESCHAN, P.E., GINN, H.E., BOURNE, J.R., WALKER, P.J., WARD, J.W.: Quantitative neurobehavioral responses to renal failure and maintenance dialysis. Trans. ASAIO 21:488, 1975.
22. TESCHAN, P.E., GINN, H.E., BOURNE, J.R., WARD, J.W.: Neuro-behavioral response to "middle molecule" dialysis and trans-plantation. Trans. ASAIO 22:190, 1976.
23. KRAMER, P., MATHAEI, D., ARNOLD, R., EBERT, P., MCINTOSH, C., SCHAUDER, P., SCHWINN, G., SCHELER, F.: Changes of plasma concentrations and elimination of various hormones by hemo-filtration. Abstract 14th Congress EDTA 1977.
24. BERGSTRÖM, J., ASABA, J., FÜRST, P., OULES, R.: Dialysis ultra-filtration and blood pressure. Proc. Europ. Dial. Trans. Asso. 1976 (in press).
25. KUNITOMO, T., LOWRIE, E., KUMAZAWA, S., O'BRIEN, M., LAZARUS, M., GOTTLIEB, M., MERRILL, J.: Controlled ultrafiltration with hemodialysis: Analysis of coupling between convective and diffusive mass transfer in a new ultrafiltration-hemodialysis system. Trans. ASAIO 1977 (in press).
26. SILVERSTEIN, M.E., FORD, C.A., LYSAGHT, M.J., HENDERSON, L.W.: Treatment of severe fluid overload by ultrafiltration. New Engl. J. Med. 291:747, 1974.
27. QUELLHORST, E.: Personal communication.
28. CHANG, T.M.S., CHIRITO, E., BARRE. P., COLE, C., HEWISH, M.: Clinical performance of a new combined system for simultaneous hemoperfusion-hemodialysis-ultrafiltration in series. Trans. ASAIO 21:502, 1975.
29. LEBER, W.: Unpublished presentation. Conference on Hemo-filtration, Gstaad, Switzerland, March 1977.

OXYSTARCH AND OTHER POLYALDEHYDES: THE PRESENT STATUS IN THE

TREATMENT OF UREMIA

Carmelo Giordano and Renato Esposito

Chair of Nephrology, I Polyclinic, University of Naples

Piazza Miraglia, 80138 Naples, Italy

Polyaldehydes, such as oxidized starch and cellulose, are in theory very potent urea and ammonia binders. However, their clinical use in the last ten years has lit some hope; their efficacy in reducing body uremic waste nitrogen accumulation has suffered, admittedly, comparable enthusiasm. In this short presentation, we wish to give some reasons and focus the possible ways for improving the clinical efficacy of these sorbents.

Experiences, duplicated in Europe and in America (1-3), demonstrate that oxystarch, when given to uremic patients, increases fecal nitrogen by binding intestinal ammonia and urea. Oxystarch and oxycellulose, in fact, react both with urea and with ammonia. Reactivity is somewhat greater with ammonia than with urea (4). However, in terms of nitrogen binding, given that urea has two nitrogen and ammonia has only one, there is no significant difference.

A critical review (5) of the reactivity of oxystarch indicated that for 1 gram of oxystarch ingested there will be 88 mg of ammonia, which is perfectly in line to the in vitro capacity of oxystarch to bind 97 mg of ammonia/gram of sorbent. The fact that oxystarch reacts very well with ammonia makes it suitable as an intestinal sorbent both in uremia and in hepatic failure.

In reality, while in the stomach there is more urea than ammonia, in the large intestine the reverse is true (6).Of course, an-

other much more important difference between the stomach and the
gut in terms of chemistry is represented by the hydrogen ion concentration, a factor this which might be of significant importance
in the clinical use of oral sorbents.

Yet, let us consider two main points: the reactivity time and
the reactivity behavior in physiologic and acidic pH. Reactivity
time: in Fig.1 is shown that polyaldehydes, such as oxystarch and
oxycellulose, are slow-reacting molecules. At 2-4 hours, less than
50% of the binding capacity has been reached; full binding capacity
requires more than 24 hours to be obtained. This means that polyaldehydes, as they have been employed so far, are suitable for
large intestine reactivity, since the intestine transit time, in
the absence of enhanced peristalsis, is of about 24 hours. However,
this also means that oral sorbents employed in clinical trials have
taken no advantage whatsoever of the acidic gastric environment,
the gastric transit time being in the order of half an hour or so.
Yet the acidic stomach conditions are of significant importance in
terms of reactivity of polyaldehydes and urea.

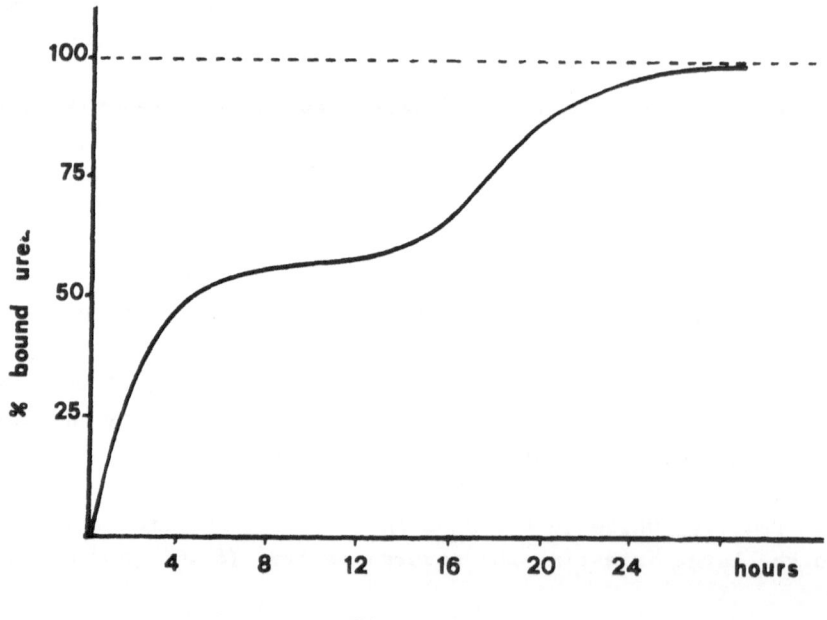

Figure 1

Let us take oxycellulose,a polyaldehyde which has been studied
later;the istotherm for urea binding at pH 7.4 is 5.18,indicating,as
shown in Fig.2,that 5.18 g. of urea are bound for each kg. of oxycellulose when urea concentration is 100 mg% at pH 1, the isotherm is 14
suggesting that the binding capacity has increased almost three times.

Oxycellulose, however, is an interesting sorbent yet not fully
appreciated in that it shows a great binding variability depending
upon the pH. This is especially true when used in the form of oxycellulose-acetate. In fact, as shown in Fig.2, while at pH 7.4 the
isotherm is 1.95 grams of urea per kilogram of oxycellulose, at pH
1 it is 60, indicating that 60 grams of urea are bound to one kilogram of oxycellulose-acetate when urea concentration is only 100 mg%.
So it is evident that in vitro polyaldehydes are the most potent

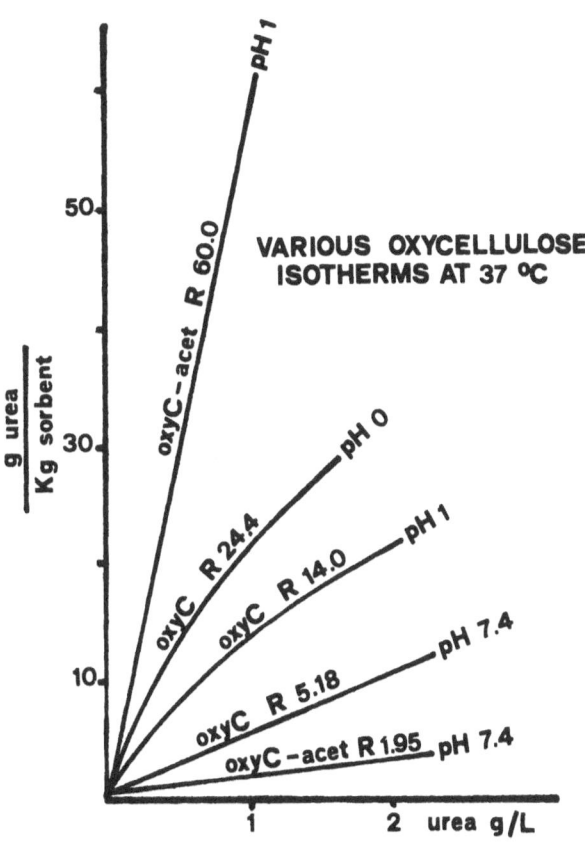

Figure 2

sorbents for binding urea and ammonia, and that clinical application so far has only used a minor part of their binding capacity.
Thus, while clinical trials have shown a binding capacity of
about 80 mg of nitrogen for 1 gram of oxystarch, in the light of
the oxycellulose isotherm, in acidic condition 600 mg of urea per
gram of sorbent would be bound.

It is therefore apparent that from now on we should work
more in acidic media than at alkaline pH. This might represent
the enhancing factor needed to make polyaldehydes the answer to
the urea removal puzzle. However, the reactivity time is too
slow to work in the stomach to a significant degree. One
significant improvement has been recently achieved in our
laboratory in preparing water-pretreated polyaldehydes and in
obtaining, by this means, a rapid reactivity curve, as shown in
Figure 3, with a maximum within 2 hours instead of 24 hours or
more, and in excess of 50% in 30 minutes. Water pretreatment of
oxystarch for 24 hours thus accelerates the activity of the
sorbent. Such accelerated activity is due to an

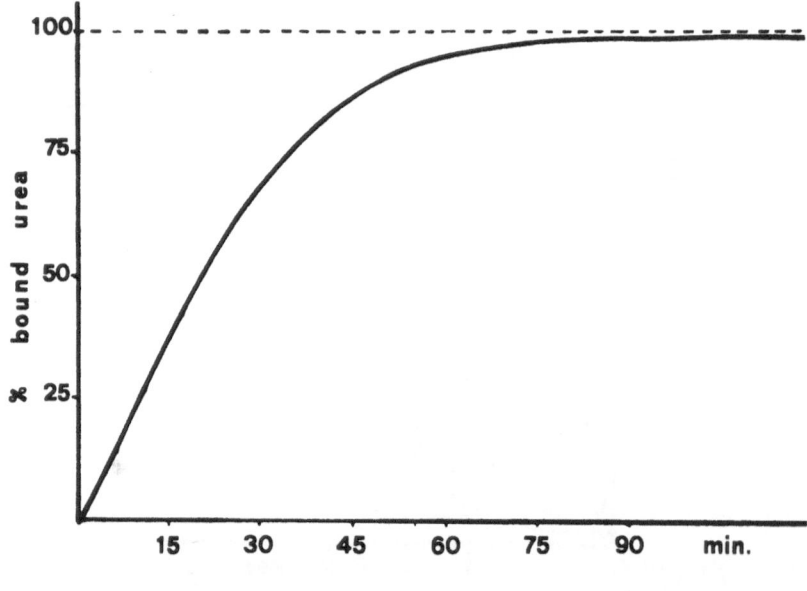

Figure 3

increase in the contact surface of the sorbent due to its swelling
with water. This observation makes it possible to utilize the polyaldehydes more as gastro sorbents than as intestinal sorbents.
In fact, the rapid binding capacity of the water-pretreated polyaldehydes allows the sorbent to work in the gastric juice, where,
in consequence of the low pH, it will bind a larger amount of urea.

A clinical trial has been accomplished in a group of uremic
patients with residual renal function characterized as in Table I.
The results obtained after oral use of oxystarch are given in Tables
II and III, from which it is apparent that there is a significant
increase in fecal nitrogen as a result of ingested water-pretreated
oxystarch (period C) in comparison to plain oxystarch (period B).
This increase exceeds by 36% the amount of nitrogen excreted when
plain oxystarch is given.

In terms of sorbent urea clearance, given by the difference
between patients' urea clearance during sorbent therapy and off
sorbent treatment, patients on pretreated oxystarch have shown an
oxystarch urea clearance higher than 3 ml/min (7). An easily improved gastro-intestinal oxystarch can thus accomplish a vicarious
activity in uremia, comparable to an amount of renal parenchyma
capable of expressing about 3 ml of urea clearance.

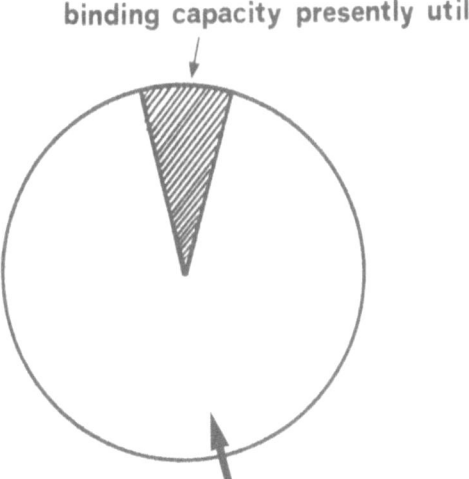

binding capacity presently utilized

further potential binding capacity

Figure 4

Table 1

	mean ± SD
creatinine (mg%)	9.16 ± 2.90
BUN (mg%)	88 ± 19

Table 2

N FECAL g/$_{24h}$

	mean ± SD
(b̄–ā)	1.20 ± .10
(c̄–ā)	1.73 ± .09
(c̄–b̄)	0.56 ± .04

a= before administration

b= on oxystarch

c= on pre-treated oxystarch

Now, has really water pretreatment of oxystarch exhausted the capability of utilization for polyaldehydes? Considering the isotherm of oxycellulose-acetate (Fig.2), it can certainly be answered no.

As a matter of fact, it looks that the actual clinical utilization of polyaldehydes, as shown in Fig.4, represents, admittedly, only a very minor sector in comparison to the rest of the circle which works in vitro, but is still unexplored in vivo.

Table III

% N CHANGE IN EXCRETION

no. cases (25)	mean ± SD	probability	t Student
$(\frac{b-a}{a})\cdot100$	143 ± 16 %	P > .005	8.93
$(\frac{c-a}{a})\cdot100$	191 ± 14 %	P > .005	13.63
$(\frac{c-b}{b})\cdot100$	36 ± 5 %	.005 < P < .01	7.20

REFERENCES

1. Giordano, C; Esposito, R; Demma, G. Possibilità di ridurre l'azo-
   temia nell'uomo mediante somministrazione di una polialdeide.
   Boll. Soc. Ital. Biol. Sper. 44: 2232-2238, 1968

2. Man, NK; Drucke, T; Paris, J; Elizalde Monteverde, C; Rondon Nu-
   cete, M; Zingraff, J; Jungers, P. Increased nitrogen removal from
   intestinal tract of uremic patients. Proc. Eur. Dial. Transpl.
   Assoc. (Pitman Medical London) 10: 143-151, 1973

3. Friedman, EA; Fastook, J; Beyer, MM; Rattazzi, T; Josephson, AS.
   Potassium and nitrogen binding in the human gut by ingested oxidized starch. Trans. Am. Soc. Artif. Intern. Organs 20: 161-167,
   1974

4. Giordano, C; Esposito, R; Pluvio, M. Oxycellulose and ammonia
   treated oxystarch as insoluble polyaldehydes in uremia. Kidney
   Internat. 7: S-380-S-382, 1975

5. Meriwether, LS; Kramer, HM. In vitro reactivity of oxystarch and
   oxycellulose. Kidney Internat. 10: S-259-S-265, 1976

6. Wrong, O. The metabolism of urea and ammonia in the alimentary
   tract. Proc. Workshop on Gastrointestinal Sorbents in Uremia.
   DHEW Publication no. (NIH) 72-78 p. 139-156, 1971

7. Giordano, C; Esposito, R; Pluvio, M. An improved oxystarch in the
   treatment of renal failure. Proc. Strathclyde Bioengineering Seminar Series, Glasgow, August, 1976.

MICROENCAPSULATED ADSORBENT HEMOPERFUSION

ARTIFICIAL CELLS FOR ARTIFICIAL KIDNEY, ARTIFICIAL LIVER

AND DETOXIFICATION

Thomas Ming Swi Chang

Artificial Organs Research Unit
McGill University
Montreal, Quebec, Canada

THE BASIS OF ARTIFICIAL CELLS FOR ARTIFICIAL ORGANS

In 1956, while a premedical student at McGill, I prepared some artificial cells mainly to demonstrate the feasibility of the principle of "artificial cells" (Chang, 1957). Their use for artificial organs came later when on calculating the total membrane area available in artificial cells (semipermeable microcapsules) of different diameters very striking results were obtained (Chang, 1964, 1966). Thus, 10 ml of 20 micron diameter microcapsules or 33 ml of 100 micron diameter microcapsules have a total surface area of about 2.5 m^2. Even 300 ml of very large microcapsules of 2 mm diameter have a total surface area of 2.5 m^2. What is more important is that membrane thickness of the microcapsules is 0.02 micron. This is 400 times thinner than the standard hemodialysis membrane. This large membrane area and the ultrathin membrane of microcapsules would, in theory, allow permeant metabolites to cross the membrane 1,250 times faster than in the standard 1 m^2 area hemodialysis machine. If something can be placed inside these semi-permeable microcapsules to trap entering metabolites then we have the basis for a miniaturized artificial organ based on artificial cells. Study carried out in this laboratory makes use of enzymes, ion exchange resin, activated charcoal and other material to retain or convert metabolites entering the microcapsules (Chang, 1964, 1966, 1972a, 1977). In this review an artificial organ based on microencapsulated charcoal will be discussed as a typical example. The other aspects of artificial cells containing enzymes, cell extracts, multienzyme system have been reviewed in detail in books (Chang, 1972a, 1977a).

MICROENCAPSULATION
IN ARTIFICIAL CELLS

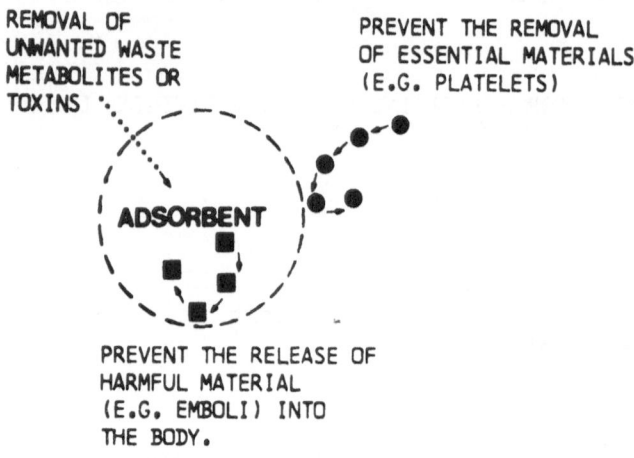

REMOVAL OF
UNWANTED WASTE
METABOLITES OR
TOXINS

PREVENT THE REMOVAL
OF ESSENTIAL MATERIALS
(E.G. PLATELETS)

ADSORBENT

PREVENT THE RELEASE OF
HARMFUL MATERIAL
(E.G. EMBOLI) INTO
THE BODY.

Figure 1

ENCAPSULATED CHARCOAL HEMOPERFUSION

Theoretical

We first proposed and demonstrated the use of the principle of
artificial cells to microencapsulate charcoal (Chang, 1966, 1972,
1975) for the following reasons. Research from the groups of
Yatzidis (1964), Kolff (1965), Schreiner (1967) and others have
demonstrated that although free activated charcoal granules can
effectively remove many uremic metabolites and drugs from perfusing
blood and release embolizing particles (Hagstam, Larsson, and
Thysell, 1966), the use of the principle of artificial cells to
encapsulate charcoal granules would retain the adsorbing properties
but prevent embolism and the adverse affect of charcoal (Figure 1)
(Chang, 1966, 1969, 1972; Chang et al., 1967, 1968).

Variations in the Encapsulated Charcoal Hemoperfusion Systems

We have made use of: nylon, collodion, heparin-benzalkonium-
complex collodion, albumin-collodion (ACAC), cellulose acetate
membrane and others for encapsulating charcoal (Chang, 1957, 1964,
1969, 1972a, 1976a; Chang et al., 1966, 1967, 1968, 1975). Of these
the Albumin-cellulose nitrate coated activated charcoal (ACAC) has
been tested here extensively in clinical trial for patients with
chronic renal failure, acute intoxication and uremia. The ACAC

approach has also been successfully reproduced by a number of other
centers (Blume et al., 1976; Odaka et al., 1976; Oka et al., 1976;
Amano et al., 1978; Odaka, 1978; Terman et al., 1977). There is
the recent development of petroleum based spherical charcoal bead
which is stronger than coconut activated charcoal granules. With
this type of spherical charcoal bead the ACAC procedure can be
used on a large scale basis with greater ease (Oka et al., 1976;
Odaka et al., 1976; Odaka, 1978; Amano et al., 1978). Other
polymers included polyhema (Andrade et al., 1972), polymethacrylate
(Gilchrist et al., 1975), gelatin (Nakabayashi, 1976). The Hemacol,
produced on an industrial scale, uses acrylic hydrogel for encapsulating charcoal granules (Fennimore et al., 1977). Adsorba 300C,
also produced on an industrial scale, is a cellulose acetate microencapsulated charcoal system (Martin et al., 1977; Thysell et al.,
1976). The principle of artificial cells or encapsulation can no
doubt be applied using an unlimited number of other polymers and
biomaterials for the encapsulation of charcoal. In addition to
encapsulation described, other modifications in the configuration
of encapsulated charcoal systems includes the following (Figure 2).
The fixed-bed charcoal system (Hill et al., 1976) consists of fine
charcoal granules fixed onto tapes previously wetted with chloro-
sulfonated polyethylene. Fiber entrapped system consists of a dis-
persion of activated charcoal powder in polymer solution which, instead of being formed into microcapsules, is extruded into fibers
(Davis, 1975). In the Enka Glantzstoff capillary encapsulated system, activated charcoal powder is used to fill hollow fiber (Nose
et al., 1976) or the outer lumen of double lumen hollow fiber (Castro et al., 1978).

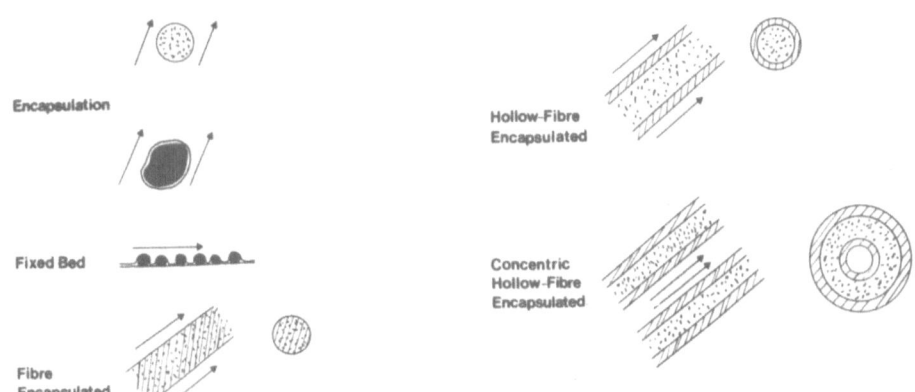

Figure 2

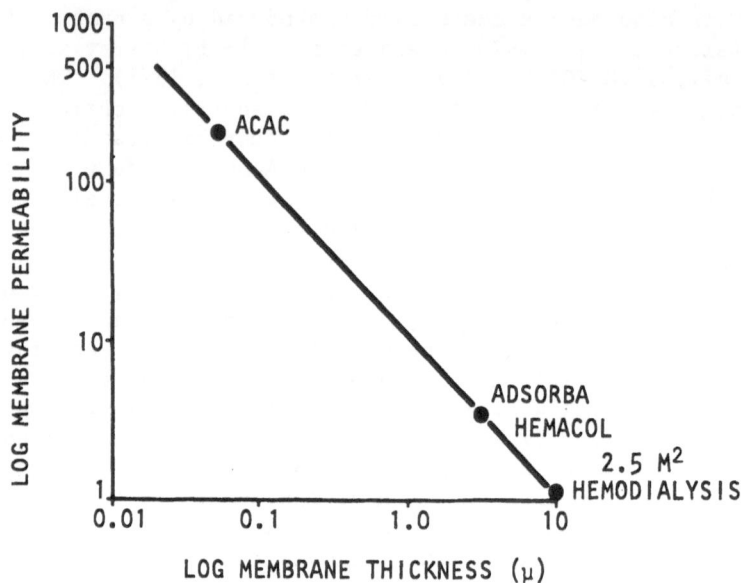

Figure 3

Permeability, Membrane Thickness and Blood Compatibility

It should be very strongly emphasized as we discuss the different hemoperfusion systems that although the membrane thickness and
the permeability of the membrane encapsulating the activated charcoal
is extremely important, and the thinner the membrane and the better
the permeability coefficient of the membrane material, the faster the
transport. However, this is only in-vitro. The most important point
in clinical situations is what happens in-vivo. If the microcapsules
are not blood compatible, when you have a thick coating of cellular
elements and fibrin on top of the membrane. If this happens no
matter how thin or permeable you membrane, the in-vivo properties
will be completely altered. For instance, let us look at the different systems. If we express the transport rate of hemodialysers
with 2.5 m^2 membrane as unity, the transport rate of the various
microencapsulated charcoal systems with different membrane thickness
can be plotted (Figure 3). The permeability of all types of microencapsulated adsorbent systems is high when compared to standard hemodialysis. However, if the system is coated with fibrin and blood
cells in-vivo, the effective membrane thickness may increase by
more than 10 microns resulting in markedly decreased transport rate
(Figure 4). Therefore, no matter whether the charcoal is uncoated
as in fixed-bed; coated with ultrathin membrane (0.05 micron) as in

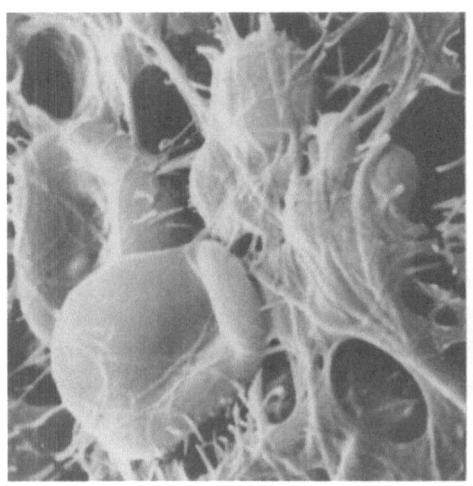
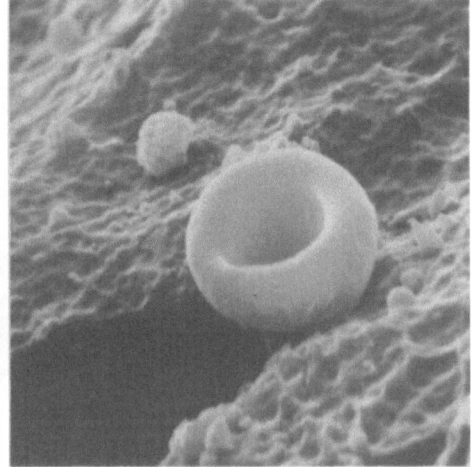

BIOCOMPATIBILITY

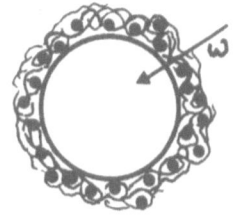
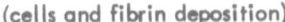
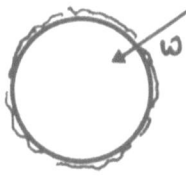

(cells and fibrin deposition)   (minimal deposition)

Figure 4

ACAC; or coated with thicker membrane (3 micron) as in Adsorba 300C
and Hemacol; a 10 micron coating will completely eliminate any major
differences in transport capacity. Unless the surface is blood compatible with minimal fibrin deposition (Figure 4).

Effects of Albumin-Collodion Coating on Blood
Compatibility and Transport Mechanism

We prepared the blood compatible system of ACAC by using an
albumin-complexed collodion membrane. This way, 2 hours of hemoperfusion in patients has resulted in no significant changes in

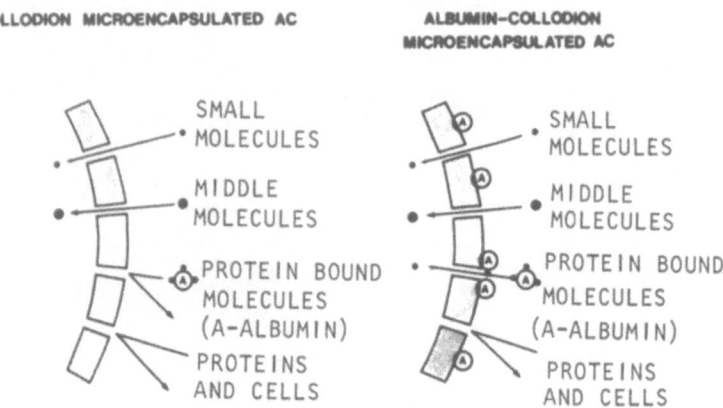

Figure 5

platelet levels (Chang et al., 1971, 1972; Odaka, 1978). Furthermore, scanning electromicroscopic examination showed that there is
no fibrin or cell entrapment (Chang, 1976a), (Figure 4). With the
incorporation of albumin into the collodion membrane there is the
possibility of the albumin extracting albumin-bound molecules from
the plasma. It may act as a facilitated transport mechanism transporting protein-bound molecules to the activated charcoal inside
the cells (Figure 5). This may explain why the clearance of the
ACAC system is much greater for protein-bound drugs like doriden,
methaqualone, etc., when compared to other hemoperfusion systems.
A further extension of the incorporation of protein onto the
microcapsule membrane is the incorporation of antigen or antibodies
onto the collodion membranes coating charcoal for in-vivo use as
immunosorbent (Terman et al., 1977).

Effects Of Albumin-Collodion Coating On Preventing Embolism

Laboratory and histological studies showed no particulate
embolism in properly prepared ACAC systems especially when using
the updated procedure (Chang, 1976a). More detailed studies using
the Coulter Counter also showed no significant release of particulates larger than 2 micron diameter (Figure 6). However, it

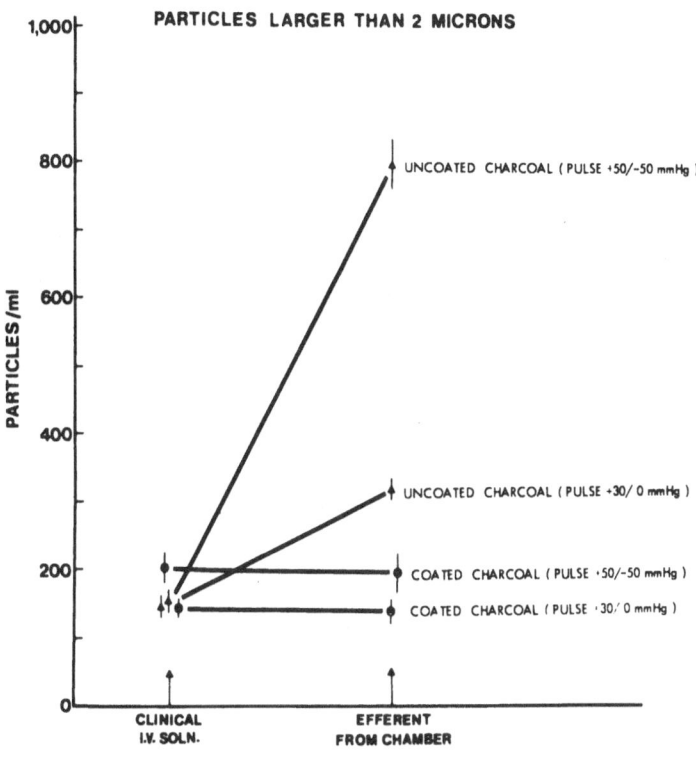

Figure 6

should be emphasized that the type of charcoal granules used for
encapsulation and the care taken before encapsulation to remove all
the fine powder before coating are extremely important factors.
For those with no experience in this technology the specially prepared spherical petroleum based charcoal beads will be easier to
prepare properly.

TREATMENT OF PATIENTS WITH CHRONIC RENAL FAILURE

Patients with chronic renal failure have been treated with
(1) ACAC hemoperfusion, (2) ACAC hemoperfusion in series with
hemodialyser and (3) ACAC hemoperfusion in series with a small
ultrafiltrator (Figure 7).

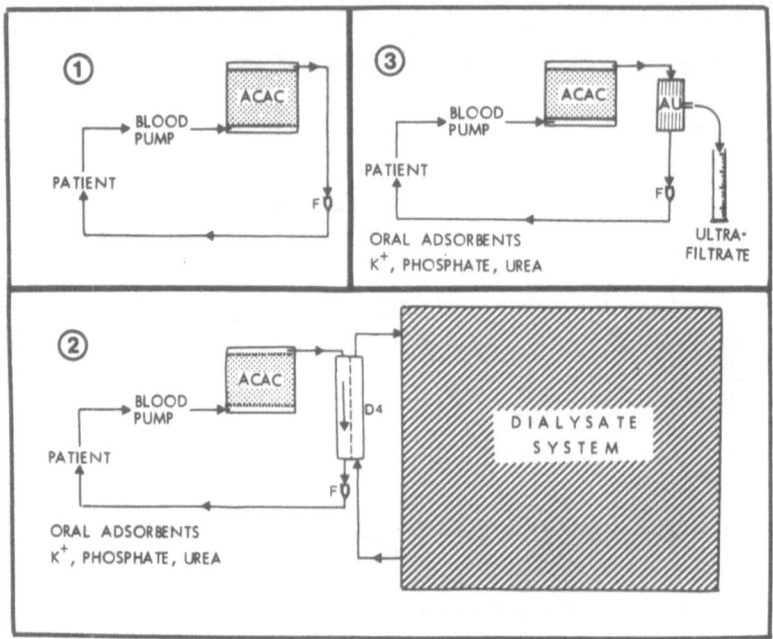

Figure 7

ACAC Hemoperfusion

Treatment using the ACAC hemoperfusion in patients with chronic
renal failure indicated that two hours of hemoperfusion maintained
patients symptom-free as effectively as the standard six to ten
hours of hemodialysis (Chang and Malave, 1970; Chang et al., 1971,
1972, 1974). In-vitro study showed that clearance of ACAC hemoperfusion remained at a high plateau for molecules of up to 1200
molecular weight. Even beyond 1200 molecular weight the clearance
remains many times higher than that for standard hemodialysis.
Based on these in-vitro results, analysis indicated that the total
amount of middle molecules removed by ACAC hemoperfusion in two
hours is comparable to the amount removed after six or more hours
of hemodialysis with the standard coil artificial kidney (Chang and
Migchelsen, 1973). Direct analysis of serum middle molecules in
patients treated with the ACAC hemoperfusion showed that two hours
of hemoperfusion removed more middle molecules than six to eight

hours treatment with the standard hemodialysis machine (Chang et al., 1974). At a blood flow rate of 300 ml/min the clearance was 144 ml/min for middle molecules (300-1500 MW) (Chang, 1977b; Chang et al., 1977) (Figure 7). PTH clearance is 62 ml/min (Q_B 200 ml) and 80 ml/min (Q_B 300 ml). Other substances like guanidines, mercaptans are also removed effectively. In addition to "middle molecules", other considerations include the more effective removal of protein-bound molecules by the ACAC microcapsule artificial kidney. Our finding has been supported by another group (Oules et al., 1978) using a more refined method for analyzing middle molecules. They have found that 2 hours of effective hemoperfusion (saturation takes place after 2 hours) with 300 gms of another type of micro-encapsulated charcoal (Adsorba 300C) is comparable to 4 hours of a high permeability hemodialysis membrane (Rhone-Proules) specially prepared for removing middle molecules.

ACAC Hemoperfusion Alternating With Hemodialysis

Although the ACAC system is more effective in maintaining patients symptom-free and in removing middle molecules, guanidines, creatinine, uric acid and protein-bound molecules, it does not remove urea, phosphates, potassium, sodium chloride and water. As a result the ACAC hemoperfusion was initially alternated with standard hemodialysis (Chang et al., 1971, 1972, 1974; Chang and Migchelsen, 1973). However, this resulted in longer intervals when patients were not treated with ultrafiltration, thus leading to water and electrolyte retention.

ACAC Hemoperfusion In Series With Hemodialysis

More recently the combined use of the ACAC in series with hemodialysers has solved these problems (Chang et al., 1974 and 1975). This approach has been supported by other centers (Winchester et al., 1975, 1976; Odaka et al., 1976; Odaka, 1977). However, this way a hemodialyser is still required although the time of treatment is greatly reduced.

ACAC Hemoperfusion In Series With a Small Ultrafiltrator

Recently an extremely effective small ultrafiltrator has become available for clinical ultrafiltration (Silverstein et al., 1974). We are investigating the combined use of the ACAC system with this small Amicon ultrafiltrator (Chang et al., 1974, 1975, 1976). Six pounds of fluid can be safely removed in two hours when the ACAC microcapsule artificial kidney is used in series with this ultrafiltrator in patients (Chang et al., 1975, 1976; Chang, 1976, 1977).

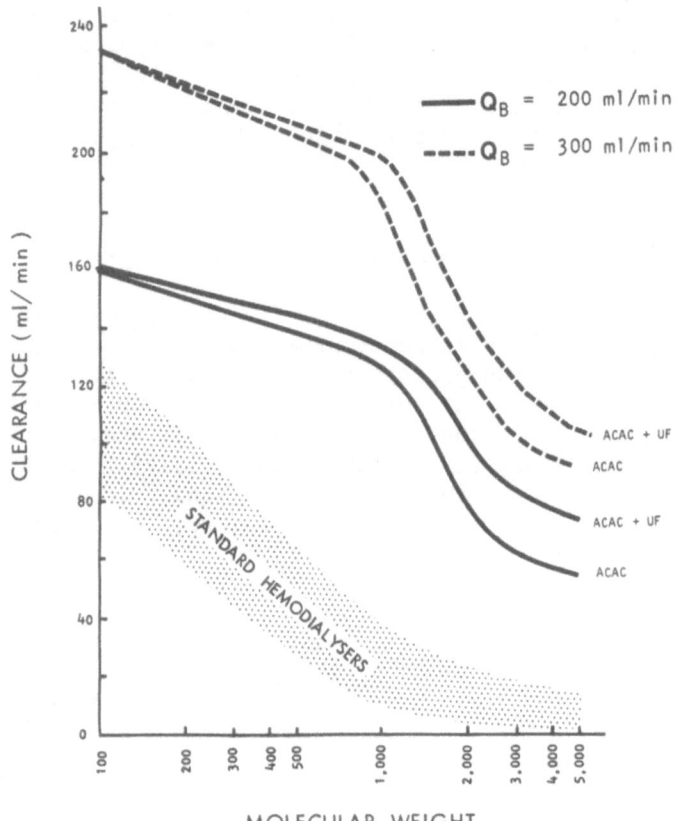

Figure 8   Clearance in patients ACAC hemoperfusion
and ACAC and Ultrafiltrator (UF) updated from
Chang et al (1977).

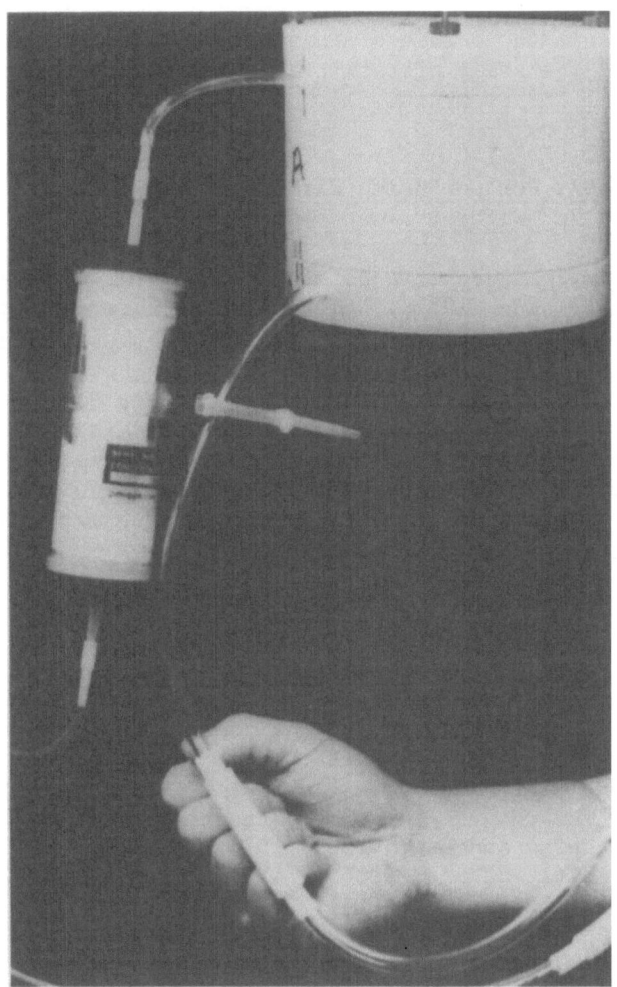

Figure 9   ACAC hemoperfusion in series
with ultrafiltrator.

Hydrostatic pressure alone is sufficient for the formation of ultrafiltrate and no other equipment except the small ultrafilter is
required (Figure 9). The ultrafiltrate can be collected directly
into a beaker. With the further development of urea adsorbent and
phosphate adsorbent, the combined miniaturized microcapsule artificial kidney and the small ultrafiltrator may result in a very
compact artificial kidney system.

ACAC Hemoperfusion With Other Means
For Water & Electrolyte Removal

More recently, the use of a gel for the removal of water has
been investigated (Chang, 1977b). A type of hydrolyzed starch-
polyacrylonitrate graft copolymer has been tested here and found to
have excellent ability to remove water with its electrolytes. However, the polymer granules tends to adhere together to form a large
sticky mass in the presence of aqueous solution making it unsafe for
oral ingestion and hemoperfusion. We have now successfully microencapsulated these granules. In the microencapsulated form they no
longer form adhesive masses in contact with aqueous solution and
can, therefore, be handled with ease.

TREATMENT OF LIVER FAILURE PATIENTS

With the first demonstration of coated charcoal hemoperfusion
as an artificial liver for improving the consciousness in a grade
IV hepatic coma patient in this Unit (Chang, 1972b) extensive
studies have been carried out in a large number of centers to assess
its possible use for the treatment of patients with acute fulminant
hepatic failure (Chang and Migchelsen, 1973; Chang, 1975, 1976a;
Gazzard et al., 1974; Odaka et al., 1978; Amano et al., 1978;
Blume et al., 1976; Gelfand et al., 1978; Silk et al., 1978). This
has resulted in an accumulation of more than 100 reported cases
around the world. These studies have conclusively supported our
initial finding (Chang, 1972b) of the effectiveness of coated charcoal hemoperfusion in improving markedly consciousness of grade IV
hepatic coma. It has been proposed that the improvement in consciousness may be related to the removal of "middle molecular weight
range" toxins and protein-bound molecules (Chang, 1972b; Chang and
Migchelsen, 1973). Unfortunately, the effects on the actual long-
term recovery of the treated patients as compared to untreated
patients are still not conclusive. Survival rates in acute fulminant hepatic failure vary according to age, etiology, grade of coma,
and other factors. This makes it extremely difficult to have
adequate control studies, since one cannot assure that the control
cases correspond exactly in age, etiologies, and grade of coma, etc.
The relatively small number of grade IV fulminant hepatic failure

patients in any one center and variations in survival rates in
different centers, further accentuates this problem to such an extent
that it would be nearly impossible to arrive at a statistical conclusion on the basis of clinical trial. A suitable animal model
system may be the only solution to this problem. As reported by us
recently (Chirito et al., 1977), galactosamine induced fulminant
hepatic rats have been used. Statistical analysis shows a significant increase in recovery for the treated group (< 0.01). Important
fundamental information can be obtained from this type of animal
model to form the basis of clinical treatment of patients. Thus,
in more recent studies it was found that if treatment is delayed
until grade IV coma, there is no statistical improvement in survival;
in addition, with low blood hemoperfusion rate there was no significant increase in survival.

TREATMENT OF PATIENTS WITH DRUG INTOXICATION

Studies carried out in this laboratory for a number of years,
both in animals and in patients, have demonstrated the effectiveness
of ACAC hemoperfusion for the removal of drugs encountered in acute
intoxications (Chang, 1969, 1972a, 1975, 1976b; Chang et al., 1973a,
1973b). Acute intoxication with Salicylate, barbiturates, placidyl,
methaqualone, methyprylon, glutethimide and others have been treated
successfully in patients with ACAC hemoperfusion. Clearance of
drugs (Table 1) is many times higher than standard hemodialysers.
The use of Hemacol, Adsorba 300C and Hemodetoxifier have also been
successfully used for the treatment of patients with acute intoxication (Vale et al., 1975; Goulding, 1976; Martin et al., 1977;
Barbour et al., 1976). The different systems differ significantly
in actual clearance but have all been found to be effective for the
treatment of patients with acute intoxication. The results obtained
so far would indicate conclusively that microencapsulated charcoal
hemoperfusion is effective for the treatment of patients with
severe acute drug intoxication. However, one should take into consideration the affinity of the drug for charcoal and the compartmental distribution of the particular drug.

FUTURE PERSPECTIVES OF ARTIFICIAL CELLS

Artificial cells containing activated charcoal for use in
artificial kidney, artificial liver, and detoxification only demonstrates the crudest possibility of the principle of artificial cells.
Ion-exchange resins have been microencapsulated alone or with enzymes
(Chang, 1966, 1972a). Resins with good adsorption for ammonium
(IONSIV) have also been microencapsulated for the removal of ammonium. However, the future perspectives of artificial cells will be
related to their uses with enzymes and other biological materials.

Table 1

ACAC Hemoperfusion for Acute Intoxication in Patients

Patients	Clinical	Drugs	Clearance	Number of Hemoperfusions	Outcome
1	Grade 4 coma	METHYPRYLON	230 ml/min	2	Recovery
2	Grade 4 coma	GLUTETHIMIDE	150 ml/min	1	Recovery
3	Grade 4 coma	METHYPRYLON METHAQUALONE	230 ml/min 230 ml/min	2	Recovery
4	Grade 4 coma	GLUTETHIMIDE PHENOBARBITAL	230 ml/min 228 ml/min	4	Recovery
5	Grade 4 coma	PHENOBARBITAL	180 ml/min	1	Recovery
6	Grade 4 coma	PHENOBARBITAL	162 ml/min	1	Recovery
7	Grade 4 coma	GLUTETHIMIDE	–	1	Recovery
8	Grade 4 coma	SALICYLATE	150 ml/min	1	Recovery
9	Grade 4 coma	MYTHYPRYLON	–	1	Recovery
10	Grade 4 coma	PHENCYCLIDINE	–	1	Recovery

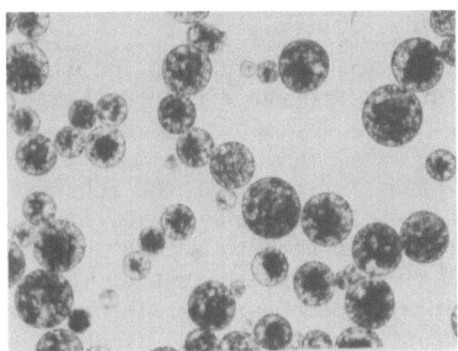

Figure 10.

Artificial Cells Containing Enzymes and Other Biological Materials

Most of the enzymes and proteins in the body function in an intracellular environment. If one were to wupplement enzymes by injecting heterogenous enzymes in free solution there may be hypersensitivity reactions, production of antibodies and rapid removal and inactivation. These problems have led to extensive research into the possible therapeutic uses of immobilized enzymes and proteins. Artificial cells (with microencapsulated enzymes) were the first reported studies of the use of immobilized enzymes and proteins for experimental therapy (Figure 10) (Chang, 1957, 1964, 1972a, 1977a; Chang and MacIntosh, 1964; Chang and Poznansky, 1968). A large number of laboratories are now seriously investigating the possible therapeutic applications of all different types of immobilized enzymes and proteins. These have been reviewed in detail in recent books (Chang, 1972, 1977a). The following is a brief review of experimental studies using artificial cells containing enzymes.

Experimental Routes of Administration

1. Local Implantation by Injection: Artificial cells containing enzymes have been implanted intramuscularly, subcutaneously, and intraperitoneally, and elsewhere (Chang, 1964, 1972, 1977a).

2. Intravenous Injection and Subsequent Localization: Intravenously injected artificial cells larger than 2 μm in diameter are filtered out by the pulmonary capillaries; smaller ones which pass through the pulmonary capillaries are subsequently removed by the reticuloendothelial system of the liver and spleen. Surface properties play an important role in the final distribution (Chang, 1972a). Intravenously injected liposomes are also removed by the liver and spleen, however, their contents can be further located in the intracellular organelles (Gregoriadis and Ryman, 1972). Erythrocyte encapsulated

enzymes have also been introduced intravenously to be removed by the
reticuloendothelial system (Ihler et al., 1973). Removal by the
reticuloendothelial system is useful for localization of enzymes
intracellularly to act on storage diseases resulting from hereditary
enzyme deficiencies.

3. Extracorporeal Shunt Systems: If the substrate to be acted on
is in the bloodstream or in the body fluid, artificial cells can be
used in an extracorporeal system to act on substrates of blood or
body fluid recirculating through the system (Chang, 1966, 1972a).
Extracorporeal shunt system containing microencapsulated urease was
used in dogs to convert blood urea into ammonium (Chang, 1966).
Heparin complexed to microcapsule membranes, shunt chamber, and
tubings avoided the necessity of systemic heparinization (Chang et
al., 1967). Extracorporeal shunts containing microencapsulated
catalase have been used to recirculate peritoneal fluid for the
removal of perborate in acatalasemic mice (Chang and Poznansky,
1968). With these demonstrations of the feasibility of extracorporeal immobilized enzymes, a large number of other extracorporeal
immobilized enzyme systems are being studied. These are reviewed
elsewhere (Chang, 1977a).

4. Local Applications: Microencapsulated enzymes may be applied
directly to local lesions to prevent absorption of the enzyme into
the body or to prevent immunological or hypersensitivity catalase
reactions (Chang, 1972a).

5. Administration into the Gastrointestinal Tract: Substrates
which equilibrate across the gastrointestinal tract might be acted
on this way. For example, microencapsulated urease was used to act
on urea either by direct introduction into the intestine or by oral
administration into animals (Chang and Poznansky, 1968; Chang and
Loa, 1970; Chang, 1972a; Gardner et al., 1971; Asher et al., 1975).

Examples of Experimental Therapy

Artificial Cells containing enzymes and proteins have been
used in a number of experimental and therapeutic conditions. Some
of these are briefly summarized.

1. Red Blood Cell Substrates: Artificial cells containing red
blood cell hemolysate have been assessed for us as red blood cell
substitutes (Chang, 1957, 1964, 1972a; Sekiguchi and Kondo, 1966,
1977). The main problem is related to removal by the reticuloendothelial systems.

2. Model Enzyme Systems for Experimental Therapy: Artificial cells
containing urease has been used as a model immobilized enzyme system
for experimental therapy (Chang and MacIntosh, 1964; Chang, 1964,

1966, 1972a). The basic result obtained paves the way for other
types of enzyme replacement therapy.

3. Hereditary Enzyme Deficiency Conditions: The first demonstration of the use of immobilized enzymes for replacement in hereditary
enzyme deficiency conditions was the use of microencapsulate catalase to effectively replace a hereditary catalase deficiency in
acatalasemia in mice (Chang and Poznansky, 1968; Poznansky and
Chang, 1974). Liposome microencapsulated enzymes have also been
used for replacement in hereditary enzyme deficiency conditions
related to storage diseases (Gregoriadis and Ryman, 1972). Red
Blood cell microencapsulated enzymes have been tested for possible
use in storage diseases (Ihler et al., 1973; Thorne et al., 1975).

4. Artificial Cells Containing Asparaginase for Substrate-Dependent
Tumors: Extensive research into the therapeutic applications of
artificial cells containing enzymes has been the use of asparaginase
for tumor suppression. Having demonstrated the effectiveness of
microencapsulated asparaginase for experimental tumor suppression
(Chang, 1969a, 1971) more detailed studies were carried out on the
various aspects of microencapsulated asparaginase (Chang, 1973b;
Mori et al., 1972, 1973; Siu Chong and Chang, 1974). Since then,
a large amount of work is being carried out by many centers using
all available types of immobilized enzymes for injection and extracorporeal shunts.

5. Extracorporeal Immunosorbent for the Specific Removal of Antigens or Antibodies: Antibodies or antigens immobilized on artificial
cells have been used for extracorporeal perfusion (Terman et al.,
1971, 1977).

6. Use of Artificial Cells for Artificial Organs: Artificial cells
have been used for the construction of artificial kidneys, artificial
livers, and detoxifiers (Chang, 1966, 1972a, 1976a, 1977a). Some
of these studies have been described above.

Multienzyme System

    Thus the biomedical application of artificial cells containing
microencapsulated enzymes have already been demonstrated experimentally using simple single enzyme systems. Unfortunately, most
metabolic functions especially those related to metabolic organs
are carried out in the body by complex multienzyme systems with
cofactor requirements. As a result, basic research is being carried
out here for the microencapsulation of multienzyme systems with
cofactor regeneration (Campbell and Chang, 1975, 1976, 1977). At
present, while still working on basic research in this area, we
are also looking into the possible applied aspects. For example,

urea (in uremia) and ammonia (in liver failure) cannot be removed
by the ACAC hemoperfusion system. We are looking into a long-term
project involving the conversion of urea and ammonia to amino acids
using sequential enzymatic reactions with microencapsulated multi-
enzyme systems. For example, in artificial cells containing multi-
enzyme systems (urease, glutamate dehydrogenase and glucose-6-
phosphate dehydrogenase) urease converts urea to ammonia which is
catalyse by glutamate dehydrogenase in the presence of α-ketoglutarate and NADPH to form an amino acid, glutamate. Glucose-6-
phosphate dehydrogenase is used to recycle the cofactor NADPH required in the reaction (Cousineau and Chang, 1977). The use of
glucose-dehydrogenase instead of glucose-6-phosphate dehydrogenase
allows blood glucose to be conveniently used for regeneration of
the cofactor NADPH (Chang unpublished).

If metabolic toxins accumulated in renal failure or hepatic
failure and other metabolic disorders can be isolated, specific
microencapsulated adsorbents or enzymes can be prepared for their
specific removal. In the longer range perspective, artificial cells
containing enzymes could be implanted directly into the body to
remove these specific toxins. These feasibilities have already been
demonstrated in experimental animal studies for simpler enzyme systems. However, an enormous amount of work will be required to put
this into actual clinical practice.

REFERENCES

Amano, I., Iwatsuki, S., Maeda, K. and Ohta, K. (1978). In this
    volume.
Andrade, J.D., Van Wagenen, R., Ghavamian, M., Volder, J., Kirkham,
    R. and Kolff, W.J. (1972). Trans. Amer. Soc. Artif. Intern.
    Organs, 18, 235.
Asher, W.J., Bovee, K.C., Frankenfeld, J.W., Hamilton, R.W., Hender-
    son, L.W., Holtzapple, P.G. and Li, N.N. (1975). Kidney Int.,
    7, S409.
Barbour, B.H., LaSette, A.M. and Koffler, A. (1976). Kidney Int.,
    10, S333.
Blume, V., Helmstaedt, D., Sybrecht, G., Baldamus, C., Sussman, P.,
    Heyer, V., Schmidt, E., Schmidt, E. (1976). Deutsche Medizin-
    ische Wochenschrift, 14, 559.
Campbell, J. and Chang, T.M.S. (1975). Biochem. et Biophys. Acta,
    397, 101.
Campbell, J. and Chang, T.M.S. (1976). Biochem. Biophys. Res. Comm.,
    69, 562.
Campbell, J. and Chang, T.M.S. (1977). In book on "Biomedical appli-
    cation of Immobilized Enzymes and Proteins", Volume 2, p.281,
    (T.M.S. Chang, ed.), Plenum Publishing Corp., New York.
Castro, L.A., Hampel, G., Gebhardt, R., Fateh, A., Gurland, H.J.
    (1978). In this volume.

Chang, T.M.S. (1957). Report of research project for B.Sc. Honours
    Physiology, McGill University, Montreal.
Chang, T.M.S. (1964). Science, 146, 524.
Chang, T.M.S. and MacIntosh, F.C. (1964). Pharmacologist, 6, 198.
Chang, T.M.S. (1966). Trans. Amer. Soc. Artif. Intern. Organs, 12,
    13.
Chang, T.M.S., Johnson, L.J. and Ransome, O. (1967). Can. J. Physiol.
    Pharmacol., 45, 705.
Chang, T.M.S. and Poznansky, M.J. (1968). Nature, 218, 243.
Chang, T.M.S., Pont, A., Johnson, L.J. and Malave, N. (1968). Trans.
    Amer. Soc. Artif. Intern. Organs, 14, 163.
Chang, T.M.S. (1969). Can. J. Physiol. Pharmacol., 47, 1043.
Chang, T.M.S. and Loa, S.K. (1970). Physiologist, 13, 70.
Chang, T.M.S. and Malave, N. (1970). Trans. Amer. Soc. Artif.
    Intern. Organs, 16, 141.
Chang, T.M.S., Gonda, A., Dirks, J., Malave, N. (1971). Trans.
    Amer. Soc. Artif. Intern. Organs, 17, 246.
Chang, T.M.S. (1972a). Artificial Cells, Charles C. Thomas, Pub-
    lisher, Springfield, Illinois.
Chang, T.M.S. (1972b). Lancet, 2, 1371.
Chang, T.M.S., Gonda, A., Coffey, J., Dirks, J., Burns, T. (1972).
    Trans. Amer. Soc. Artif. Intern. Organs, 18, 465.
Chang, T.M.S. and Migchelsen, M. (1973). Trans. Amer. Soc. Artif.
    Intern. Organs, 18, 314-319.
Chang, T.M.S., Coffey, J.F., Barre, P., Gonda, A., Dirks, J., Levy,
    M. and Lister, C. (1973a). Can. Med. Assoc. J., 108, 429.
Chang, T.M.S., Coffey, J.F., Lister, C. Stark, R. and Taroy, E.
    (1973b). Trans. Amer. Soc. Artif. Intern. Organs.,
Chang, T.M.S., Migchelsen, M., Coffey, J.F., Stark, R. (1974).
    Trans. Amer. Soc. Artif. Intern. Organs, 20, 364.
Chang, T.M.S. (1975). Kidney Int., 7, S387-S392.
Chang, T.M.S., Chirito, E., Barre, P., Cole, C. (1975). Trans. Amer.
    Soc. Artif. Intern. Organs, 21, 502.
Chang, T.M.S. (1976a). J. Kidney International, 10, S218.
Chang, T.M.S. (1976b). J. Kidney International, 10, S305.
Chang, T.M.S. (1977a). Biomedical Application of Immobilized Enzymes
    and Proteins, Vol. 1, pp. 428, Vol. 2, pp. 352. Plenum
    Publishing Corp., New York.
Chang, T.M.S. (1977b). J. Dialysis and Transplantation, 6, 50.
Chang, T.M.S., Chirito, E., Barre, P., Cole, C., Lister, C.,
    Resurreccion, E. (1977). J. Dialysis, 1(3), 239.
Chirito E., Reiter, B., Lister, C. and Chang, T.M.S. (1977).
    Artificial Organs, 1, 76-83.
Cousineau, J. and Chang, T.M.S. (1977a). Proc. Can. Fed. Biol. Soc.,
    20.
Cousineau, J. and Chang, T.M.S. (1977b). Biochem, Biophys. Res.
    Commun. (in press).
Davis, T.A. (1975). Kidney Int., 7, S406.
Fennimore, J., Kolthammen, J.C., and Lang, S.M. (1977). In Arti-
    ficial Organs (T. Gilchrist, ed.).

Gardner, D.L., Falb, R.D., Kim, B.C. and Emmerling, D.C. (1971).
     Trans. Amer. Soc. Artif. Intern. Organs, 17, 239.

Gazzard, B.G., Weston, M.J., Murray-Lyon, I.M., Filax, H., Record,
     C.O., Portman, B., Langley, P.G., Dunlop, E.H., Mellon, P.J.,
     Ward, M.D. and Williams, R. (1974). Lancet, 1(7870), 1301.

Gelfand, M.C., Knepshield, J.H. and Schreiner, G.E. (1978). In
     this volume.

Gilchrist, T., Jonsson, E., Martin, A.M., Naucler, L., Cameron, A.,
     Courtney, J. (1975). In "Artificial Liver Support", p.319.
     (R. William and I. Murray-Lyon, ed.). Pitman Medical Publisher,
     U.K.

Goulding, R., (1976). Kidney International, 10, S338.

Gregoriadis, G., Leathwood, P.D. and Ryman, B.E. (1971). FEBS
     Letters, 14, 95.

Gregoriadis, G. and Ryman, B.E. (1972). Eur. J. Biochem., 24, 485.

Hagstam, K.E., Larsson, L.E. and Thysell, H. (1966). "Experimental
     Studies on Charcoal Hemoperfusion in Phemobarbital Intoxication
     and Uremia Including Histological Findings". Acta Med. Scand.,
     180, 593-603.

Hill, J.B., Palaia, F.L., McAdams, J.L., Palmer, P.J., Skinner, J.T.
     and Marel, S.M. (1976). Kidney International, 10, S328.

Hill, J.B., Palaia, F.L. and Horres, C.R. (1977). In "Artificial
     Organs" (R.M. Kenedi, J.M. Courtney, J.D.S. Gaylor and T.
     Gilchrist, ed.), p. 123. MacMillan Press Ltd.

Ihler, G.M., Glew, R.H. and Schnure, F.W. (1973). Proc. Nat. Acad.
     Sci. U.S., 70, 2663.

Martin, A.M., Gibbins, J.K., Jonsson, E. and Trinder, P. (1977).
     In "Artificial Organs", (R.M. Kenedi, J.M. Courtney, J.D.S.
     Gaylor and T. Gilchrist, eds.), p. 196. MacMillan Press Ltd.

Mori, T., Sato, T., Matuo, G., Tosa, T. and Chibata, I. (1972).
     Biotechnol. Bioeng., 14, 663.

Mori, T. Tosa, T. and Chibata, I. (1973). Biochim. Biophys. Act,
     321, 653

Nakabayaski, N. (1976). In "Proc. 3rd International Symposium on
     Microencapsulation 1976", (in press).

Nose, Y., Malchesky, P.S., Castino, F., Koshino, T., Schwischer, K.
     and Nokoff, R. (1976). Kidney Int., 10, S244.

Odaka, M., Kobajash, H., Tabata, Y., Soma, M. (1976). Kidney Int.,
     10, 197.

Odaka, M. In this volume.

Oka, K., Ohta, T., Kobayashi, M. Yoshida, S., Kaneko, I., Agishi, T.
     and Sugihara, M. (1976). Kidney Int., 10, 197.

Østergaard, J.C.W. and Martiny, S.C. (1973). Biotechnol. Bioeng.,
     15, 561.

Oules, R., Furst, P. and Bergstrom, J. (1978). In this volume.

Poznansky, M. and Chang, T.M.S. (1974). Biochim. Biophys. Acta,
     334, 103.

Sekiguchi, W. and Kondo, A. (1966). J. Japan. Soc. Blood Trans-
     fusion, 13, 153.

Silk, D. and Williams, R. (1978). In this volume.

Silverstein, M.D., Ford, C.A., Lysaght, M.J., Henderson, C.W. (1974).
  New Eng. J. Med., 291, 747-751.

Siu Chong, E.D. and Chang, T.M.S. (1974). Enzyme, 18, 218.

Terman, D.S., Petty, D., Ogden, D., Pefley, C. and Buffaloe, G.
  (1971). J. Clinical Investigation, 57, 1201.

Terman, D.S., Tavel, T.,Petty, D., Racic, M.R. and Buffaloe, G.
  (1977). Clin. Exp. Immunol., 28, 180.

Thorne, S.R., Fiddler, M.B. and Desnick, R.J. (1975). Pediat. Res.,
  9, 918.

Thysell, H., Lindholm, D., Meinegard, N., Jonsson, E., Nylem, U.,
  Suensson, T., Berjkirst, G., Gullberg, G.A. (1976). Proc. 2nd
  Ann. Meeting Europ. Soc. Artif. Organs.

Vale, J.A., Rees, A.J., Widdop, B., Goulding, R. (1975). Brit.
  Med. J., 1(5948), 5-9.

Winchester, J.F., Apiliga, M.T., MacKay, S.M., Kennedy, A.C. (1975).
  Proc. Eur. Dialysis Transplant. Assoc., 12.

Winchester, J.F., Apiliga, M.T., MacKay, J.M., Kennedy, A.C. (1976).
  Kidney Int., 10 (supp. 7), S315.

CLINICAL EXPERIENCE OF BEAD-SHAPED CHARCOAL HAEMOPERFUSION IN CHRONIC RENAL FAILURE AND FULMINANT HEPATIC FAILURE

Michio Odaka, Yoichiro Tabata, Hirotada Kobayashi,
Yoichi Nomura, Hiromitsu Soma, Hiroyuki Hirasawa and
Hiroshi Sato

Department of Surgery (II), School of Medicine
Chiba University, Chiba, Japan

SUMMARY

A new dialysis system using direct haemoperfusion with collodion-micro-encapsulated, albumin-coated, bead-shaped petroleum activated carbon and artificial kidney in series has been devised. This new system has been applied to the purpose of treatment of patients in chronic renal failure, fulminant hepatic failure and intoxication.

For the purpose of an artificial kidney, about 400 dialyses have been performed on 3 patients as a chronic haemodialysis (19, 16 and 3 months). This system is available to cut off regular haemodialysis time to 3 hours with good results. During 3 hours dialysis, reduction ratio of BUN was 48.1%, that of creatinine 49. 6%, and that of uric acid 61.6%. Blood cells were slightly increased in 3 hours dialysis and adjustment of blood pH and base excess were done well with excellent removal of water approximately 2.5 liters in each dialysis.

For the purpose of artificial liver assist in fulminant hepatic failure, this system was applied to 10 patients. Fourty-five dialyses have been done on 10 patients with hepatic coma due to viral hepatitis and drug hepatitis. As a result, 3 of 7 patients, who improved their conciousness, were alive.

INTRODUCTION

The principle of the haemodialysis depends on the phenomena of both diffusion and ultrafiltration, using the semipermeable membrane across the blood and dialysate. In these phenomena, the

small weight molecules of metabolites in the blood are easily removed, but the middle weight molecules of the endogenous substances
of metabolites can little be dialyzed even in long time dialysis.

Since the report by Muirhead and Reid in 1948, many works of
haemoperfusion using resins have been done for removal of exogenous
toxins and endogenous metabolites. On the other hand, Yatzidas reported in 1964 that a column of granular activated charcoal could
efficiently remove barbiturates from perfusion blood.

Unfortunately, there were a number of problems preventing
their widespread clinical application. When resin or activated
charcoal were used to the blood directly, the blood coagulate as a
result of absorbed platelets and leucocytes on the surface of absor-
bents.

In 1970, Chang and his co-workers developed clinical use of
the direct haemoperfusion system, using collodion microencapsulated
albumin-coated activated coconut charcoal to prevent platelet adhesion and particulate embolism. In our case the coconut charcoal we
used had an irregular shape with many sharp edges and a complete
encapsulation with thin membrane was difficult. This factor led to
release of some fine particles from the encapsulated charcoal.

METHODS AND PATIENTS

We have used the new petroleum activated carbon, treated in
high temperature. This carbon has no volatile organic substances

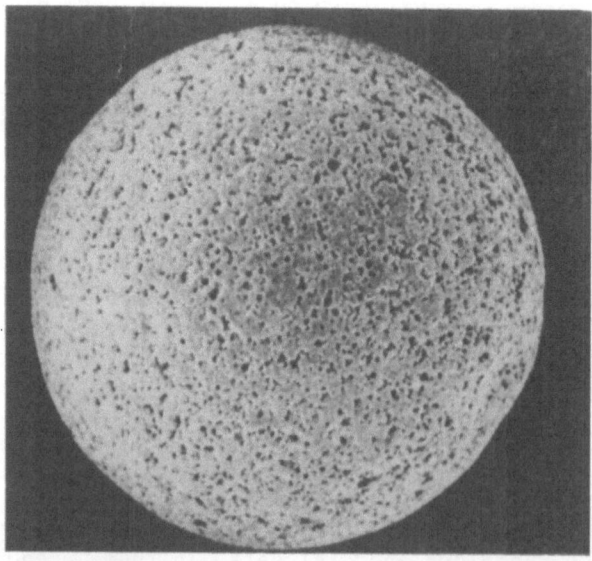

Figure 1. Scanning electron microscope photograph of the
surface of bead-shaped carbon before encapsulation

after this treatment, the ash is less than 0.03% by weight and includes traces of Co, Ni, Cr, Cu, Fe and Mg. The carbon particles
are 0.6mm in average diameter and have 1,000 M^2 per g of adsorption
surface area(by BET method). Other characteristics are spherical
form, considerable hardness and high absorption capacity.

Due to this spherical form, it is easy to coat with a thin
and homogenous film on the surface. In this series, collodion is
used for micro-encapsulation by Chang's method. This material is
coated with albumin solution after collodion encapsulation.

Figure 1 shows the surface of this carbon particle before
micro-encapsulation, viewed with scanning electron microscope.

Figure 2 shows the cut surface of this material after micro-
encapsulation, viewed with scanning electron microscope. The thickness of this film encapsulated is approximately 0.5µ.

An activated charcoal absorbs creatinine, uric acid and middle
molecular weight substances except urea, electrolytes and water.
For the purpose of an artificial kidney, adjustments of electrolytes
and water during haemodialysis are inevitably requested. Therefore,
an ordinary artificial kidney is applied in this purpose. In the
course of this study, a new dialysis system has been devised, in
combining direct haemoperfusion with collodion-micro-encapsulated,
albumin-coated, bead-shaped petroleum carbon and haemodialysis in
series (Figure 3).

The module is made by the following procedure: sieving (> 32
mesh), acid and alkaline treatment, washing and drying, micro-encapsulation with collodion, drying, autoclaving and filling a column
with 130g of capsulated carbon under sterile condition.

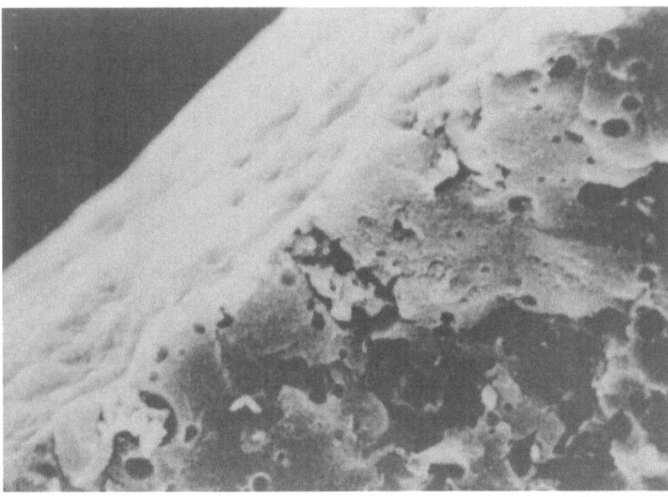

Figure 2. Scanning electron microscope photograph of the
cut surface of bead-shaped carbon after encapsulation

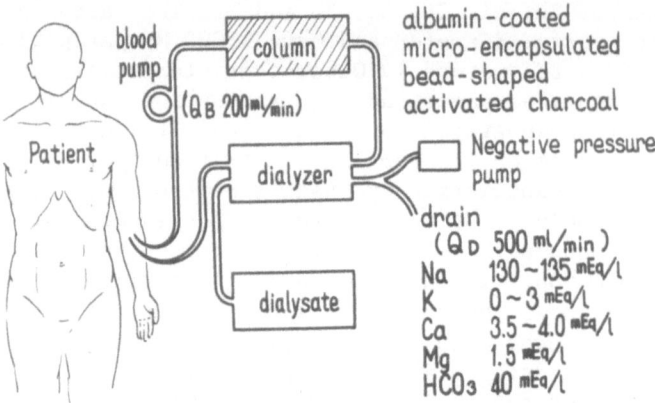

Figure 3. Diagram of our newly devised dialysis system combining direct haemoperfusion and haemodialysis

        The constitution of dialysate for this system used to chronic
maintenance dialysis was as follows; Na:130-135 mEq/l, K:0-3.0 mEq/l,
Ca:3.5-4.0 mEq/l, Mg:1.5 mEq/l and bicarbonate:40 mEq/l. Bicarbonate
used here was very important for prevention of disequilibrium syn-
droms during very rapid dialysis. Flow of dialysate was 500 ml/min.
in single pass method and applied negative pressure was 400-500mmHg.
Duration of dialysis applied was only 3 hours.
        The constitution of dialysate used to artificial liver assist
was as follows; Na:130-145 mEq/l, K:2.5-4.0 mEq/l, Ca: 3.5-4.5 mEq/l,
Mg:1.5 mEq/l, bicarbonate:25-35 mEq/l, and glucose:600-800 mg%. Flow
of dialysate was 500 ml/min in single pass method and applied negative pressure depends upon water balance of each patient.

                                RESULTS

        This 3 hours maintenance dialysis was applied to 3 patients.
The first patient was a 47 year-old male, who had received about 8
years of chronic haemodialysis 3 times a week without urinary output. The second was a 27 year-old male with history of only 2.5
months chronic haemodialysis twice a week with 1,200-1,400 ml/day
urinary output and the last was a 24 year-old female having received
about 7 years of chroinc haemodialysis treatment twice a week with
1,200-1,500 ml/day urinary output.
        For the purpose of artificial liver assist, this system was
applied to 10 patients. Their ages were between 25 and 76 years old.
There were 7 males and 3 females in sex incidence.

Three hundred and ninty-nine dialysis were performed on 3 patients. The first case was treated with this system in 16 months, the second in 19 months and the third in 3 months without any treatment of ardinary artificial kidney during this period. These three patients were kept well with good blood chemical data. During 3 hours dialysis, an average of 2,400 ml of water was removed in each dialysis with symptom-free condition. The average blood flow was 213 ml/min.

Figure 4 shows the blood cell changes during 3 hours perfusion. RBC changes from $150.1 \times 10^4 \pm 34.5 \times 10^4$ to $165.7 \times 10^4 \pm 37.5 \times 10^4$, a 6.1% increase. WBC changes from $3,835 \pm 1,277$ to $4,291 \pm 1,427$, a 11.9% increase and platelet count changes from $178,277 \pm 63,891$ to $184,840 \pm 72,777$, a 3.7% increase.

The reduction in urea, creatinine and uric acid are shown in Figure 5. BUN; 87.2 ± 33.0 to 54.0 ± 28.1 mg/dl or 38.1% with 100g of charcoal, 72.2 ± 23.9 to 37.5 ± 20.4 mg/dl or 48.1% with 130g of charcoal, creatinine; 13.0 ± 3.1 to 6.6 ± 2.3 mg/dl or 49.8% with 100g of the charcoal, 10.7 ± 2.9 to 5.4 ± 1.6 mg/dl or 49.2% with 130g charcoal; uric acid; 10.2 ± 1.6 to 4.1 ± 1.4 mg/dl or 59.3% with 100g of charcoal, 8.6 ± 1.1 to 3.3 ± 0.8 mg/dl or 61.6% with 130g of charcoal column.

The changes in total protein was from 7.1 ± 0.7 to 7.4 ± 0.7 g/dl or a 2.8% increase. The changes in albumin was from 3.8 ± 0.4 to 4.0 ± 0.4 g/dl, a 4.7% increase. The effect on the blood electrolytes was as follows: Na 138.2 ± 2.8 to 138.8 ± 2.7 mEq/l; K 5.3 ± 1.5 to 3.6 ± 0.8 mEq/l; Ca 7.9 ± 1.2 to 9.5 ± 1.2 mg/dl and phosphate 4.6 ± 1.4 to 3.5 ± 1.1 mg/dl.

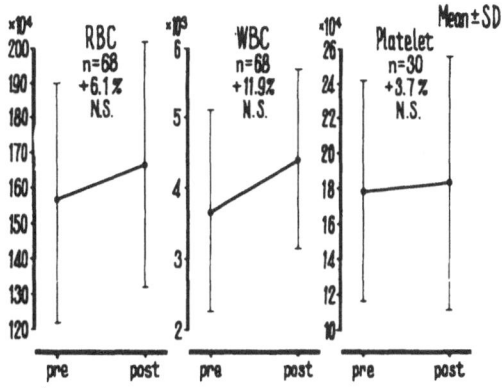

Figure 4. Changes of blood cells during 3 hours perfusion

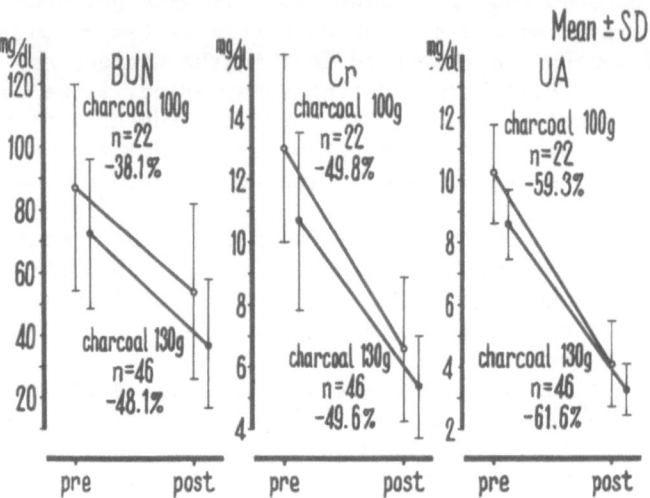

Figure 5. Reduction of BUN, creatinine and uric acid during
        3 hours perfusion

The blood pH changed from 7.361±0.037 to 7.461±0.03 and base excess changed from -4.2±4.1 to 2.4±4.6, however, pH changed from 7.315±0.03 to 7.313±0.08 with charcoal column perfusion only and base excess showed the same results; they changed from -9.4±2.7 to -8.5±3.4.

During this 3 hours dialysis, 6,000 units of heparin were used in each dailysis for systemic heparinization.

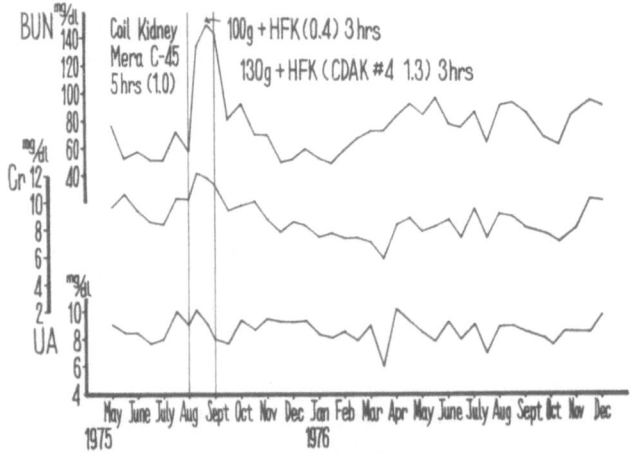

Figure 6. BUN, creatinine and uric acid pre-dialysis levels
        in case 1, 47 year-old male 58 kg

Figure 6 shows predialysis BUN, creatinine and uric acid level for case 1 from May 1975 to December 1976. Before August he was treated with the Mera coil kidney (surface area $1.0M^2$) for 5 hours at a time. From the begining of August 1975 he was treated with this new system over 3 hours. At the begining of this study, 100g of charcoal and the Asahi hollow fiber kidney (surface area 0.4 M^2) were used. The level of BUN increased to 145-155 mg/dl. This suggested that the capacity of this system was too small for him. Then we changed to 130g of charcoal and the 1.3 M^2 hollow fiber kidney. After this, his level of BUN, creatinine and uric acid decreased significantly to the usual maintenance level.

During 399 dialyses in these 3 patients, there have been only 3 episodes of complaint, one of headache, and two of chills and fever at the begining of this series due to mechanical defect of the column used.

Artificial liver assist

A total of 45 haemoperfusion were performed on 10 patients with fulminant hepatic failure (Table 1): 7 with hepatitis B, 2 with hepatitis A and one with drug induced hepatitis. One of them had had no effect with treatment of exchange transfusion.

Seven of the 10 patients improved their conciousness with the perfusion and 3 of 7 patients, who improved their conciousness were discharged to their home.

Duration of the perfusion by this system applied was 4 to 6 hours in each perfusion. The hollow fiber kidney or disposable parallel type dialyzer were used as artificial kidney.

Case No.	Name	Age	Sex	Etiology	GOT mU/ml	GPT mU/ml	T.Bil. mg/dl	D.Bil. mg/dl	Pro.Time sec.	NH_3 /dl	Grade of Coma	Recovered Consciousness	Outcome
1	KM	37	F	Hepatitis B	4410	5160	9.6	4.2		179	III	-	dead
2	TS	71	M	Hepatitis A	903	1332	11.0	6.0		272	IV	+	dead
3	TA	36	F	Hepatitis B	360	1464	12.7	8.0	24.9	130	III	+	alive
4	TS	25	M	Hepatitis B	612	1122	32.8	27.3	25.1	166	IV	+	alive
5	YA	39	M	Hepatitis B	2020	2700	39.2	25.4	28.6	135	IV	+	dead
6	NS	46	M	Hepatitis B	3140	3110	8.7	4.4	48.5	130	IV	+	dead
7*	TT	26	M	Hepatitis B	1680	3110	10.3	5.0	49.0	103	III	-	dead
8	HT	37	M	Drug Hepatitis	1225	750	9.4	7.4	20.5	131	III	+	alive
9	HM	76	M	Hepatitis B	1218	1194	7.4	2.2	37.3	171	IV	-	dead
10**	IH	25	F	Hepatitis A	67	106	10.9	7.6	22.9	309	III	+	dead

* with exchange transfusion
** no effect of exchange transfusion

Table 1. Clinical cases of hepatic coma treated with perfusion

During this perfusion sGOT, sGPT, total bilirubin, direct bilirubin, anmonia and alkaline-phosphatase were not significantly decreased: sGOT decreased 22.6%, sGPT decreased 20.4%, total bilirubin
decreased 10.6%, direct bilirubin decreased 14.7%, anmonia decreased
23.1% and alkaline-phosphatase decreased 11.3%.

However, in serum aminograms, there was a decreased of free
amino acids after the perfusion such as: aspartic acid, isoleucine,
threonine, serine, proline, glycine, cysteine, methionine, tryosine,
phenylalanine, histidine and tryptophan.

Figure 7 shows a clinical course of case 4. He was a 25 years
old male, having received surgery of pyelolithotomy without blood
transfusion on July 4, 1975. In the middle of October 1975, his
liver function was disturbed in spite of no complaints. In the middle of November 1975, the level of sGOT increased up to 820 mU/ml
and sGPT to 790 mU/ml, then he was admitted in a hospital and received ordinary therapy. But on 28 November, jaundice appeared and total bilirubin increased up to 32.8 mg/dl. On 1 December, he had a
grade IV encephalopathy, and therefore, he was transferred to our
University Hospital for treatment with direct haemoperfusion.

His data of blood chemistry and liver function tests are as
follows: sGOT 612 mU/ml, sGPT 1,122 mU/ml, total bilirubin 32.8 mg/
dl, direct bilirubin 27.3 mg/dl, serum anmonia 166 g/dl and prothrombin time 25.1 sec.

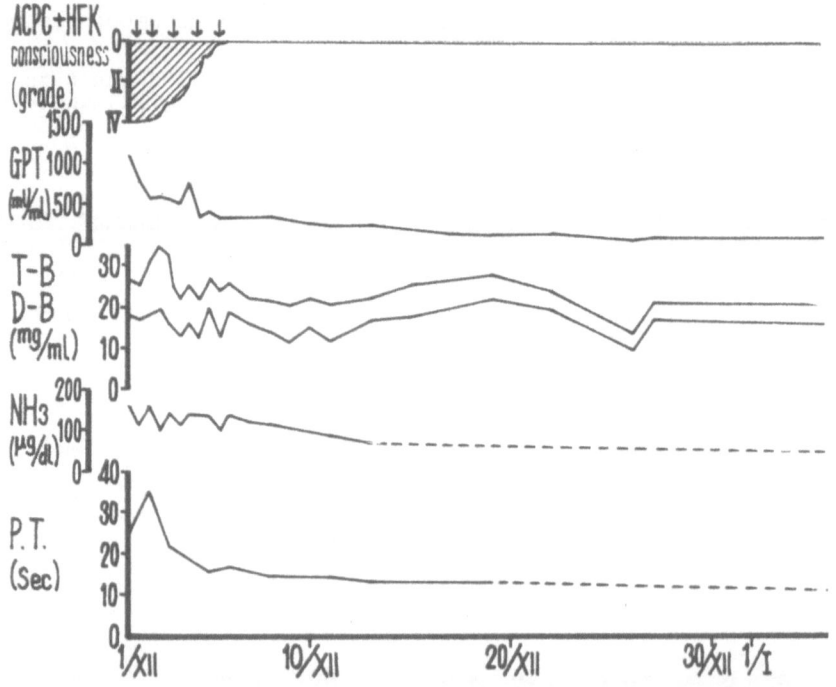

Figure 7 Clinical course of case 4, 25 years old male

In the night of December 1, 1975 an arterio-venous cannula was inserted into his left arm and then the direct haemoperfusion was started through the cannula. After 3 times perfusion, his pain sensation recovered. After the 4th perfusion , he could count numbers. Total 5 times haemoperfusion was performed before complete recovery of his conciousness. His liver biopsy specimen in 2 months after the haemoperfusion suggested strong degenerations of liver cells with severe intistitial fibrosis.

DISCUSSION

In maintenance dialysis, removal of water and adjustment of electrolytes and acid-base balance are essential. For this reason, we applied both direct haemoperfusion and haemodialysis with ordinary artificial kidney to patients with chronic renal failure. Although Chang and his co-workers were afraid of the reduction in platetlets during haemoperfusion with charcoal, in our series there is no platetlet depletion but platetlet increase. Our bead-shaped charcoal protected with perfect membrane prevents platetlet adhesion.

By using 130g of charcoal and 1.3 M^2 surface dialyzer in 3 hours perfusion, the removal capacity of urea, creatinine and uric aicd increases to 1.5 to 2.5 times than ordinary dialyzer. Besides this, middle molecular weight substances may be adsorbed by this system. This character enables us to cut dialysis time by half. Three hours maintenance dialysis helps patients to easy rehabilitation. We are able to use one artificial kidney machine in 2 or 3 shifts in one day.

An absorbent type of artificial organs with charcoal has more effective capacity of excluding endogenous metabolites like middle

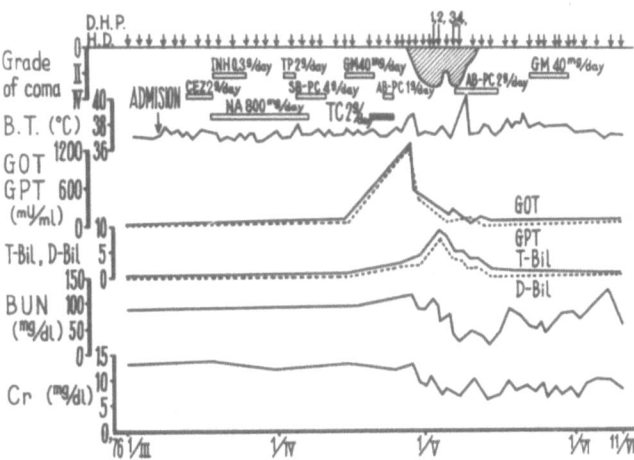

Figure 8 . Clinical course of case 8, 37 years old male

weight molecular substances than ordinary dialyzer. Our charcoal
does not reduce blood elements and coagulation factors, and the
newly devised dialysis system combined with direct haemoperfusion
and haemodialysis is useful to dialyze for all kinds of chronic
renal failure patients, not only for maintenance but also for introduction.

Figure 8 shows the clinical course of a case with fulminant
hepatic failure induced by drug. He had been receiving chronic
maintenance haemodialysis since November 1974. On March 5, 1976 he
was admitted to a dialysis center, with a slight fever. In spite
of the administration of antibiotics, his temperature did not fall.
Finally, after urine culture, we found oxytetracycline was effective
to him. Three days after injection of oxytetracycline 2g/day, jaundice appeared and sGOT increased up to 1,224 mU/ml and total bilirubin was 9.4 mg/dl. After the appearance of his jaundice, haemodialysis with ordinary dialyzer was performed 3 to 4 hours daily.
However, his consciousness did not recover. After 4 times of haemodialysis, a charcoal column was inserted into haemodialysis line just
before the dialyzer. After the 4th haemoperfusion, he recovered
from Grade IV to Grade II. After this he was returned to his standard chronic haemodialysis treatment using a standard dialyzer.

This case suggested to us that our new system devised had more
effective clinical results than ordinary haemodialysis. Autopsy was
carried out on 7 patients, who died from fulminant hepatic failure
despite treatment with our new system. There was evidence of liver
regeneration in the 4 patients who recovered their consciousness
after treatment. However, in those patients who did not recover consciousness, there was diffuse necrosis in their livers. These observations suggest that this system is useful for the treatment of fulminant hepatic failure, although the clinical indication for the use
of this system is a very important problem which has to be worked out.

ACKNOWLEDGEMENTS
We wish to thank for cooperation in this study of Teijin Co.,
Ltd. Tokyo. They supplied all columns of both clinical and animal
use. This work is supported in part by grants from the Ministry of
Health and Welfare in Japan and from The Research Development
Corporation of Japan.

REFERENCES

Chang,T.M.S. Removal of endogenous and exogenous toxin by a microencapsulated adsorbent. Canad. J. Physiol. Pharm. 47:1043, 1969.
Odaka, M. et al: Medical application of albumin-coated activated
granular petroleum carbon. 1975 Symposium on Biomaterials. 185, Soc.
Materials Science Kyoto, 1975.
Odaka, M. et al: Three-hour maintenance dialysis combining direct
haemoperfusion and haemodialysis. Proc. E.D.T.A. 13:257, 1976.

HEPATIC ASSIST SYSTEM USING BEAD-TYPE CHARCOAL

I. Amano, H. Kano, H. Takahira, Y. Yamamoto, K. Itoh,
S. Iwatsuki, K. Maeda, and K. Ohta

Chukyo Hospital and The Biodynamics Research Institute
Chukyo Hospital: 1-23 Sanjyo-cho, Minami-ku
Nagoya, Japan

SUMMARY

Our hepatic assist system consists of a combination of hemoperfusion (200Gm of bead-type charcoal coated with 0.5μm collodion
in a column) and hemodialysis against 35 liters of acetate-free recirculating dialysate. Totally, 55 perfusions have been performed
in 15 patients with acute liver failure (viral hepatitis 13, and
halothan-associated 2) and 3 patients with post-hepatic cirrhosis
(1 with porto-caval shunt). The most frequently treated patient
underwent 9 perfusions, each for 3 hours. Of the above 15 patients,
6 patients partially recovered consciousness. The EEG findings after
hemoperfusion improved in 3 patients, remained unchanged in 3 and
were impaired in 3. Three patients with acute liver failure has
survived. Complications in the other 12 patients were; G.I. bleeding 5, renal failure 2, respiratory failure 3, and cerebral edema
4. The total plasma amino acids had been 245.1mg/100ml (normal
control 47.1mg/100ml) on an average, and they decreased by 26.2%
after hemoperfusion. The total amino acids in cerebro-spinal fluid
(CSF) was 81.9mg/ml (normal control 7.8mg/100ml) on an average, in
which glutamine, methionine, tyrosin and phenylalanine were significantly high. The total CSF amino acids soon after perfusion decreased by 4.1%. And, in patients with improved EEG grades, the total
CSF amino acids were further lowered by 18.2% in 5 hours.

INTRODUCTION

The clinical application of charcoal hemoperfusion (c-HP) as a
new attempt in treating liver failure, especially hepatic coma, had

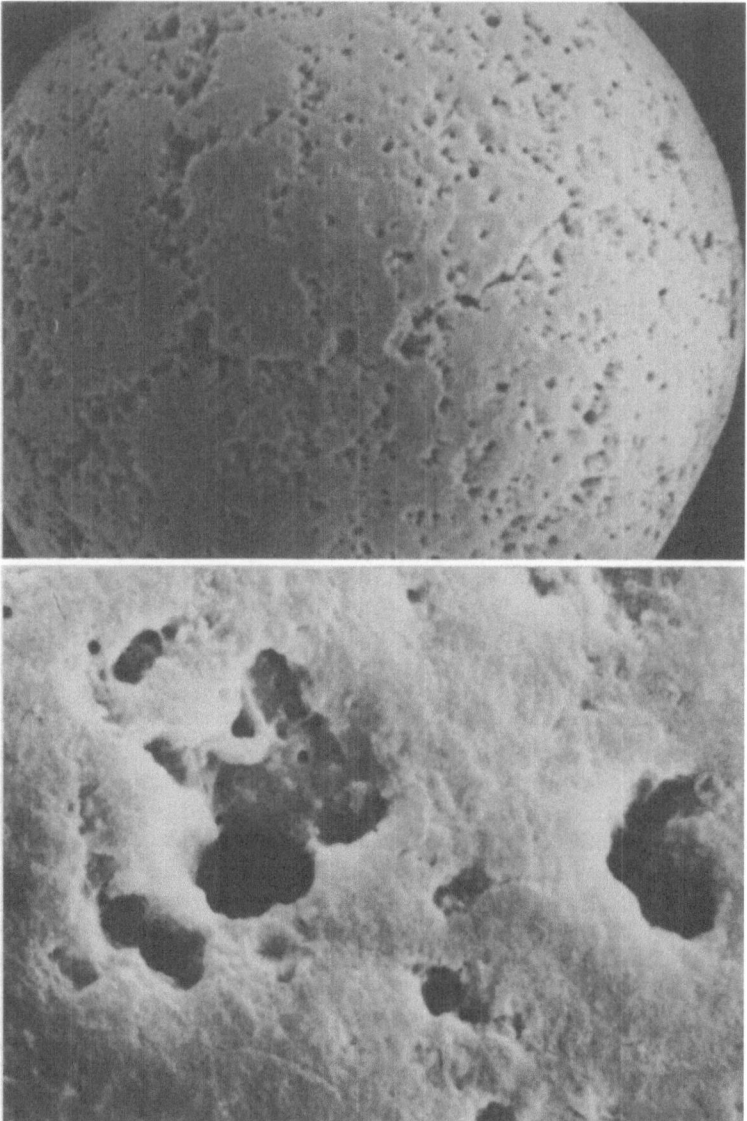

Figure 1. 0.5µm (thickness) collodion coated petroleum charcoal.

Top: 200 X $\frac{2}{3}$ X $\frac{9}{10}$ Bottom: 3000 X $\frac{2}{3}$ X $\frac{9}{10}$

already been reported by Chang, in 1972, Gazzard[2], in 1974, Gelfand[3], in 1975 and others. Its application to acute liver failure, which is a loosely-defined clinical syndrome, entails the consideration of considerably more complicated factors than those associated with the treatment of uremia or drug intoxication. Different and difficult as the situation may be, we have tried the treatment of 15 acute liver failure patients on a hepatic assist system that we have developed on our own, in which bead-type charcoal plays the central role. It should be parenthetically noted here that it is of extreme importance that, in the process of this particular treatment, not only the changes in mental state and electro-encephalogram (EEG), but those in the various amino acids in plasma and cerebro-spinal fluid (CSF) be monitored for the purpose of inferring the toxicity of the amino acids themselves, as well as that of their metabolic products.

MATERIALS AND METHODS
Properties of Micro-Encapsulated Bead-Type Charcoal

Use has been made of bead-type charcoal derived from petroleum pitch (called BAC-LQ or T601) as a detoxicator which forms the core of our hepatic assist system[4]. The bead-type charcoal was coated with a 0.5μm (thickness) collodion membrane, for use in direct hemoperfusion, by spraying a 0.1% pyroxylin ethanol solution using 3.75Gm of pyroxylin per 1Gm of charcoal. (Figure 1)

150-200Gm of this micro-encapsulated bead-type charcoal was steralized in an antoclave and then was sealed in a polycarbonate column whose priming volume being 129ml and pressure drop, 3.7mmHg at a blood flow rate of 200ml/min. The column is filled with a physiological saline solution. Figure 2 shows the numbers of carbon particles that exudes into this saline solution. The numbers of the charcoal particles were determined by a coulter counter immediately after the fabrication of the column, after an overland shipping distance of 4000Km by truck, and also after washing in 0.5L and 1L of physiological saline solution. The counting was carried out only on those particles larger than 2μm, with the result of: 1/ml, 5μm and larger; 5/ml, 2μm and larger.

On the other hand, we have conducted a comparative study on the adsorption capacity of 5 different types of micro-encapsulated activated charcoal (1. 0.5μm collodion-coated BAC-LQ, 2. 1.5μm collodion-coated BAC-LQ, 3. uncoated BAC-LQ, 4. Haemocal--in England 5. Defoxyl-1--in Italy). Selected as adsorbabale susbtances were Vitamin B_2(MW 376 daltons), sodium sulfo-bromophthalein (838), Vitamin B_{12}(1578), and insulin (6,000), which were all tested under the experimental perfusion conditions of: 1. sorbent, 1 gm; 2. total circuit volume, 10ml; flow rate, 1ml/min. (Figure 3)

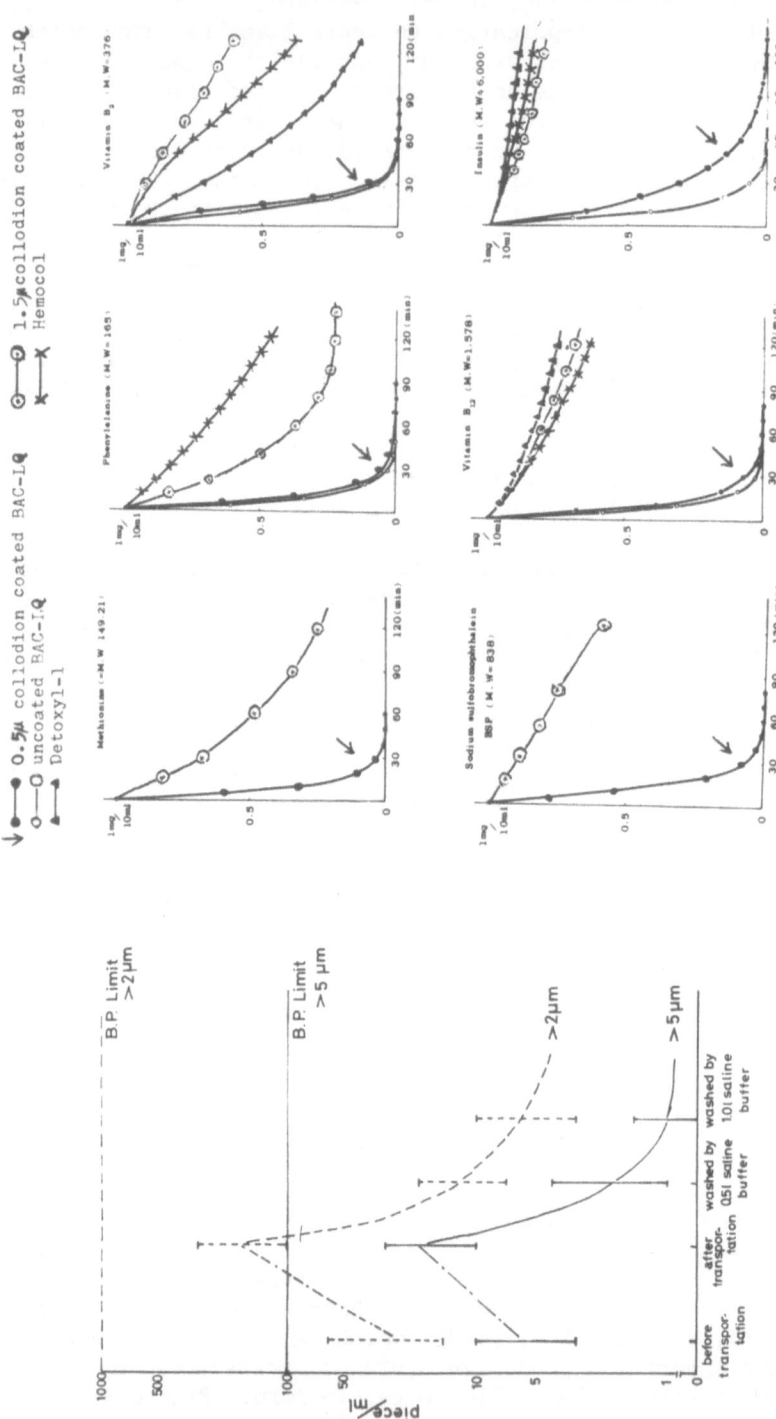

Figure 3. Adsorption capacity of microencapsulated charcoals for different molecular
substances

Figure 2. The numbers of pulverized carbon
particles in the 200Gm of charcoal column

The results have made it clear that both 0.5μm collodion-coated BC-LQ and uncoated BAC-LQ have almost the same adsorption capacity, but that the former enjoys a better performance in the so-called middle molecular range.

Clinical Approach

Our hepatic assist system combines bead charcoal hemoperfusion and hemodialysis by a cuprophane membrane in which 35L of acetate-free dialysate is recirculated, the total priming volume being about 300ml.

The patient's blood passes through the charcoal column and the dialyzer at a flow rate of 200ml/min. During perfusion, 0-1,000 units/hr of sodium heparinate is used to control the clotting time (Lee-White) to 30-60min. One perfusion takes 3hrs, and requires approximately 400ml of fresh blood or fresh frozen plasma.

A total of 55 perfusions had been performed between May, 1975 and March, 1977 on 15 acute liver failure patients--viral hepatitis 13, halothan-associated 2, and 3 patients with post-hepatic cirrhosis (1 with porto-caval shunt). By our definition, liver failure is considered "acute" when it involves fulminant hepatitis and the patient has fallen in coma within 8 weeks of the onset of the hepatitis.

For the purpose of evaluating the effectiveness of the system, observation was made of changes in mental state and EEG, which were divided into 5 levels, 0-V, and 5 grades, A-E, respectively. (0: normal, I: depression or euphoria, II: drowsiness, III: stupor, IVa: coma--response to painful stimuli, IVb: coma--hyperextension and pronosupination after painful stimuli, IVc: coma--no response to painful stimuli, V: clinical decerebration)/(A: slow α waves, bursts of θ waves, B: continuous θ waves or prevalent θ waves, C: continuous slower and irregular δ waves, E: flat). Biochemical examinations were conducted on prothrombin time, s-GOT, s-GDT, s-bilirubin, RBC, Hts, WBC, s-electrolytes and the blood gas was analyzed, while measurements by auto-analyzer JLC-6AH were made of plasma amino acid concentrations in 4 aucte liver failure patients before and after 9 perfusions, where 8 normal men were used as controls. Simultaneous measurements were also made of cerebro-spinal fluid amino acids in 4 of the patients before and after 8 perfusions, where 5 non-metabolic disease patients free of consciousness disorders were used as controls. Furthermore, additional measurements were made on CSF amino acids five hours after the perfusions.

CLINICAL RESULTS
Consciousness Level & Biochemical Tests
The changes in the consciousness level of the 15 acute liver

Table I. List of hepatic coma patients treated with our hepatic assist system.

case	age sex	etiology	prothrombin time (sec)	bilirubin (mg/100ml)	GOT GPT (K unit)	ammonia (μg/100ml)	pH PO₂ PCO₂ (mmHg)	Na K (mEq/l)	coma level	EEG grade	No. of perfusion	complication	cause of death	liver weight (grm)
1	40 ♀	cirrhosis with portal caval shunt	22.8	1.8	56	216	7.410 / 66.79	140 / 3.5	III→0	C	2			
2	63 ♂	cirrhosis	15.0	2.0	44 / 12	206	7.360 / 90.28	128 / 3.9	III→0	C	2		G I bleeding	
3	58 ♀	viral hepatitis	21.4	23.0	376 / 202	310	7.500 / 66.26	136 / 2.8	IVa→0	C	9	pneumonia	respiratory failure	660
4	38 ♂	viral hepatitis							III→0	C	1	acute renal failure	G I bleeding	
5	44 ♀	viral hepatitis	16.4	33.8	483 / 516	184	7.390 / 76.28	128 / 3.2	IVa→I	B	7		cerebral edema	730
6	64 ♂	viral hepatitis	19.2	4.2	823 / 144	212	7.500 / 92.32	148 / 3.0	III→0	C	2			
7	27 ♀	viral hepatitis(B) chronic renal failure	51.3	6.6	16000 / 8060		7.202 / 66.30	133 / 6.1	III→I	C	3	DIC	G I bleeding	823
8	58 ♀	viral hepatitis	19.1	22.6	2450 / 1320	79	7.412 / 76.42	137 / 5.2	IVa>IVb	D	2		cerebral edema	920
9	32 ♂	halothan	20.0	4.6	3780 / 4250	200	7.450 / 68.46	148 / 3.9	III→0	C	2	alive →	heart failure	
10	25 ♀	viral hepatitis	40.2	13.6	1320 / 480		7.420 / 68.36	136 / 3.2	IVa→IVa	B	5	DIC	respiratory failure	1000
11	46 ♂	cirrhosis	17.4	2.4	42 / 32	148	7.420 / 94.28	138 / 3.6	III→0	C	2			
12	32 ♂	viral hepatitis	22.1	15.2	820 / 690		7.470 / 92.29	136 / 3.2	IVa>Na	C	4	acute renal failure	cerebral edema	820
13	36 ♂	viral hepatitis	21.0	8.4	1250 / 1340		7.480 / 76.32	140 / 3.8	III→0	B	3			
14	56 ♂	halothan	34.4	5.5	3500 / 4200		7.430 / 65.30	138 / 3.2	IVa>IVb	D	3	DIC	respiratory failure	
15	28 ♂	viral hepatitis(B)	20.2	4.2	890 / 780		7.460 / 66.46	134 / 3.6	III→0	C	3			
16	26 ♂	viral hepatitis	28.2	8.8	1280 / 1040		7.550 / 72.42	138 / 3.0	IVa<IVb	D	2		G I bleeding heart failure	
17	50 ♀	viral hepatitis	19.2	18.6	642 / 452	82	7.490 / 82.34	138 / 3.0	II→I	B	2			
18	59 ♂	viral hepatitis	25.4	20.4	2042 / 1864		7.550 / 92.39	142 / 5.0	Na→Na	C	1		cerebral edema G I bleeding	720

failure patients treated on the system were as follows: recover of
consciousness level, 6 (III→0, 5, IVa→0), mental state and EEG
grade improved 3 (IVa→I, 1, III→I, 1, II→I, 1), unchanged 3 (IVa→
IVa, 3), impaired 3 (IVa→IVb, 3).

Of the above 15 patients, 3 has survived (liver functions returned to normal)--(Table 1). Changes after a single perfusion
were: platelet counts dropped by 0-50%, s-bilirubin was elevated
0-5%, and WBC showed no change. No appreciable changes were observed in prothrombin time, s-GOT and s-GDT immediately after perfusion.

Amino Acids Analysis

The plasma total amino acids of the acute liver failure patients was 245.1mg/100ml (n=9), which was extremely high compared
with the 47.1mg/100ml (n=8) of the normal controls. A single
application of the present method resulted in an average drop of
26.2%, which breaks down into: aspartic acid 33.3%, threonine 9.8%,
serine 7.3%, asparagine, 4.1%, glutamic acid 34.8%, glutamine 23.1%,
proline 21.3%, glycine 21.4%, alanine, 28.7%, valine 2.0%, cystine
11.1%, methionine 38.2%, isoleucine 27.2%, leucine 11.1%, tyrosin
40.3%, phenylalanine 33.9%, triptophane 14.8%, lysine 36%, histidine
31.2%, and arginine 43.0%. (Figure 4)

Also, the CSF total amino acids registered an extremely high
average value of 81.90mg/100ml (n=8) compared with the 7.75mg/100ml
of the controls (n=5). Of these, abnormally high were glutamine
68.50mg/100ml, methionine 1.66mg/100ml, tyrosine 1.80mg/100ml,
phenylalanine 1.89mg/100ml. (Figure 5) Even immediately after the
application of the system, the CSF total amino acids dropped by an
average of no more than 4.1% (n=8). But when tested again 5hrs
after the perfusion, an average drop of 18.2% (n=3) was observed
when the calculation was limited to only those patients who had
shown improvements in their EEG grade. (Figure 6)

Complications

The complications in the 11 deaths were: G.I. bleeding 5,
renal failure 2, respiratory failure 3, heart failure 2, pneumonia
1, metabolic acidosis 1, increased jaundice 5, and autopsic cerebral edema 3.

DISCUSSION

Attempts have been made to treat 15 acute hepatic failure
patients on our hepatic assist system, of whom 3 have been saved,
and 1 is still under treatment. As regards the relationships
between treatment results and the time of the commencement of

	Before perfusion	After perfusion	P
Aspartic acid	0.3 ± 0.2	0.2 ± 0.2	NS
Threonine	8.1 ± 2.2	7.3 ± 2.0	0.001
Serine	4.1 ± 0.9	4.4 ± 1.4	0.001
Asparagine	4.8 ± 0.5	4.6 ± 0.6	0.001
Glutamic acid	9.2 ± 7.4	6.0 ± 5.0	0.02
Glutamine	78.1 ± 12.2	60.2 ± 20.1	0.001
Proline	14.1 ± 6.2	11.1 ± 5.1	0.05
Glycine	11.2 ± 1.2	8.8 ± 0.8	0.001
Alanine	23.7 ± 6.3	16.9 ± 8.1	0.05
Valine	4.8 ± 1.6	4.7 ± 2.3	0.05
Cystine	4.5 ± 2.0	4.0 ± 2.3	0.02
Methionine	13.1 ± 6.9	8.1 ± 3.1	0.01
Isoleucine	1.1 ± 0.9	0.8 ± 0.2	NS
Leucine	1.8 ± 0.9	1.6 ± 0.2	NS
Tyrosine	10.4 ± 6.6	6.2 ± 3.0	0.001
Phenylalanine	12.1 ± 3.9	8.0 ± 2.4	0.02
Tryptophane	2.7 ± 1.7	2.3 ± 1.1	NS
Lysine	17.5 ± 2.5	11.2 ± 4.8	0.01
Histidine	9.3 ± 3.9	6.4 ± 2.0	0.001
Arginine	14.2 ± 1.2	8.1 ± 1.1	0.01

mg/100ml

Figure 4. Plasma amino acids in patients with acute liver failure (n=9)

		normal control (n=5)
Aspartic acid	0.82 ± 0.24	0.00 ± 0.00
Threonine	1.30 ± 0.20	0.31 ± 0.10
Serine	0.84 ± 0.08	0.28 ± 0.06
Asparagine	0.29 ± 0.16	0.17 ± 0.07
Glutamic acid	0.04 ± 0.04	1.46 ± 0.24
Glutamine	68.5 ± 20.5	1.95 ± 0.26
Proline	0.00 ± 0.00	0.00 ± 0.00
Glycine	0.24 ± 0.22	0.17 ± 0.12
Alanine	0.71 ± 0.20	0.42 ± 0.24
Valine	0.15 ± 0.02	0.11 ± 0.05
Cystine	0.00 ± 0.00	0.00 ± 0.00
Methionine	1.66 ± 1.21	0.00 ± 0.00
Isoleucine	0.11 ± 0.09	0.10 ± 0.04
Leucine	0.10 ± 0.04	0.28 ± 0.11
Tyrosine	1.80 ± 0.75	0.19 ± 0.08
Phenylalanine	1.89 ± 0.89	0.22 ± 0.10
Tryptophane	1.28 ± 0.60	0.94 ± 0.44
Lysine	0.66 ± 0.22	0.39 ± 0.10
Histidine	0.62 ± 0.40	0.22 ± 0.08
Arginine	0.90 ± 0.22	0.48 ± 0.16

mg/100ml

Figure 5. Cerebro spinal fluid amino acids in patients with acute liver failure (n=8)

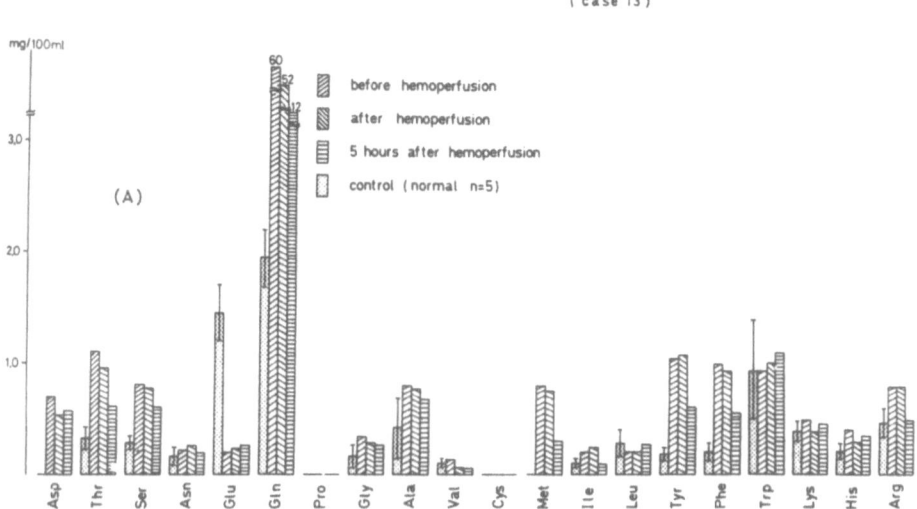

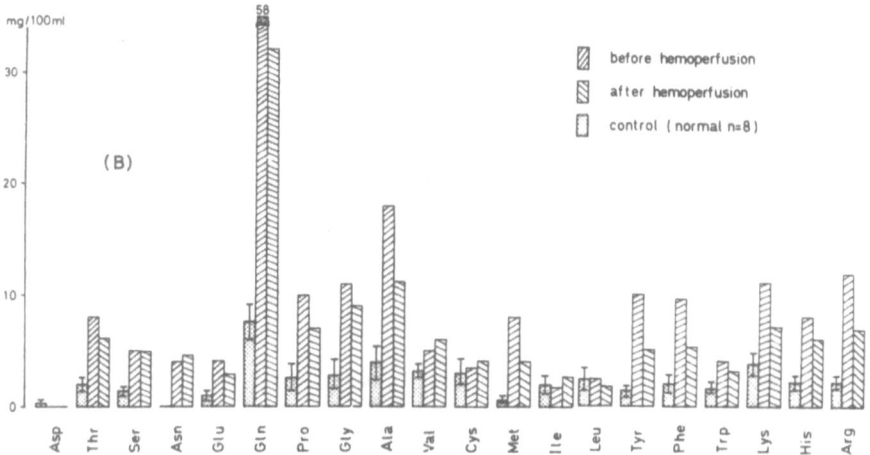

Figure 6.   Results of amino acid analysis of cerebrospinal
fluid (A) and plasma (B) pre- and post- application of our hepatic assist system.   (case 13)

treatment by the system and the patients' mental state, all the
cases saved had commended at II-III,while those commencing at IVa-
IVb all died eventually.

However, of the 11 deaths, partial recovery of consciousness
was observed in 5, whose possible causes of death had been thought
to be various complications, especially hemorrhage, cerebral edema,
infections, renal failure; rather than genuine hepatic failure. In
fact, when autopsies were conducted on 7 of the deaths, regeneration of hepatic cells was observed with a hepatocyte volume fraction of 45-60%. All these findings are in agreement with the reports by Gazzard et al.[5]

It should also be noted here that our use of 400ml fresh blood
or fresh frozen blood seemed to be more effective in controlling
bleeding tendency and blood pressure.

The CSF amino acids compensation by the application of the
system was delayed compared with plasma amino acids compensation
with a net result that CSF amino acids were not always compensated
for. This may well have been influenced by the severity of the
disease.

The present system, with its life-saving rate of 20%, is in
no way superior to blood exchange, but holds open the possibility
of saving more lives if consideration is to be given to: 1) commencing treatment before consciousness level deteriorates, 2) taking
appropriate measures against serious complications, and 3) simultaneously using fresh blood.

REFERENCES

1. Chang, T.M.S., and Migchelsen, M. Trans. Amer. Soc. Artif.
    Int. Organs 19:213, 1973.
2. Gazzard, B.G., Weston, M.J., Murray-Lyon, I.M., Flax, H.,
    Mellon, P.G., Ward, M.B., and Williams, R. Lancet I: 1301,
    1974 c.
3. Gelfand, M.C. Kidney International, Vol. 10, Suppl. 7, 1976.
4. Amano, I., Kano, H., Saito, A., Manji, T., Yamamoto, Y.,
    Iwatsuki, S., Takahira H., Ohta, K., and Maeda, K. Proc.
    Europ. Dial. Transplant Ass. pp. 262, 1976.
5. Gazzard, B.G. et al.: Q. J. Med. 44:615, 1975.

EXTRACORPOREAL IMMUNOADSORBENTS FOR SPECIFIC EXTRACTION

OF CIRCULATING IMMUNE REACTANTS

David S. Terman, M.D. and George Buffaloe, M.S.

Baylor College of Medicine

Houston, Texas 77030

INTRODUCTION

Considerable evidence has accumulated to substantiate the role of immune reactants in many experimental and human diseases.[1,2] Therapy for many of these immunologically mediated diseases has been dependent upon the use of pharmacologic agents that widely and non-specifically suppress host immunity leading to numerous undesirable effects.[3] In addition, there has been an increasing awareness of the etiologic factors in many immunologically mediated diseases and the concomitant development of many sensitive radioimmunological techniques to measure them. Therefore, we have focused our attention on a specific therapeutic measure, i.e., the development of solid phase immunoadsorbents to specifically remove pathogenic immune reactants from the circulation. For this purpose we have developed several immunoadsorbents consisting of immobilized antigens, antibodies and enzymes. When placed in an extracorporeal circuit, these immunoadsorbents have shown a capacity to specifically extract or hydrolyze immune reactants in the circulation with no demonstrable release of immobilized substances and no significant immediate or long-range toxicity to the host.

MATERIALS AND METHODS

Mongrel dogs, 15 to 25 kg were employed for these studies. Preparation and purification of antigens, antibodies and enzymes have been previously described.[4-9] Preparation of collodion-charcoal and nylon microcapsule immunoadsorbents for each system herein described have been detailed in previous communications.[4-9] For extracorporeal circulation studies, dogs were anesthetized, antico-

aglutated and either an arteriovenous fistula or the femoral artery
and vein were cannulated with wide bore polyethylene catheters. Arterial blood was pumped directly through immunoadsorbent chambers or
into a continuous flow plasma-cell separator (American Instruments
Company, Silver Springs, Maryland). When the plasma-cell separator
was employed, arterial blood was partitioned into plasma and formed
elements and plasma was pumped at 40 ml/min through immunoadsorption
chambers. Plasma was then recombined with formed elements and was
then returned to the femoral vein. Schematic representation of the
extracorporeal circulation system is shown in Figure 1.

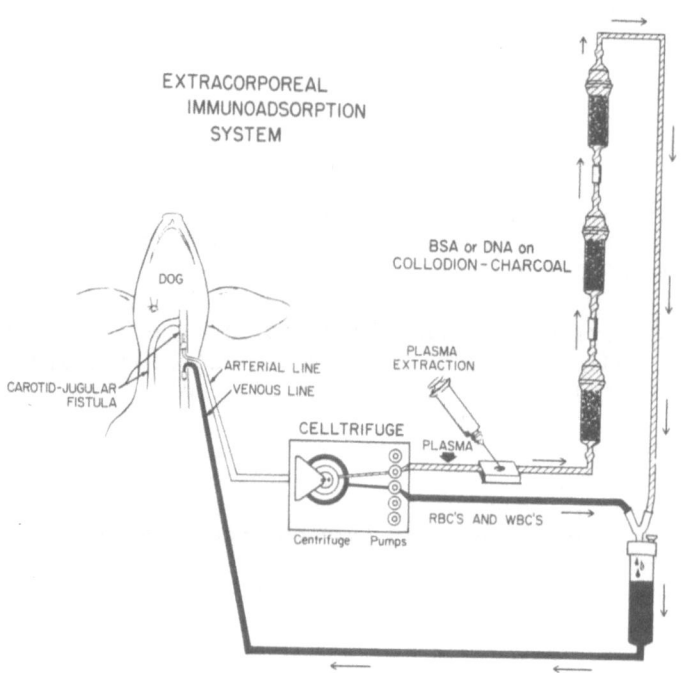

Figure 1   Schematic representation of extracorporeal immunoadsorption system is depicted.

RESULTS AND CONCLUSIONS

The protein antigen bovine serum albumin (BSA) was immobilized
in collodion-charcoal as previously described.[4] Employing ^{125}I BSA
as a marker in the entrapment procedure, we were able to demonstrate
a 47% uptake of unlabelled antigen in collodion-charcoal representing
43 mg of BSA bound. To determine whether BSA would retain its anti-

genicity once immobilized in collodion-charcoal, it was placed in an
extracorporeal circulation system in vivo on line with the plasma-
cell separator. This unit was employed in order to permit contact of
plasma alone with the immunoadsorbent surface and to increase the
efficiency of immunoadsorption. Rabbit anti-HSA and anti-BSA was
passively infused into adult mongrel dogs and after an equilibration
period of 15 minutes, canine plasma was pumped over BSA collodion-
charcoal at a flow rate of 50 ml/min. This resulted in an abrupt
and specific decline in BSA binding by sera with no significant
change in HSA binding over the same time period.[4](Figure 2)

Mongrel dogs were then actively immunized to BSA and HSA. After perfusion of plasma over BSA collodion-charcoal there was an 80%
decline in BSA binding with a slow tempo of rebound in the postperfusion period that reached preperfusion levels in 7 days. Retreat-
ment of this animal in the postperfusion period resulted in a similar specific decline in BSA binding that was further augmented by
the interjection of a second BSA collodion-charcoal column. The
pattern of postperfusion rebound was similar to that in the initial
study. HSA binding was unchanged over the same time period. In
neither study was there any evidence of release of ^{125}I BSA from the
immunoadsorbent into the circulation or evidence of acute or chronic
host toxicity.[4]

Up to 3 mg of purified rabbit antibodies to BSA were immobilized
in collodion-charcoal and placed in parallel with control columns
having normal rabbit gamma globulin entrapped in collodion-charcoal.
Both systems were placed on line with the plasma-cell separator. The
capacity of the immobilized anti-BSA to specifically remove circulating antigen was tested by passively infusing ^{125}I BSA intravenously.
The resultant uptake of ^{125}I BSA was up to 9 fold greater on the anti-BSA collodion-charcoal compared to control charcoal.[5](Table 1)

The capacity of the collodion-charcoal system to specifically
remove DNA antibodies was investigated. DNA antibodies when combined
with specific antigen, i.e., DNA, form immune complexes which deposit
in tissues and create inflammation. Indeed, DNA:anti-DNA immune
complexes are considered to be the major pathogenic immune complex
system in systemic lupus erythematosus (SLE). Up to 7 mg of native
DNA antigen were immobilized in collodion-charcoal which were capable
of specifically removing anti-DNA antibodies that were passively infused into the circulation of mongrel dogs. After an equilibration
period of 20 minutes there was an abrupt and specific decline in DNA
binding by plasma after passage over DNA collodion-charcoal with
minimal change in BSA binding over the same time period.[6](Figure 3)

We then approached the question of eliminating DNA, circulating
free or as part of a DNA anti-DNA immune complex. For this purpose
the enzyme deoxyribonuclease (DNAase) which rapidly degrades DNA was
immobilized on activated nylon microcapsules. Employing ^{131}I DNAase

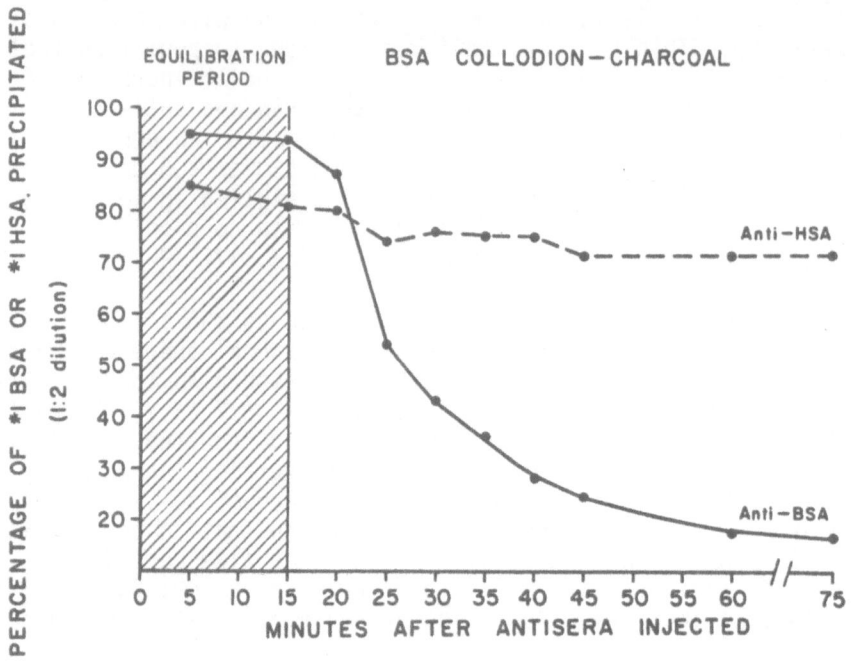

Figure 2   Dog was infused with rabbit anti-BSA and rabbit anti-HSA antisera. After an equilibration period of 15 minutes, plasma was circulated over BSA collodion-charcoal which resulted in a specific reduction in BSA binding by dog sera compared to minor changes in HSA binding over the same time periods.

as a marker, 4.7 mg of DNAase was covalently conjugated to the nylon microcapsules.[7,8] For in vivo studies DNAase nylon microspheres were placed in siliconized glass chambers and ^{125}I DNA was then administered intravenously to mongrel dogs. Whole blood was pumped over DNAase microspheres at a flow rate of 200 ml/min. After a control period of circulation over untreated microcapsules, DNAase microcapsules were then introduced into the extracorporeal circuit. This resulted in an abrupt acceleration in the pattern of DNA decay compared to the control period and to the extrapolated slope of normal decay into the experimental period.[7] In a second series of studies, DNA:anti-DNA immune complexes were prepared at 6 times equivalence and injected intravenously into mongrel dogs. After a control period of 8 minutes, DNAase microcapsules were introduced into the circulation period which resulted in an abrupt change in the slope of decay of DNA:anti-DNA complexes compared to the control period and to the extrapolated control slope into the experimental period thus suggesting that hydrolysis of DNA in the complexes was

TABLE I

Uptake of ^{125}I-BSA on Collodion-Charcoal[a]

Dog No.	Anti-BSA Collodion-Charcoal		Normal Gamma Globulin Collodion-Charcoal	
	cpm	Ug	cpm	Ug
in vitro	52,334	1.30	6,441	0.16
1	388,688	9.71	43,358	1.08
2	271,689	6.79	37,688	0.94
3	251,826	6.29	88,838	2.22

Approximately 1.5 x 10^6 cpm of BSA were found to be circulating in each animal based on cpm in 1-ml plasma sample taken 5 min after injection of ^{125}I-BSA extrapolated for total plasma volume of each dog calculated at 4.98% of total body weight. At the conclusion of in vitro or in vivo circulation studies, collodion-charcoal was washed with 400 ml of 0.15 M NaCl and counted in a gamma scintillation counter.

was occurring.[7] This DNAase microcapsule system coupled with the DNA collodion-charcoal adsorbent, described above,[6] may provide a dual approach to the specific removal or hydrolysis of the major pathogenic immune reactants in the circulation of patients with SLE.[7]

We then sought to extend our extracorporeal immunoadsorbent studies to the immobilization of a tissue antigen in order to determine whether it would be capable of attenuating or arresting the development of an autoimmune disease by specifically removing a pathogenic antibody. For this purpose we chose to study the model of passively induced nephrotoxic glomerulonephritis in dogs. Antibody to canine glomerular basement membrane (GBM) was raised in rabbits and then it was isolated and purified.[8] This anti-GBM antibody was employed to create glomerulonephritis in mongrel dogs. Up to 4 mg of GBM antigen was prepared and was incorporated into collodion-charcoal in a fashion similar to BSA.[8] In each experimental and control dog open renal biopsies were performed prior to extracorporeal pertusion and again just before the termination of the extracorporeal procedures. In each animal, histologic and florescent findings were graded at the conclusion of each experiment and results were compared with the animal's own preperfusion biopsy.

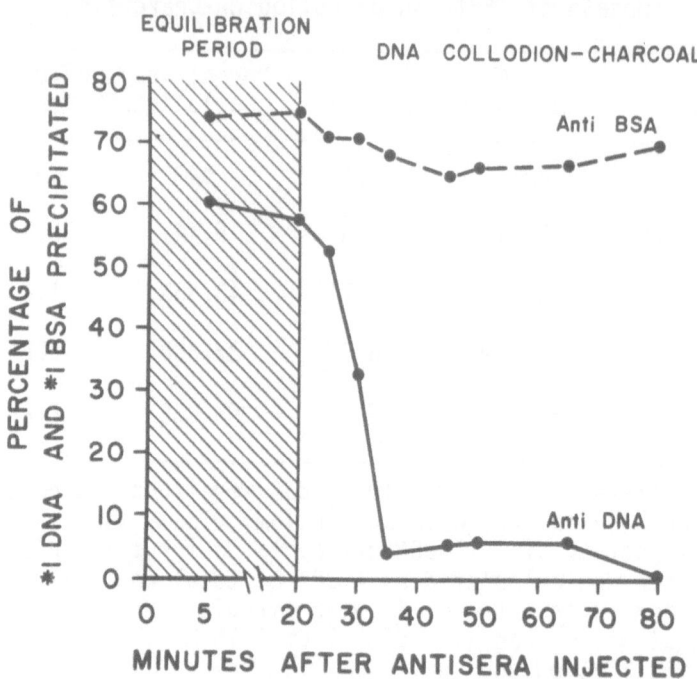

Figure 3   Human anti-DNA and rabbit anti-BSA antibodies were
injected intravenously and after an equilibration period of 20 minutes plasma was pumped over DNA-collodion-charcoal. There was an
abrupt and specific decline in DNA binding over the ensuing 15 minutes with minimal change in BSA binding over the same time period.

Anti-GBM antibody was infused intravenously into dogs and whole blood
was pumped over GBM collodion-charcoal. In control dogs, blood was
pumped over collodion-charcoal in which no antigen or an irrelevant
antigen was physically entrapped in collodion-charcoal. In the first
series, a significantly more rabbit IgG was deposited in control
glomeruli in a diffuse linear pattern compared to deposition in experimental glomeruli.[8](Table 2)   Light microscopic grades to include findings such as neutrophil exudation and mesangial hypercellu-
larity showed considerably more inflammation in the controls compared
to experimental kidneys.[8]

In conclusion we herein describe the development of two new extracorporeal immunoadsorbents. In one system several antigens including BSA, DNA and GBM were immobilized in collodion membranes ad-
herent to small charcoal particles. The immobilized BSA was capable

TABLE II
GBM Immunoadsorbent Histology

Immobilized Antigen	Cumulative Histologic Grade	Major Pathologic Pattern
HSA	***	Neutrophil exudation Mesangial hypercellularity
HSA	**	Mesangial hypercellularity
GBM	0	-
GBM	0	-

of specifically removing circulating BSA antibodies from the sera of both passively and actively immunized dogs. DNA similarly immobilized may specifically remove circulating DNA antibodies. Canine glomerular basement membrane antigen was also physically entrapped in collodion membranes. Mongrel dogs injected with heterologous anti-GBM antibody and whose blood was perfused over GBM collodion-charcoal showed less deposition of gamma globulin and less inflammation in kidneys compared to controls. Deoxyribonuclease covalently coupled to activated nylon microspheres showed the capability of hydrolyzing DNA circulating free or bound in an antigen antibody complex. The latter system employed together with DNA-collodion-charcoal in an extracorporeal circuit may be capable of extracting or hydrolyzing the major pathogenic immune reactants in the circulation of patients with SLE. The present findings suggest that extracorporeal immunoadsorbents are capable of specifically removing actual or potentially pathogenic immune reactants from the circulation and may be potentially useful in the therapy of numerous immunologically mediated diseases in man.

REFERENCES

1. Cochrane, C.C., and D. Koffler. 1973. Immune complex disease in experimental animals and man. Adv. Immunol. 16:185.

2. Vaughan, J.H. 1971. Autoallergic diseases: concepts and general considerations. Immunological Diseases. 2:987.

3. Decker, J.L., Bertino, J.R., Hurd, E.R. & Steinberg, A.D., 1973. Cytotoxic drugs in rheumatic diseases. Arth. and Rheum. 16:79.

4. Terman, D.S., Petty, D., Pefley, C., Buffaloe, G. Specific re-
    moval of circulating antibody by antigen immobilized in collo-
    dion-charcoal. Clin. Exp. Immunol. In Press.

5. Terman, D.S., Petty, D., Ogden, D., Pefley, C. and Buffaloe, G.,
    1976. Specific extraction of antigen in vivo by extracorporeal
    circulation over antibody immobilized in collodion-charcoal. J.
    Immunol. 117:1971.

6. Terman, D.S., Petty, D., Ogden, D., Harbeck, R., Buffaloe, G.,
    and Carr, R. 1976. Specific removal of DNA antibodies in vivo
    by extracorporeal circulation over DNA immobilized in collodion-
    charcoal. Clin. Immunol. Immunopathol. In Press.

7. Terman, D.S., Tavel, A., Tavel, T., Petty, D., Harbeck, R.,
    Buffaloe, G., and Carr, R. 1976. Degradation of circulating
    DNA by extracorporeal circulation and nuclease immobilized on
    nylon microcapsules. J. Clin. Invest. 57:1201.

8. Terman, D.S., Tavel, T., Petty, D., Tavel, A., Harbeck, R.,
    Buffaloe, G. and Carr, R. 1976. Specific removal of bovine
    serum albumin (BSA) antibodies by extracorporeal circulation
    over BSA immobilized in nylon microcapsules. J. Immunol. 116:
    1337.

9. Terman, D.S., Durante, D., Buffaloe, G. and McIntosh, R. 1977.
    Attenuation of canine nephrotoxic glomerulonephritis with an ex-
    tracorporeal immunoadsorbent. Scand. J. Immunol. 6:195.

EVALUATION OF CHARCOAL HEMOPERFUSION IN UREMIA

James F. Winchester, M.B., M.R.C.P.

Royal Infirmary, Glascow, Scotland
Presently at Georgetown University Hospital
Nephrology Division, Washington, D.C.

This paper deals primarily with the evaluation of activated charcoal hemoperfusion in the management of the uremic patient. The studies were performed on a short-time basis (1, 2), and no long term studies of the particular charcoal hemoperfusion device used in these studies have been performed. Chang, et al (3, 4) have published the only long-term studies of charcoal hemoperfusion in the management of uremia.

Modern hemodialysis therapy has been remarkably successful in the maintenance of many thousands of end-stage kidney disease patients throughout the world (5, 6). The introduction of dialysis in a workable form by Kolff in 1944 (7), and its refinement in modern times, have dramatically improved the prognosis for acute and chronic renal disease. It is, however, clear that the metabolic consequences of renal failure are not completely reversed, and a search has been made for alternatives to dialysis, adjuncts to dialysis and improvements in dialytic techniques. Charcoal hemoperfusion, offers a new approach to the removal of metabolic waste products by the process of physical adsorption; activated charcoal does not remove significant quantities of plasma water, urea, or electrolytes (1-4) and hemoperfusion requires combination with dialysis or ultrafiltration in order to correct the fluid/electrolyte problems present in end-stage kidney disease.

METHODS AND RESULTS

Three stable end-stage renal disease patients underwent 6 combined hemodialysis-hemoperfusion treatments, on a thrice weekly

basis; using standard dialysis apparatus and a charcoal column
containing 300 G acrylic hydrogel coated activated charcoal (Smith
and Nephew Research, Ltd., Harlow, Essex, England). Comparison of
2 hrs of combined hemodialysis/hemoperfusion (HP/HD), after which
dialysis alone was continued, was made with a standard 5 hr hemodialysis (HD), normally employed in these patients. Seven
patients underwent 2 hrs of charcoal hemoperfusion alone (HP), and
a further 2 patients with the syndrome of dialysis encephalopathy
underwent at least two 4-hr treatment periods of combined hemo-
dialysis/hemoperfusion (HP/HD). Blood flow was maintained at 300
ml/min, except in the dialysis encephalopathy patients (150-200
ml/min). Measurements of coagulation and hematological status
were taken, in addition to biochemical determination of plasma,
urea, phosphate, creatinine, and uric acid at timed intervals
during each procedure. Free amino acids and serum middle molecular
weight substances (MMs) (8) were determined before and after the
procedures, and hormone concentrations (Total T3 and T4, HGH,
insulin) determined before and after, and across the dialyzer/hemo-
perfusion apparatus after 15 minutes of treatment. Solute
clearance (ml/min) was calculated from the formula

$$\text{Clearance} = \text{Blood Flow Rate} \times \frac{\text{Inlet plasma conc.} - \text{outlet plasma conc.}}{\text{Inlet plasma conc.}}$$

Total solute removal was calculated from the area between inlet
outlet concentration curves (9). Clinical observations were also
made.

     No significant differences were observed in terms of solute
clearance from siting the hemoperfusion device proximal (in 6
treatments) or distal to the dialyzer and the results are combined.
No additional phosphate or urea removal was observed during
combined HD/HP. Mean solute clearances of creatinine and urate
(Table 1) were significantly greater during combined HD/HP than
during HD or HP alone; for HP alone there was an observed fall in
creatinine and urate clearances after 2 hrs treatment. Total
creatinine and urate removal (Table 2) was slightly greater for 2
hr combined HD/HP than for 2 hr HD alone, but significantly less
than 5 hr HD alone. Two hr HP alone removed quantities of
creatinine and urate equivalent to 2 hr HD. Total solute removal
during HD/HP agrees well with solute removal reported by Chang,
et al, 1975 (10). Middle molecular weight substances were reduced
by HP alone, and from visual appreciation of the chromatograms
after HD/HP the middle molecular weight peaks appeared lower than
after HD alone.

     Changes in amino acids and hormones are respectively shown in
Tables 3 and 4; free amino acid concentrations were decreased with
HD or HP/HD, the combined HP/HD treatment being associated with

TABLE 1

Solute Clearance (Ml/Min) (M ± SD) Blood Flow Rate 300 Ml/Min

		Creatinine	Urate
Standard HD	15 Min	114 + 59	107 + 29
(n = 18)	3 Hr	113 ± 46	105 ± 52
2 Hr HD/HP	15 Min	275 + 38	165 + 43
(n = 18)	2 Hr	227 ± 44	144 ± 76
2 Hr HP	15 Min	181 + 7	116 + 29
(n = 6)	2 Hr	123 ± 14	71 ± 17

TABLE 2

Solute Removal (G) (M ± SD)

		Creatinine	Urate
Standard HD	2 Hr	1.6 + 0.4	0.7 + 0.3
(n = 18)	5 Hr	3.1 ± 1.3	1.6 ± 0.5
2 Hr HD/HP		1.7 + 0.6	1 . + 0.5
(n = 18)		(2.0)	(0.7)
	HD	1 + 0.6	0.5 + 0.2
	HP	0.8 ± 0.2	0.4 ± 0.3
2 Hr HP (n = 6)		1.3 + 0.6	0.6 + 0.2

(   ) From Chang, et al, TRANSACTIONS ASAIO, 1975

greater percentage changes in cystine, glycine, histidine, valine, and threonine, than HD alone. In contrast HP alone was associated with a significant fall only for cystine, and significant rises in serine. Hemoperfusion was associated with greater changes in total T4, T3, and insulin than HD alone, and HGH was reduced with all therapeutic modalities.

Table 5 is a summary of the hematological and coagulation changes associated with hemodialysis and/or hemoperfusion in the patients studied. Platelet count decreased only during HD/HP (30%) or during HP alone (20%), but no associated changes in screen filtration pressure (a measure of platelet-white cell aggregates) (11) during dialysis alone or hemoperfusion alone occurred. Small changes in total fibrinogen occurred with the addition of HP to dialysis, and HP alone, but no changes in coagulation tests nor coagulation factor concentrations occurred.

TABLE 3

Changes in Amino Acids

(Amino acids examined were ala, cys, gly, his, ileu,
leu, lys, met, phe, ser, thre, tyr, val)

	Fall	Rise
Standard HD (n = 4)	ala*, cys*, gly* met*, thre*	—
HD/HP (n = 6)	ala*, cys**, gly** thre**, val*, his**	—
HP (n = 7)	cys*	ser*

*p < 0.05   **p < 0.025

In the two dialysis encephalopathy patients, although increased solute clearance and solute removal occurred with the addition of HP to HD, associated with a greater removal of MMs, no observable clinical change occurred over a two week study period, and both patients subsequently died.

No significant clinical problems arose with hemodialysis, although in the first patient in whom a large volume dialyzer was used (Travenol Ultraflo 145) on two occasions significant hypotension was observed when HP was used additionally. In the other 2 patients in whom a Cordis-Dow dialyzer was used and in the patients undergoing HP alone, no hypotensive episodes were observed.

TABLE 4

Changes in Hormones (Total T3, Total T4, Insulin, HGH)

	Fall	Rise
Standard HD (n = 12)	HGH**	T4**
HD/HP (n = 12)	T4**†, HGH**	
HP (n = 6)	T3**, Insulin** HGH*	

*p < 0.05   **p < 0.01

†(Removal at 15 mins p < 0.01)

Table 5

Hematological Changes with Hemoperfusion in Uremia

	Standard HD	HD/HP	HP
WBC	Transient	Transient	Transient
Platelets	—	30% ↓	20% ↓
SFP	—	Not measured	—
Coag Tests	—	—	—
Fibrinogen	—	10% ↓	30% ↓
Coag Factors (II-XII)	—	—	—

DISCUSSION

Activated charcoal hemoperfusion possesses useful sorbent properties for medical application of which the most widely used and accepted is in the field of acute drug intoxication (12-14). Charcoal hemoperfusion is, however, capable of removing many uremic toxins, such as creatinine, uric acid, middle molecular weight substances, organic acids, phenols, indoles, polyamino acids, small polypeptides, amino acids (15) and recently the hormones T3 and T4 (16). Hemoperfusion has also given encouraging results in the treatment of hepatic coma (4, 17, 18), although further study is necessary to define its role in this field.

Charcoal hemoperfusion using 200-300 G charcoal is incapable of removing significant quantities of water, electrolytes, and urea, a disadvantage which imposes major restrictions on its use, as a sole measure, in renal failure and necessitates its combination with dialysis or ultrafiltration in this respect (1-4, 10).

Although this study and many others have shown that charcoal hemoperfusion can increase the efficiency of hemodialysis, it must be demonstrated to have additional properties (19) which would validate its use as an alternative to dialysis. In this respect, hemoperfusion has been shown to remove middle molecules more efficiently than standard hemodialysis (3), although in this study only minor additional middle molecule removal was seen on combining hemoperfusion with hemodialysis. Middle molecules may be responsible (20, 21) for the continuing metabolic disturbances seen in maintenance dialysis patients, such as anemia, pericarditis, and neuropathy, etc., and the long-term studies of Chang, et al (3, 4, 10) show that neuropathy may be improved to some extent. It has been proposed that a 2 hr hemoperfusion time (alone or in combination with dialysis or ultrafiltration) is sufficient repetitive therapy in uremia, and although small solute removal (creatinine and urate) in this study was less than standard 5 hr hemodialysis, there is only circumstantial evidence implicating

urea (23) or creatinine (24) in the pathogenesis of the uremic
state.

Recently Oules, et al (25) have demonstrated that middle
molecule (peaks 7a, b, c, d) removal by charcoal hemoperfusion for
3 hrs in uremia, is equivalent to 4 hrs of hemodialysis, and
substantiate the findings in this study. They (25) also showed
that phenylalanine, tyrosine, and arginine were removed, and that
serine, glycine, and alanine were released after initial adsorption
on charcoal. The rise in serine concentrations with HP alone in
this study may reflect serine release from charcoal.

Free T3 and free T4 (not measured in this study) are known to
be adsorbed in patients undergoing charcoal hemoperfusion for
thyrotoxicosis (16), and the falls in total T3 and T4 seen in this
study could be accounted for by removal of the free components.
The falls in insulin, and HGH seen in this study were unexpected,
with hemoperfusion alone; during dialysis or dialysis/hemoperfusion
the dialysate concentration of glucose was 206 mg%, which may be
responsible for pituitary HGH suppression. HGH concentrations are,
however, known to fall during glucose free dialysis in diabetic
subjects, the mechanism of which is obscure, although heparin
induced rise in free fatty acids may suppress HGH (26). Dialysis
is known to remove insulin inefficiently (27) and hemoperfusion may
be responsible for removal of insulin, although this requires
further investigation.

Hemostatic changes occurring with hemoperfusion have recently
been reviewed (28), and in this study it was felt that although
minor changes in platelets and fibrinogen did occur, these changes
are acceptable. No observable changes in SFP were recorded,
although dramatic rises in SFP have occurred with charcoal hemoperfusion in the treatment of hepatic coma (29), suggesting that
the platelet defects in hepatic coma may differ from the known
platelet defects in uremia (30).

It is not yet possible to define the role of charcoal hemoperfusion in uremia, but combination with dialysis or ultrafiltration is desirable; it would also seem that if efficiency in terms
of solute removal of the devices presently available (including
the device used in this study) is to be improved, that different
charcoal preparations or alternative sorbents would be necessary
for repetitive use in the maintenance of uremic patients.

SUMMARY

The studies reported in this paper were designed to assess
quantitatively the effect of hemoperfusion (HP) on total solute
removal, middle molecular weight substance removal (MMs) and

effect on coagulation status in uremic patients. A HP column containing 300 G acrylic hydrogel coated activated charcoal was used alone (6) or combined with hemodialyzer (18) for periods of 2 hrs, at blood flow rates of 300 ml/min. HP alone removed 1.3 ± 0.6 G creatinine, and 0.6 ± 0.2 G urate, while combined HP and HD removed 1 ± 0.5 G creatinine and 0.6 ± 0.2 G urate. Both treatment schedules removed less solute than conventional 5 hr HD, but were associated with increased MMs removal. A 30% fall in platelet count was observed with HP but no association changes in coagulation factors occurred. Changes in amino acids and hormones also occurred.

HP has considerable potential for use in uremia but this study suggests that the HP device used may require modification to increase efficiency.

ACKNOWLEDGEMENTS

This work was made possible by the help and guidance of several colleagues, and particular thanks is made to Professor A.C. Kennedy, Drs. J.M. Mackay and M.T. Apiliga, and Sister E.A. McAllister of the Dialysis Unit. Smith and Nephew Research, Ltd., kindly donated hemoperfusion columns; and the advice of J. Fennimore and P. Watson is gratefully acknowledged.

Secretarial assistance was received from Mrs. P. Werr.

REFERENCES

1. Winchester, J.F., Apiliga, M.T., Mackay, J.M., Kennedy, A.C. Haemodialysis with charcoal haemoperfusion. Proc Eur Dial Transplant Assoc 12:526-533, 1975.

2. Winchester, J.F., Apiliga, M.T., Kennedy, A.C. Short-term evaluation of charcoal hemoperfusion combined with dialysis in uremic patients. Kidney Int 10:S315-S319, 1976.

3. Chang, T.M.S., Migchelsen, M., Coffey, J.F., Stark, A. Serum middle molecule levels in uremia during long-term intermittent hemoperfusions with the ACAC (coated charcoal) microcapsule artificial kidney. Trans Amer Soc Artif Int Organs 20:364-371, 1974.

4. Chang, T.M.S. Hemoperfusion alone and in series with ultrafiltration or dialysis for uremia, poisoning, and liver failure. Kidney Int 10:S305-S311, 1976.

5. Bryan, F.A. Sixth Annual Progress Report, National Dialysis Registry, 1973-1974.

6. Brunner, F.P., Giesecke, B., Gurland, H.J., Jacobs, C.,
    Parsons, F.M., Scharer, K., Seyffart, G., Spies, G., Wing,
    A.J. Combined report on intermittent dialysis and transplan-
    tation in Europe. Proc Eur Dial Transplant Assoc 12:3-64,
    1975.

7. Kolff, W.J., Berk, H.T.J. Artificial kidney: Dialyzer with
    great area. Acta Med Scan 117:121-134, 1944.

8. Dall'Aglio, P., Buzio, C., Cambi, V., Arisi, L., Migone, L.
    La retention de moyennes molecules dans le serum uremique.
    Proc Eur Dial Transplant Assoc 9:409-415, 1972.

9. Winchester, J.F., Edwards, R.O., Tilstone, W.J., Woodcock,
    B.G. Activated charcoal hemoperfusion and experimental
    acetaminophen poisoning. Toxicol and Appl Pharmacol 31:120-
    127, 1975.

10. Chang, T.M.S., Chirito, E., Barre, B., Cole, C., Hewish, M.
    Clinical performance characteristics of a new combined system
    for simultaneous hemoperfusion-hemodialysis ultrafiltration in
    series. Trans Amer Soc Artif Int Organs 21:502-508, 1975.

11. Swank, R.L., Roth, J.G., Jansen, L. Screen filtration pres-
    sure method and adhesiveness and aggregation of blood cells.
    J Appl Physiol 19:340-346, 1964.

12. Chang, T.M.S., Coffey, J., Lister, C., Stark, A., Taroy, E.
    The efficiency of the ACAC microcapsule artificial kidney for
    the removal of glutethimide, methyprylon, and methaqualone in
    patients with acute intoxication. Trans Amer Soc Artif Int
    Organs, 19:87-91, 1973.

13. Vale, J.A., Rees, A.J., Widdop, B., Goulding, R. Use of
    charcoal hemoperfusion in the management of severely
    poisoned patients. Br Med J 1:5-9, 1975.

14. Gelfand, M.C., Winchester, J.F., Knepshield, J.H., Hanson,
    K.M., Cohan, S.L., Strauch, B.S., Geoly, K.L., Kennedy, A.C.,
    Schreiner, G.E. Charcoal hemoperfusion in severe drug over-
    dosage. Trans Amer Soc Artif Int Organs 23 (In press), 1977.

15. Winchester, J.F. Clinical Application of haemoperfusion in
    uraemia. In Artificial Organs (Ed. R.M. Kenedi, J.M. Courtney,
    J. Gaylor, T. Gilchrist), Macmillan Press, Ltd., London &
    Basingstoke, 1977 (In press).

16. Hermann, J., Rudorff, K.H., Gockenjan, G., Konigshausen, Th.
    Grabensee, B., Kruskemper, H.L. Charcoal haemoperfusion in

thyroid storm. Lancet 1:248, 1977.

17. Gazzard, B.G., Portmann, B.A., Weston, M.J., Langley, P.G.
     Murray-Lyon, I.M., Dunlop, E.H., Flax, H., Mellon, P.J.,
     Record, C.O., Ward, M.B., Williams, R. Charcoal haemoper-
     fusion in the treatment of fulminant hepatic failure.
     Lancet 1:1301-1307, 1974.

18. Gelfand, M.C., Knepshield, J.H., Cohan, S., Ramirez, B.,
     Schreiner, G.E. Treatment of hepatic coma with hemoperfusion
     through polyacrylamide hydrogel coated charcoal. Kidney Int
     10:S239-S243, 1976.

19. Kennedy, A.C. In Discussion, Proc Eur Dial Transplant Assoc
     13:270, 1976.

20. Babb, A.L., Popovich, R.P., Christopher, T.G., Scribner, B.H.
     The genesis of the square meter hypothesis. Trans Amer Soc
     Artif Int Organs 17:81-91, 1971.

21. Furst, P., Asaba, M., Gordon, A., Zimmerman, L., Bergstrom, J.
     Middle molecules in uremia. Proc Eur Dial Transplant Assoc
     11:417-426, 1974.

22. Yatzidis, H. A convenient haemoperfusion micro-apparatus
     over charcoal for the treatment of endogenous and exogenous
     intoxications. It use as an artificial kidney. Proc Eur
     Dial Transplant Assoc 1:83-97, 1964.

23. Johnson, W.J., Hagge, W.W., Wagoner, R.D., Dinapoli, R.P.
     Rosevear, J.W. Toxicity arising from urea. Kidney Int
     7:S288-S293, 1975.

24. Jones, J.D., Burnett, P.C. Creatinine metabolism and
     toxicity. Kidney Int 7:S294-S298, 1975.

25. Oules, R., Asaba, H., Baum, A, Furst, P., Gunnarson, B.,
     Bergstrom, J. The removal of uremic small and middle
     molecules and free amino acids by charcoal hemoperfusion.
     Trans Amer Soc Artif Int Organs 23 (In press), 1977.

26. Avram, M.M., Lipner, H.I., Sadiqali, R., Iancu, M., Gan, A.C.
     Metabolic changes in diabetic uremic patients on hemodialysis.
     Trans Amer Soc Artif Int Organs 22:412-418, 1976.

27. Pavone-Macaluso, M., Alexander, R.W., Goering, R.B., Galletti,
     P.M. Parabiotic dialysis. Trans Amer Soc Artif Int Organs
     10:285, 1964.

28. Winchester, J.F. Haemostatic changes induced by adsorbent
     haemoperfusion. In Artificial Organs, Ed. R.M. Kenedi, J.M.
     Courtney, J. Gaylor, T. Gilchrist, Macmillan Press, Ltd.,
     London & Basingstoke, (In press), 1977.

29. Weston, M.J., Williams, R., Experience with haemoperfusion in
     fulminant hepatic failure. Proc First International Symposium
     on Gastrointestinal Emergencies. (In press), 1975.

30. Winchester, J.F., Forbes, C.D., Lang, S., Courtney, J.M.,
     Prentice, C.R.M. Platelet function regulating agents-experi-
     mental data relevant to renal disease. In Thromboembolism
     A New Approach to Therapy. Academic Press (In press), 1977.

CHARCOAL HEMOPERFUSION: GEORGETOWN UNIVERSITY HOSPITAL EXPERIENCE

Michael C. Gelfand, M.D.

Nephrology Division, Georgetown University Hospital

3800 Reservoir Road, NW, Washington, DC 20007

At Georgetown University Hospital, interest in charcoal hemoperfusion as a means of facilitating toxin removal from blood has
shown a doubled peaked history. After the pioneering work of
Yatzidis, et al (1) in 1965 in the treatment of barbiturate
poisoning, DeMyttenaere, Maher, and Schreiner in 1967 demonstrate
the effectiveness of charcoal hemoperfusion in the treatment of
glutethimide overdosage in dogs (2). Unfortunately, because of
the significant and potentially life threatening dangers of
thrombocytopenia and charcoal embolization, charcoal hemoperfusion
was not pursued as an attractive therapeutic modality for toxin
removal in clinical practice.

In 1974, Smith and Nephew, Ltd. (London, England) developed
a method of coating activated charcoal with an acrylic hydrogel
material (3). This coating process enhanced biocompatibility and
eliminated the danger of charcoal embolization. The Smith and
Nephew device called the Haemacol rekindled interest in charcoal
hemoperfusion at Georgetown in 3 areas: drug overdosage, hepatic
coma, and uremia. Dr. Winchester will describe some of the work
done in charcoal hemoperfusion in uremia in a separate paper (4),
therefore, this communication will review our second generation
experience in the treatment of drug overdosage and hepatic coma.

The methods used for charcoal hemoperfusion have been
published previously (5) and will only be briefly referred to here.
After obtaining informed consent, an A-V shunt is created
surgically for vascular access. Heparin is used for anticoagulation and the blood is pumped at approximately 200 ml/min in an
antigravity direction through the Haemacol column. Vital signs

are monitored at frequent intervals and biochemical and hematological parameters are followed during and after the procedure.

EXPERIENCE IN DRUG OVERDOSAGE

It has been demonstrated that the vast majority of patients
with drug overdosage will survive if given good supportive care,
nevertheless, 5 to 38% of patients in Stage IV coma from drug
overdosage die (6). Because of this very high risk of mortality
in the severely poisoned patient, we advocate some form of
facilitated drug removal in certain cases. The criteria we have
followed in considering a patient for use of charcoal hemoperfusion
in the treatment of drug overdosage are shown below.

Criteria

1) Severe clinical intoxication leading to hypoventilation,
hypothermia, hypotension, and non-responsiveness to supportive
clinical measures.

2) Plasma concentrations of one or more drugs in highly
toxic range.

3) In the absence of clinical "Time-dose-cytotoxic relationship", intoxication with toxic levels of potentially adsorbable
compounds.

4) Prolonged coma associated with pneumonitis or known
severe chronic pulmonary disease.

In the past year, six patients in Stage IV coma from drug
overdosages met these criteria and were treated with charcoal
hemoperfusion. Clinical data and the agents ingested by these
patients are summarized here: Three patients ingested glutethimide alone, 1 glutethimide plus acetylsalicytic acid, 1 phenobarbital, 1 pentobarbital plus secobarbital, and 1 ethchlorvynol. All
6 patients survived, moreover, complications in patients were not
common and when seen were not severe. Modest decreases in platelet counts were seen averaging approximately 25%, however, since
these patients were in generally good health prior to hemoperfusion,
the platelet levels were satisfactory post hemoperfusion and no
significant bleeding was encountered. Mild hypotension or
exacerbation of already existing hypotension was observed on 3
occasions. Saline infusion in those patients not already on an
anti-hypotensive agent or increasing the rate of infusion of the
anti-hypotensive agent resulted in maintenance of adequate blood
pressure. Mild hypothermia was observed but was easily treated
by warming blankets.

TABLE 1

Clearances of Various Drugs by Charcoal Hemoperfusion

Clearance (ml/min) $\pm$ SE

	Initial (1/2 hr)	2 Hr	4 Hr	Mean
Glutethimide	140 + 19	132 + 33	139 + 31	137 + 3
Phenobarbital	76	105	128	103 + 15
Pentobarbital	48	44	100	64 + 18
Secobarbital	30	67	60	52 + 11
Aspirin	93	28	113	78 + 26
Ethchlorvynol	114	67	Not done	91*

*Mean for 2 hours of perfusion

Clearance calculations for the various agents seen in our
patients are shown in Table 1 at the initiation of perfusion,
mid-way, and at the end. At blood flow rates of about 200 ml/min,
there is satisfactory clearance throughout the four hours of the
usual perfusion in all cases where data are available. Initial
clearances for glutethimide for the 3 patients and 5 hemoperfusions
were 100 ml/min or greater in every case. At 4 hrs, in only one
instance was the clearance significantly below 100 ml/min (76
ml/min). The clearances of the other agents are quite satisfactory as shown by comparison to peritoneal and hemodialysis in Table
2. To our knowledge, no other data on charcoal hemoperfusion
from ethchlorvynol intoxication is available for comparison.

We have also examined the effect of charcoal hemoperfusion on

TABLE 2

Measured Drug Clearances (ml/min)

	P.D.	H.D.	Charcoal H.P.
Glutethimide	*	24-149	135.4 + 50.8
Pentobarbital	<10	35	63 - 80
Secobarbital	<10	15	30 - 75
Phenobarbital	<10	22	50 - 72
Ethchlorvynol	18	64	36 - 114
Aspirin	25	100	92 + 23.6
Acetaminophen	< 3	120	190 - 315
Paraquat	*	0-8.5	109 + 28.6

*Ineffective or insufficient data

removal of digoxin in vitro and in vivo in intoxicated dogs (7).
In vitro clearances from outdated whole blood ranged from 33 ml/
min at the initiation of hemoperfusion to 30 ml/min at 2 1/2 hrs.
Moreover, the adsorptive capacity of the column was not saturated.
In dogs, clearances for digoxin ranged from 55 ml/min at the
initiation of hemoperfusion to 37 ml/min at 2 1/2 hrs. Thus,
hemoperfusion may represent a helpful addition to the available
methods of treating digoxin intoxications.

EXPERIENCE WITH HEPATIC COMA

After publication of the very exciting results of hemoperfusion in hepatic coma from King's College Hospital (8), we became
interested in this problem. Fortunately, our first patient was
treated and awoke (5) giving us the enthusiasm to proceed in this
very difficult condition. We have now treated 9 patients in
Stage IV hepatic coma. All patients received standard supportive
medical care and in spite of this had been in Stage IV coma for
at least 24 hours before initiating treatment. The clinical data
on these patients is shown in Table 3. Eight of the 9 patients
awoke after hemoperfusion. In all but one instance, awakening
from coma required 2 perfusions. One patient failed to respond.
There was no apparent correlation between duration of coma pre-
perfusion and the rapidity of awakening.

Although 8 of 9 patients awoke, only 3 patients survived.
Two were young men aged 13 and 18 and one was a female age 58.
The 13 year old had sustained hepatic failure secondary to sepsis

TABLE 3

Etiologies of Fulminant Hepatic Failure for
Patients Treated with Charcoal Hemoperfusion

Pt#	Age/Sex	Etiology of Hepatic Failure	Outcome	
			Awoke	Survived
1	34/M	Nutritional cirrhosis	Yes	No
2	48/M	Metastatic carcinoma and abdominal sepsis	Yes	No
3	56/M	Chronic aggressive hepatitis	No	No
4	13/M	Halothane and sepsis	Yes	Yes
5	46/F	Acute hepatitis non-B	Yes	No
6	16/M	Metastatic carcinoma Drug toxicity	Yes	Yes
7	64/F	Hepatitis A	Yes	No
8	28/M	Hepatitis B	Yes	No
9	59/F	Acetaminophen overdose	Yes	Yes

and possibly drug sensitivity. He had received 2 exchange trans-
fusions and 2 hemodialyses without result prior to attempting
hemoperfusion. The other boy sustained hepatic failure consequent
to metastatic juvenile hepatoma and associated with chemotherapy.
He awoke from coma and was able subsequently to tolerate
additional chemotherapy which was successful in inducing enough
of a remission in his neoplastic process to allow him to leave
the hospital and return home. The third patient's fulminant
hepatic failure resulted from overdosage of acetaminophen. This
lady is of particular interest in that she demonstrated very
little activity on EEG on admission but has fully recovered.

The mechanism by which hemoperfusion was able to reverse
hepatic coma has been studied preliminarily by examining the effect
of hemoperfusion on blood ammonia levels and on plasma, and
cerebrospinal fluid amino acid levels.

Blood ammonia levels were elevated in all patients prior to
beginning hemoperfusion. Although post perfusion levels never
became normal (< 65 ug/100 ml), they were lower after 8 of 13
perfusions. The mean pre-perfusion level was 315 ± 33 ug/100 ml
decreasing to 241 ± 25 ug/100 ml post perfusion ($p < 0.05$).

Blood amino acid levels were grossly deranged in most of the
patients with fulminant hepatic failure. Zieve has suggested that
elevations in levels of the amino acid tyrosine, methionine,
histidine, and phenylalanine might play roles in the pathogenesis
of hepatic coma. Table 3 shows the effect of charcoal hemoperfusion on these amino acids comparing pre and post hemoperfusion
levels. There is considerable clearance of these amino acids with
values ranging from 126 ml/min for methionine to 135 ml/min for
histidine and blood flow rates of 200 ml/min (Table 4).

TABLE 4

Alterations in Plasma Amino Acid Levels
during Charcoal Hemoperfusion

Amino Acid	No. of patients with elevated levels		Clearance*
	Pre-Perfusion	Post-Perfusion	(ml/min)
Tyrosine	3	0	130
Methionine	5	1	126
Histidine	3	2	135
Phenylalanine	4	0	134

*Calculated for patient #3

Cerebrospinal fluid amino acid levels also undergo considerable change during hemoperfusion. In one patient examined, pre and
post perfusion, 20 amino acids decreased in concentration with
tyrosine decreasing 23%, methionine 65%, phenylalanine 33%, and
histidine 64%. In a second patient, 8 amino acids decrease in
concentration in the CSF comparing pre and post perfusion levels
while only one increased in concentration.

Complications of hemoperfusion were considerably more
significant in this group of patients compared to those otherwise
healthy patients with drug ingestions. Platelet levels decreased
dramatically (33%) in the first two patients as did clotting
factors V, VII, X, and XI in one patient studied. We, therefore,
have routinely administered platelet packs (7-10 units) and
fresh frozen plasma (5-10 units) at the termination of each
perfusion. This procedure has resulted in the decrease of platelet loss to approximately 9%.

Hypotension is also a more significant problem in these
patients. One reason for this might be that there is already a
large cardiac output in these patients and the added stress of an
extracorporeal circulation is not well tolerated. We have
measured the cardiac output in one patient (#8) and found it to be
15-18 L/min.

In summary, the results reported here indicate that charcoal
hemoperfusion is effective in reversing the encephalopathy of
hepatic failure. Eight of nine patients treated regained full
consciousness with complete orientation to time, place, and person.
The lucid periods lasted up to 25 days in the 4 who eventually
succumbed and continue in the 3 survivors. The coma reversal was
associated with some decrease in blood ammonia and amino acids
such as methionine, tyrosine, phenylalanine, histidine. These
results are similar to those reported by Gazzard, et al (8) and
support Chang's earlier suggestion of the use of hemoperfusion in
attempting to reverse hepatic coma (9).

Although the capacity to reverse coma in a large proportion
of patients may represent a major adjunct in the support and
treatment of hepatic coma, the overall survival of patients with
this disease remains poor. Nevertheless, all patients who died
had little or no regenerating liver tissue, suggesting that a
careful selection of patients with acute, reversibly problems
such as toxic hepatic necrosis, might provide more encouraging
results.

In the area of drug intoxications, our experience has
convinced us that charcoal hemoperfusion is the preferred treatment for adsorbable substances in patients fitting into the

criteria outlined above.

ACKNOWLEDGEMENTS

The author wishes to acknowledge all the members of the
Hemoperfusion Team at Georgetown University Hospital including
Drs. Knepshield, Schreiner, Cohan, Strauch, Geoly, as well as
Ms. K. Hanson, W. Barnard, and S. Briddell.

REFERENCES

1. Yatzidis, H., Oreopoulos, D., and Triantaphyllidis, D. Treat-
    ment of seven barbiturate poisonings. Lancet 1:216-217,
    1965.

2. DeMyttenaere, M.M., Maher, J.F., Schreiner, G.E. Hemoperfu-
    sion through a charcoal column for glutethimide poisoning.
    Trans Am Soc Artif Int Organs, 13:190, 1967.

3. Fennimore, J. and Munro, G.D. Design and development of the
    Smith and Nephew Column. 1, Proceedings of an International
    Symposium on Artificial Support Systems for Acute Hepatic
    Failure, 330, 1974.

4. Winchester, J.F. Evaluation of charcoal hemoperfusion in
    uremia (In press).

5. Gelfand, M.C., Knepshield, J.H., Cohan, S., Ramirez, B., and
    Schreiner, G.E. Treatment of hepatic coma with hemoperfusion
    through polyacrylamide hydrogel coated charcoal. Kidney Int
    10:S239, 1076.

6. Arieff, A.I, and Friedman, E.A. Coma following non-narcotic
    drug overdosage. Management of 208 adult patients. Am J
    Med Sci 266:405-426, 1973.

7. Carvallo, A., Ramirez, B., Honig, H., Knepshield, J.H.
    Schreiner, G.E., and Gelfand, M.C. Treatment of digitalis
    intoxication by charcoal hemoperfusion (CHP). Tran Am Soc
    Artif Int Organs 22:718-722, 1976.

8. Gazzard, B.G., Portmann, B.A., Weston, M.J., Langley, P.G.,
    Murray-Lyon, I.M., Dunlop, E.H., Flax, H., Mellon, P.J.,
    Record, C.O., Ward, M.B., Williams, R. Charcoal hemoperfusion
    in the treatment of fulminant hepatic failure. Lancet
    1:1301-1307, 1974.

9. Chang, T.M.S. Haemoperfusions over microencapsulated adsorbent
    in a patient with hepatic coma. Lancet 2:1371-1372, 1972

TREATMENT OF FULMINANT HEPATIC FAILURE BY CHARCOAL HAEMOPERFUSION AND POLYACRILONITRILE HAEMODIALYSIS

D. B. A. Silk and Roger Williams

Senior Lecturer and Consultant, and Director
Liver Unit, King's College Hospital & Medical School
London, SE5, England

INTRODUCTION

Despite the considerable regenerative capacity of the liver, mortality from fulminant hepatic failure is as high as 80% in most reported series (1-3). Few of the patients who recover develop cirrhosis, however (4), and it is for this reason that a temporary means of liver support has been sought to tide these patients over the acute phase of their illness.

Early attempts at liver support systems were based on exchange transfusion and later on the clinically complex procedure of circulation of the patient's blood through an animal's liver. Improvement in conscious levels were observed in some instances (5,6), but few of the patients survived to leave hospital. The exact nature of the toxic metabolites that accumulate in acute hepatic failure and form the basis of the encephalopathy and other multisystem disorders is uncertain, but they are likely to be low to middle molecular weight (up to 5000) compounds that are either water soluble, thus existing in the free form in plasma, or protein bound. With respect to the latter group of compounds, removal from the circulation can be achieved by haemoperfusion through a variety of exchange resins. So far, however, application of such techniques to the clinical situation has been hampered by severe biocompatibility problems. With regard to water soluble substances, Chang and his colleagues demonstrated experimentally that these could be removed during perfusion of blood through activated charcoal (7), and when we perfused the blood of animals with surgically induced liver failure through columns packed with activated charcoal, plasma levels of several potentially toxic metabolites were reduced and survival prolonged (8). Encouraged by these results we went on to

use charcoal haemoperfusion in patients with fulminant hepatic
failure, and report here on 71 patients so treated, all of whom
had deteriorated to grade IV coma. We have also taken the opportunity
to test the efficacy of the new Rhone-Poulenc haemodialysis system
as a means of artificial liver support. The polyacrilonitrile
dialysis membrane differs from standard cupraphane and cellaphane
membranes previously used during renal haemodialysis in that it is
permeable to water soluble compounds with molecular weights of up to
15,000 (9). This enables the membrane to remove the same range of
compounds from the circulation of patients with liver failure as are
removed during charcoal haemoperfusion. We report here our
experiences of polyacrilonitrile membrane haemodialysis in the
treatment of 24 patients with fulminant hepatic failure.

Finally, during the course of these studies 53 patients with
fulminant hepatic failure who deteriorated to grade IV coma have
been treated by conservative measures alone. For comparison, our
results of conservative therapy alone are also presented in this
communication.

PATIENTS AND METHODS

The series includes 148 consecutive patients with fulminant
hepatic failure treated by standardised therapy in a purpose-built
liver failure unit opened in 1973. Fifty-three patients received
conservative treatment alone, in 71 patients conservative treatment
was supplemented by repeated periods of charcoal haemoperfusion and
in 24 patients by repeated periods of polyacrilonitrile haemodialysis.
All patients had deteriorated to grade IV coma before charcoal
haemoperfusion or haemodialysis was instituted, and all patients
treated conservatively developed signs of grade IV coma at some stage
in their illness. The clinical details of the patients are
summarised in Table 1.

All patients were treated with full supportive measures,
including intravenous glucose, lactulose, neomycin, magnesium
sulphate enemata, and vitamin supplementation. Seventeen of the
24 patients treated by haemodialysis received cimetidine as part of
a controlled clinical trial of the prophylactic use of this drug in
the prevention of upper gastrointestinal haemorrhage (10). Hypotension was treated with fresh frozen plasma or whole blood transfusion. EEG tracings were monitored continuously using a bipolar
EEG amplifier (Simonsen and Weel Ltd, EAP 205).

Technique of haemoperfusion

The first 5 patients were treated using plastic chromatography
columns filled with 200 g of charcoal, the perfusion in 62 of the
remaining patients being carried out with the pre-packed and washed,
sterilised disposable columns containing 300 g of charcoal, produced

TABLE 1   Survival of patients with fulminant hepatic failure in grade IV coma

Treatment	Total number of cases	Overall survival	Aetiology & survival					
			Hepatitis		Paracetamol		Other	
			n	% survival	n	survival	n	survival
Conservative alone	53	15.1%	22	3 (13.6%)	22	2 (9.1%)	9	3 (33.3%)
Charcoal haemoperfusion	71	23.9%	26	8 (30.8%)	28	5 (17.9%)	17	4 (23.5%)
Haemodialysis	24	33.3%	8	1 (12.5%)	16	7 (43.8%)	-	-

by Smith & Nephew Research Ltd. The charcoal was covered with a 4%
by weight coating of an acrylic hydrogel polymer and was washed
thoroughly in normal saline just prior to use. Charcoal columns
manufactured by Becton Dickinson & Co containing 120 g charcoal
immobilised on a polyester film were used in the treatment of 4
patients. Blood from an arterio-venous shunt was pumped through
the column at a constant flow rate of between 100 and 300 ml/minute,
using a Watson-Marlow peristaltic pump, and the patient was
heparinised so as to maintain the Lee-White clotting time at between
10 and 20 minutes. The plan of treatment was to perfuse each patient
for up to 4 hours per day until recovery of consciousness (grade II
encephalopathy) or death occurred.

Technique of haemodialysis

After insertion of an arteriovenous shunt, heparin was given
intravenously in a loading dose of 15,000 units, with further doses
during the haemodialysis period to maintain a Lee-White clotting
time of greater than 20 minutes. Standard dialysis lines were used
to connect the shunt to the polyacrilonitrile membrane (RP6, Rhone-
Poulenc, Paris, France) which had been washed and primed with
heparinised saline before use. Dialysis was carried out using a
Rhone-Poulenc Rhodial 75 apparatus. In this closed circuit system,
75 litres of dialysis fluid (final concentration in mmol/l: sodium
130, calcium 1.55, potassium 1.53, magnesium 0.5, chloride 102.5,
acetate 33) were recirculated at a flow rate of 500 ml/min. Blood
flow, measured by bubble transit time was maintained between 180 -
250 ml/min. As with charcoal haemoperfusion, the aim was to start
treatment immediately the patient showed signs of grade IV coma and
dialyse each patient for 4 hours per day until recovery of
consciousness or death occurred.

Biochemical monitoring

Arterial blood was sampled daily for standard liver function
tests, full blood count, prothrombin time, serum creatinine, and
plasma electrolyte estimations. To investigate platelet losses
arterial blood was sampled immediately before and after charcoal
haemoperfusion or haemodialysis. In addition blood was drawn
simultaneously from input and output lines 30 minutes after starting
charcoal haemoperfusion and haemodialysis when blood pressure and
the clinical condition of the patient was stable. At this and later
time periods samples were also examined for microaggregates using
the Swank filtration technique (11).

RESULTS

Conservative therapy alone

Twenty-five of the 53 patients who were treated by conservative

therapy alone were seen before the charcoal haemoperfusion programme
was started. Only four of these survived to leave hospital. Out
of a further group of 28 patients who were treated conservatively
when charcoal haemoperfusion was discontinued and before the
programme with haemodialysis had been instituted, 4 (14.3%) survived.
In our experience therefore only 8 of a total of 53 patients (15.3%)
with fulminant hepatic failure who were treated conservatively
survived.

Charcoal haemoperfusion

     Of the first 37 patients treated by repeated periods of charcoal
haemoperfusion 14 (37.8%) survived. However, many of the subsequent
34 patients developed severe unresponsive hypotension during treatment
and only three of these (8.8%) survived, so that overall survival in
the 71 patients treated was 23.9%. As with the patients treated by
conservative measures alone, neither age, sex, or aetiology of the
hepatic necrosis influenced survival. Based on initial observations
that the hypotensive reactions were associated with variable losses
of circulating platelets, detailed studies of platelet function in
8 patients treated by repeated charcoal haemoperfusion were performed
(12).

     Four hours charcoal haemoperfusion resulted in a significant
drop in the arterial platelet count (154.4 $\pm$ 25 to 124 $\pm$ 24 x 10^9/1,
p$<$ .02, n = 13). In addition to these changes there was a
significant reduction in median platelet volumes (6.42 $\pm$ 0.68 to
5.46 $\pm$ 1.15 fl, p$<$ .02). Marked elevation in the Swank filtration
pressure of blood leaving the columns (greater than 200 mmHg) were
found during 5 of the 13 perfusions.

     Reductions of arterial platelet counts were greater during
perfusions when the screen filtration pressure rose (59.6% reduction
of initial arterial count at end of perfusion) compared to when no
rises in screen filtration pressure were observed (20.4%). There
was a close temporal relationship between rise in screen filtration
pressure and fall in blood pressure, and in three of these perfusions
blood pressure became unrecordable.

Haemodialysis

     Eight of the 24 patients survived to leave hospital. Again, as
with the other two forms of therapy, neither age, sex or aetiology
of the hepatic necrosis affected outcome.

     In all, the 24 patients underwent 71 periods of haemodialysis
for a total of 245 hours. Platelet loss, measured during 15 periods
of dialysis during a single passage of blood past the membrane,
averaged 16.9 $\pm$ SD 19.5%, p$<$ .02 of the original level, but in
contrast to charcoal haemoperfusion the mean platelet volume was

unaltered. Microaggregate formation, as evidenced by a rise in the Swank filtration pressure, was detected on only one occasion in blood drawn from the output dialysis lines, and was associated with reversible hypotension.

Including the above hypotensive reaction, a systolic blood pressure of less than 80 mmHg was recorded at some stage during 20 out of the 71 periods of haemodialysis (28.2%). All but 4 of these episodes occurred within 1 hour of starting the procedure, and they occurred more frequently in the treatment of those that eventually died (16 episodes in 12 patients during a total of 42 periods of dialysis) than in those who survived (4 episodes in 4 patients during 29 periods of dialysis) ($p < .05$). All but 4 of the hypotensive reactions settled spontaneously or responded to volume expansion.

DISCUSSION

Analysis of our results has been restricted to the 148 patients treated by standardized therapy in a purpose-built liver failure unit which was opened in 1973. Compared to the results of conservative therapy alone (15.3% in 53 patients) the initial results of charcoal haemoperfusion (37.8% in 37 patients) were encouraging. During the early stages of the programme the procedure was well tolerated clinically and no untoward side-effects occurred. As mentioned, however, several of the later patients developed severe unresponsive hypotension, which in some cases necessitated cessation of perfusion.

Early on during our investigations of the hypotensive reactions, variable losses of platelets were noted. In subsequent more detailed studies (12) we have been able to show that the onset of hypotension during charcoal haemoperfusion was associated with a selective loss of large platelets and an increase in screen filtration pressure of blood leaving the columns. Such increases in filtration pressure are indicative of microemboli formation, and it is tempting to speculate that these microemboli in fact represent aggregates of large-sized platelets which have formed as a result of damage caused to the platelet membranes during passage through the charcoal columns. There was a close temporal relationship between rise in screen filtration pressure and fall in blood pressure which suggests a cause and effect relationship. At present this remains unproven, but in this context it is of interest that similar changes have been seen experimentally in dogs on oxygenators (13) and release of vasoactive materials from platelets was suspected as the cause of the hypotension. Why these problems were only encountered during the later series of perfusions is unclear. It is possible that some hitherto unidentified changes occurred in the activation process of the charcoal used, or that the clinical condition of the patients treated changed.

So far the results of haemodialysis using the polyacrilonitrile
membrane are also encouraging (33.3% survival in 24 patients) and
compare favourably not only with conservative therapy alone but also
with the initial results of charcoal haemoperfusion. These results
were achieved despite the fact that the present patients had
longer prothrombin times than either the initial patients treated
by charcoal haemoperfusion (p < .005) or the patients treated
conservatively alone (p < .001) (Table 2).

Seventeen of the present patients received cimetidine, but
there is no evidence that results were influenced by the use of
this drug as survival amongst those who received cimetidine (6 of
17) was not significantly different from those who did not (2 of
7) (p = 0.36).

The dialysis procedure was well tolerated clinically, and all
but 4 of the 71 treatment periods were completed successfully. The
only untoward side-effect observed was hypotension. Most episodes,
however, occurred early on during dialysis, were transient and
either settled spontaneously or responded to simple volume expansion
alone. As such, these episodes have the characteristics of the
hypotension commonly encountered during haemodialysis in patients
with acute renal failure and were quite unlike the severe unresponsive hypotensive reactions observed during the later series of
charcoal haemoperfusions. Microaggregate formation was noted on
only one occasion and there was no selective loss of large platelets.

TABLE 2   Prothrombin time (seconds prolonged) in patients at
           the start of treatment by charcoal haemoperfusion and
           haemodialysis or within 24 hours of grade IV coma
           developing in patients managed conservatively. Values
           are mean ± SE, numbers of patients in brackets

	Conservative management	Charcoal haemoperfusion	Haemodialysis
Complete group	51.2 ± 4.8 (53)	53.3 ± 7.6 (22)	83.4 ± 7.0 (24)
Survivors	25.6 ± 8.1 (8)	54.3 ± 12.0 (10)	65.5 ± 12.9 (8)
Non survivors	55.6 ± 5.2 (45)	52.5 ± 10.2 (12)	92.3 ± 7.7 (16)

In contrast to present results with the polyacrilonitrile membrane little benefit has been observed with haemodialysis using cellaphane and cupraphane membranes (14,15). This difference is likely to be related to the permeability characteristics of the dialysis membranes. One explanation therefore for the difference in results is that water soluble compounds in the middle molecular weight range (500 - 5000), which can only be removed during polyacrilonitrile haemodialysis, may be involved in the pathogenesis of the coma (16). However, elevation of plasma amino acid levels has also been implicated in the pathogenesis of hepatic coma (17-19) and during haemodialysis up to 8 pretreatment pools were removed during four hours haemodialysis, so we cannot exclude the possibility that the beneficial effects of this treatment are related to more rapid clearance of these compounds.

Finally, it is important to consider how survival can be improved further. It is now clear that no form of liver support therapy will be effective if it is instituted at a preterminal stage in the illness. Indeed, experience with haemodialysis and charcoal haemoperfusion suggests that such patients should not be included in future evaluations of liver support systems. A retrospective analysis of 92 of our cases has shown that more than 90% of those admitted in grade III ultimately progressed to grade IV coma. It would therefore seem logical to institute treatment much earlier in the course of the illness, and this could both improve survival and lower the incidence of cerebral oedema. Towards this end we are now instituting haemodialysis whenever possible in grade III coma, and 3 out of 4 patients so treated have survived.

ACKNOWLEDGEMENTS

This study represents part of a research programme into the development of an artificial liver support system supported by the Medical Research Council. We are grateful to the Wates' Foundation, the National Research Development Corporation, the Department of Health and Social Security, and Rhone Poulenc Ltd for their generous support. The Departments of Anaesthesia, Haematology, Chemical Pathology, and Radiology provided valuable assistance. We are particularly grateful to the numerous research fellows, past and present, who have participated in these studies, and to the nursing staff, the house-physicians, and other clinical staff involved in the coma rota, without whom this study would not have been possible.

REFERENCES

1. Benhamou, J.P., Rueff, B., Sicot, C. Rev. Franc. Etud. Clin. Biol., 1968, 12, 651.

2. Trey, C., Davidson, C.S. Progress in Liver Disease, vol 3, edited by H. Popper and F. Schaffner. p 282. Grune and Stratton, New York, 1970.

3. Saunders, S., Hickman, R., MacDonald, R., Terblanche, J. Progress in Liver Disease, vol 4, edited by H. Popper and F. Schaffner. p 333. Grune and Stratton, New York, 1972.

4. Karvountzis, G.G., Redeker, A.G., Peters, R.L. Gastroenterology, 1974, 67, 870.

5. Kennedy, J., Parbhoo, S.P., MacGillivray, R. Quarterly J. Med., 1973, 42, 549.

6. Winch, J., Kolthammer, J.C., Hague, R. Scand. J. Gastro., 1973, 8, 725.

7. Chang, T.M.S. Artificial Cells, Springfield, Illinois, 1972.

8. Weston, M.J., Gazzard, B.G., Buxton, B.H., Winch, J., Flax, H., Machado, I., Williams, R. Gut, 1974, 15, 482.

9. Sausse, A., Granger, A., Mann, N.K., Funck-Brentano, J.L. Nouv. Presse med., 1974, 3, 957.

10. Macdougall, B.R.D., Bailey, R.J., Williams, R. Lancet, 1977, 1, 617,

11. Swank, R.L. Series Haematologica, 1968, 1, 146.

12. Weston, M.J., Langley, P.G., Rubin, M.H., Hanid, A., Mellon, P., Williams, R. Gut, 1977, in press.

13. Allardyce, D.B., Yoshida, S. H., Ashmore, P.G. J. Thorac. Cardio. Surg., 1966, 52, 706.

14. Kiley, J.E., Pender, J.C., Welch, H.F., Welch, C.J. New Eng. J. Med., 1958, 259, 1156.

15. Sherlock, S. Gastroenterology, 1961, 41, 1.

16. Delorme, M.L., Rapin, J.R., Bloch, P., Bloschat, M., Opolon, P. Proceedings of the European Society for Artificial Organs, vol 3, in press.

17. Record, C.O., Buxton, B., Chase, R.A., Curzon, G., Murray-Lyon, I.M., Williams, R. Eur. J. Clin. Invest., 1976, 6, 387.

18. Fischer, J.E., Funovics, J.M., Aguirre, A., James, J.H., Keane, J.M., Wesdorp, R.I.C., Yoshimura, N., Westman, T. Am J. Surg., 1975, 78, 276.

19. Schenker, S., Breen, K.J., Hoyumpa, A.M. Gastroenterology, 1974, 66, 121.

USE OF ACTIVATED ABSORBENT HAEMOPERFUSION IN ACUTE INTOXICATION

Roy Goulding

B.Sc., M.D., F.R.C.P.

Poisons Unit, Guy's Hospital, London, U.K.

INTRODUCTION

In reporting on this work devoted to the treatment of acute
drug overdosage and carried out over the past four years at the
Poisons Unit, Guy's Hospital, London, U.K., my colleagues and I
claim no credit as innovators. Indeed, we are mindful of the
sound basis to haemoperfusion that was hewn out by Yatsidis and,
above all, by Professor Chang here in Montreal, to whom as host
I should like to take this opportunity to express my appreciation
and gratitude, not only for conceiving and organising this current
symposium but also for inviting me personally to participate and,
in so doing, facilitating my attendance.

Turning to our own endeavours, what we do contend is that
we have been instrumental in the clinical realisation of extracorporeal haemoperfusion as a safe and effective procedure in
the management of severe cases of poisoning from drug overdosage
in circumstances in which no other form of active intervention
would either avail or succeed. There is no doubt that from the
outset we have been greatly assisted by the provision of equipment by commercial firms, whose extensive bio-engineering resources
more than made good our amateur deficiencies in this respect. At
this juncture I should acknowledge our indebtedness primarily to
Smith & Nephew Research in the U.K. and, subsequently, to Becton,
Dickinson in the U.S.A. and Gambro in Sweden.

ACUTE POISONING IN THE UNITED KINGDOM

Not that we have ever regarded haemoperfusion as a universal panacea in the practice of clinical toxicology. Rather have we regarded it as a technique to be employed discriminately and, to this end, we have propounded and adhered to strict indications which take their bearings from the overall epidemiology of acute poisoning as it confronts us in the United Kingdom at the present time.

We have no reliable data on the extent of poisoning in our country insofar as the patients fail to reach hospital. We can only conclude that these cases fall into two extreme categories; those in which the intoxication is so mild that recovery is spontaneous or takes place with the simple ministrations of the general practitioner and those, on the other hand, who are so mortally afflicted that they are found dead and consequently are beyond the reach of any measures of recovery that might be extended to them in the wards. Figures in fact suggest that of all the deaths from acute poisoning in Britain, three-out-of-four happen in this way, i.e. found dead.

At the same time, through the ongoing Hospital In-Patient Enquiry System that operates through our National Health Service we are aware that, each year, some hundred-thousand admissions are recorded with a diagnosis of poisoning, among which are approximately twenty-thousand children. The great majority of those patients are in no physical danger at all and emerge medically, if not psychologically, in a short space of time with no more than simple supportive management, so it is only a small minority that constitutes a challenge to the physician to whose care they are entrusted. For a very few of these people are substantive measures practicable, e.g. forced alkaline diuresis for profound salicylate or phenobarbitone overdose, specific antidotes for paracetamol (acetominophen), opiates, etc. Reluctant, moreover, as I am to admit this in the presence of Professor Kolff himself, haemo-dialysis has revealed itself to us, on critical, objective and quantitative scrutiny, to be disappointing in this context. Hence our interest and enthusiasm became directed at other techniques that might substantially and readily remove substantial amounts of toxin from the body without entraining corresponding hazards. This is where, we are convinced, haemoperfusion has now vindicated itself.

HAEMOPERFUSION - BASIC PRINCIPLES

At this juncture, however, pharmacokinetics cannot be neglected. Among the drugs popular among those indulging at the present time in self-poisoning are the tricyclic and pharmacologically related antidepressants. For these the 'volume of distribution' is inordinately large and so the plasma level and, by the same token, the proportion of the body level that is circulating in the plasma is disproportionately small. Complete clearance of the offending material from the circulation will accordingly be relatively unrewarding. Haemoperfusion has no place here. Similarly, with paracetamol (acetominophen) the natural 'half-life' is brief and the hepatic damage, if it is to be sustained, is afflicted early on. Again, haemoperfusion is then pointless.

HAEMOPERFUSION - INDICATIONS

We are nevertheless left with a number of drugs, still widely available (albeit on medical prescription) to patients intent on deliberately taking an excess that can readily prove lethal and the distribution of which in the body is such that their active elimination from the plasma can rapidly deplete their accumulation in the central nervous system where, lingering, they may prolong coma and respiratory depression, so militating against recovery. These are listed in Table 2.

This, I admit, is an arbitrary classification, as are the critical levels. Yet experience over the past four years has not dictated any radical revision and, for the time being at least, we see no reason for easing these standards.

In fact, we do not pay attention solely to the pharmacological indices. Clinical features are also taken into account and the criteria by which we accept patients for this advanced form of treatment are set out in Table 3.

Hospital Admissions		Deaths	
Analgesics & Soporifics	31,190	Psychotherapeutics	223
Barbiturates	11,310	Barbiturates	1,657
Salicylates & Congeners	14,570	Salicylates & Congeners	232
Carbon Monoxide	1,180	Carbon Monoxide	1,263
Total	99,800	Total	4,011

Table 1.   Poisoning in England and Wales - England and Wales 1971

Phenobarbitone and barbitone	Over 100 mg/litre
Other barbiturates	" 50 "/ "
Glutethimide	" 40 "/ "
Methaqualone	" 40 "/ "
Ethchlorvynol	" 50 "/ "
Meprobamate	" 100 "/ "
Trichloroethanol	" 50 "/ "
Salicylates	" 800 "/ " *

(or over 500 mg/litre if the arterial pH is below
7.34 more than 4 hours after ingestion)

Table 2.   Criteria for Patient Selection - Drug Levels

THE TECHNIQUE

To an audience such as that assembled here today it would be
superfluous to describe the technique in detail. You, naturally,
are familiar with the circuit and the manner in which we tap the
arterial outflow in the arm and make connection with the venous
return through the same limb. At the same time I need hardly
remind you that adequate, but no excessive, heparinisation is
indispensable and this we can monitor conveniently in our hospital
by actively and repeatedly measuring the heparin levels in the
blood.

1.   Severe clinical intoxication, e.g. grade 4 coma,

     hypotension, hypothermia, hypoventilation.

2.   Progressive deterioration or failure to improve

     inspite of good supportive management.

3.   Prolonged coma with complications, e.g. pneumonia,

     chronic respiratory diseases.

Table 3.   Criteria for Patient Selection - Clinical Features

So far, we have adhered to perfusion columns in which the active absorbent material has been activated charcoal, coated or otherwise rendered non-embolic. Early on we did essay clinically some resin circuits, which we had prepared ourselves, but with these we were not too happy and we have not ourselves used in practice the commercial device about which Dr. Rosenbaum is going to report to you subsequently in this programme.

RESULTS

In the space of this lecture I can do no more than briefly summarise our results. These are tabulated, so far as drug overdose has been involved, in Table 4.

To date, as you will notice, we have carried out this procedure in altogether 29 patients, mostly with the Smith and Nephew 'Haemocol' device and, more recently, with the Becton, Dickinson and Gambro equipment. Not quite every patient has survived, but we would argue that those who have succumbed, despite haemoperfusion, were in all probability doomed anyway, owing to irreversible brain damage having already been suffered, most likely owing to prolonged cerebral anoxia.

	No. of Patients	Deaths	Average Clearance
'Tuinal' (Amylobarbitone + Quinalbarbitone)	7	1	87 ml/min
Phenobarbitone	6	1	80 "/"
Butobarbitone	6	2	100 "/"
Amylobarbitone	2	–	100 "/"
Pentobarbitone	2	2	41 "/"
Mixed Barbiturates	2	–	–
Glutethimide	1	–	125 "/"
Methyl Salicylate	1	–	57 "/"
Meprobamate	1	–	153 "/"
Ethchlorvynol	1	–	120 "/"

Table 4.   Summary of Drug Overdose Cases

As you will observe, "clearances" have been calculated as a
product of perfusion flow rate and drug level differences in the
blood before and after the passage through the column. Pharma-
cokinetically I know that the argument can be raised that this is
not an absolutely valid function, as so derived. Nevertheless,
it seems a reliable enough guide and allows us to contend that,
in most instances, a substantial amount of drug has been removed.
Occasionally, a poor performance in terms of "clearance" will be
revealed. This can sometimes be explained by a poor flow rate and
one is compelled to admit that, if the head of arterial pressure
in the patient is feeble, then no energetic priming of the extracorporeal pump will effect any improvement. It is possible, too,
that occasionally the absorptive power of the column may be relatively defective. That is why we continue to place equal emphasis
on assuring the utmost supportive care to the patient, simultaneously with maintaining the circuit.

The length of the perfusion cycle is variable and a matter
of judgement. In general the decision about discontinuance has
been a clinical one, in relation to overall response. What has
impressed us has been the often quite remarkable and dramatic
lightening of coma and dispensing with supplementary ventilating
support, notwithstanding an apparently quite modest fall in the
measured plasma level of drug by this stage.

For reasons, mainly ethical, on which I need not expatiate
to you today, we have never contemplated a controlled trial, -
not that it could ever be 'double-blind'. Fortuitously, though,
we were furnished with a striking comparison, the features of
which are depicted in Figure 1. The two patients bore a close
resemblance, in sex, age, drug taken, clinical condition and
drug levels. Their progress and survival was, however, quite
distinct. Two cases alone may not carry total conviction; at
least they are extremely suggestive.

PARAQUAT

As you will be aware, the herbicide paraquat is invaluable
in terms of crop husbandry and economics. Regrettably, though,
the acute oral mammalian toxicity of this chemical is very high.
While we have discerned no alarming hazards from its proper use
in agriculture there have been instances of accidental ingestion
and, more so, of deliberate self-poisoning with this agent. A
single dose by mouth of more than about 10-15 ml of the 20%
concentrate is usually fatal and, once the morbid processes are
initiated in the tissues, there is no redress.

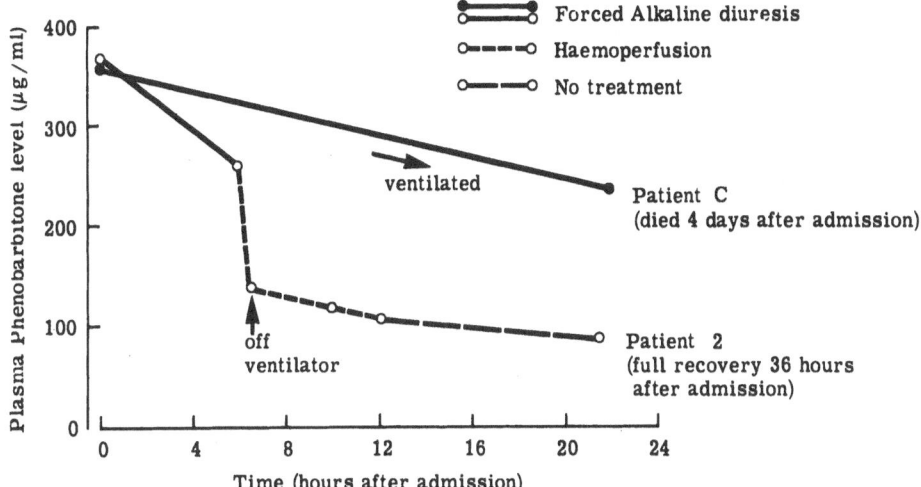

Figure 1.   Comparison of Two Patients Suffering from Severe
Phenobarbitone Poisoning

    Almost in desperation we have turned to haemoperfusion in
this baleful condition and the outcome in 12 such cases is shown
in Table 5, with 1 survival. From this we can gain neither
confidence nor credit. The 'clearances' are in some degree
encouraging and experimental work in dogs is proceeding using a
resin in preference to a charcoal absorbent. But hopes are not
high. Characteristically, in self-poisoning with paraquat, such
enormous overdoses are swallowed that early multi-organ
destruction ensues. Therapeutically, it is virtually beyond
belief that any counter-measures could stem this toxic onslaught.

ADVERSE REACTIONS AND COMPLICATIONS

    Gratifyingly our ventures into haemoperfusion have been
accompanied by no devastating adverse reactions at all. Bleeding,
apart from oozing at the site of cannulation, has been negligible,

so long as heparinisation has been meticulously controlled.
Platelet depression, though marked, is no greater than that
encountered in other extra-corporeal manoeuvres and is neither
progressive nor a prelude to clinical complications. Embolic
phenomena have been absent, despite careful checks, and alterations
in the blood constituents have been absent, except perhaps for
lowering of urate and sometimes of phosphate values.

CONCLUSION

We continue to insist that, in serious cases of overdosage
with certain drugs, haemoperfusion can be an effective and safe
form of treatment that can be carried out in any properly run
intensive care or renal, unit in hospital. With informed
supervision, moreover, it is an eminently safe technique and one
which, today, we as clinical toxicologists would not like to be
denied. Nevertheless, in the proper selection of cases and,
to some extent, in their ongoing management, it is imperative to
have at one's command a laboratory analytical service for drug
detection and levels that, besides being reliable, can function
on demand throughout the 24 hours. At the Poisons Unit at
Guy's Hospital, London, U.K. we are well-placed for this purpose;
not everyone else is so fortunate.

I would not care to conclude today giving the impression that
I, alone, should take credit for the work I have just described.
Much more is this due to my colleagues and associates, individually
and collectively, in the Unit, for whose inspiration, continuing
efforts and unselfishness I have come to depend.

Male 10   Female 2

Age 17 - 76 (Mean 44.2 years)

Amount ingested 30-300 ml   (Mean 90 ml)

Survivors - 1

Table 5.   Summary of Paraquat Cases

CLINICAL EXPERIENCE WITH CELLULOSE-COATED CARBON HEMOPERFUSION

A.M. Martin, J.K. Gibbins, A. Oduro, R. Herbert

Dept. of Medicine, Medical Renal Unit

Royal Infirmary, Sunderland

This presentation defines the specifications of the hemoperfusion system used - The Adsorba 300[1], outlines its role and performance in severe drug and chemical intoxication and describes some effects of short term use in chronic uraemia.

SPECIFICATIONS

The column consists of 300 gms of carbon, coated with a 3 to 5 micron thickness cellulose membrane. The fine release prior to clinical use is 15 particles/ml bigger than 5 micron and 140 particles/ml bigger than 2 micron. The priming volume of the column without lines is 260 mls. Since the most frequently encountered drug in serious poisoning in our series has been glutethimide and the published dialysis clearance figures vary widely[2] we have assessed the in vitro clearances across a Gambro Lundia Ontima 13,5 dialyser and the Adsorba 300 C. At a blood flow rate of 200 ml/min the mean clearances were 63 and 156 ml/min respectively. Similar results were obtained for phenobarbitone. The heparinisation regime used has been a wash through solution primed with 10,000 units and a single patient injection of 5000 units at the start of perfusion, followed up with clotting times.

INDICATIONS AND TECHNIQUES

Hemoperfusion has been used in any patient in grade IV
coma who has lost a vital function and this clinical
assessment is correlated with blood level measurements
of the drugs in question. Clinical deterioration even
in the face of lower blood levels than defined in the
table would also indicate the need for perfusion. This
is quite justified if one considers that 1/3 of all
cases have taken a mixture of drugs whose identity
may not be known. In cases of intoxication by tricyclic
antidepressants and chemicals such as herbicides, a
history alone is an indication for action. Tricyclics
rapdily enter the tissues, clearance even with hemo-
adsorption is low and should be commenced immediately
if a dose of 10 mgs/kg or more has been ingested. 2
our of 3 cases that we have treated have died almost
certainly as a result of delay.

Table 1

1. Clinical state
              - Grade IV coma
              - BP   90 mmHg
              - Hypoventilation (3 ltr/min)
              - Hypothermia
              - Overall deterioration within 24 hours of
                instituiting conservative measures

2. Blood levels
              - Glutethimide   30 mg/ltr
              - Short acting barbiturates 30 mg/ltr
              - Long acting barbiturates 80 mg/ltr
              - Methaqualone   30 mg/ltr
              - Paracetamol   180 mg/ltr at 12hrs
              - Salicylates   800 mg/ltr
              - Tricyclic antidepressants 2 mg/ltr

3. History alone
              - Paraquat any quantity liquid or granules
              - Tricyclics   10 mg/Kg dose ingested
              - Unknown mixture grade IV coma

4. I.V.C. cannulation when possible. Duration of
   perfusion depends on clinical response up to 4 hours
   procedure repeated if no response or deterioration.
   Combined perfusion and dialysis when unknown drugs
   ingested.

Indications on using Hemoperfusion in Drug Intoxication

In both cases the patients were admitted in a drowsy
state but after about 4 hours lost consciousness in
association with cardio-respiratory arrest and
convulsions and never regained consciousness despite
immediate resuscitation. We would hemoperfuse any
patient in whom the drug history was unknown or
uncertain. Vessel access is by I.V.C. cannulation
when possible, this being the only useful method in
hypotensive patients. The duration of perfusion
depends on the clinical response. We have been
perfusing for up to 4 hours then repeating the
procedure depending on response and blood levels.
There is a place for combined hemoperfusion and
hemodialysis when confronted with severe poisoning
by unknown drugs or chemicals.

Case Data

About 400 patients are admitted to the unit each year.
1 to 3 % have been treated by hemoperfusion or a
combination of perfusion and dialysis.

Table 2
Charcoal Hemoperfusion in Acute Drug Intoxication

Year	Hemoperfusion ± Dialysis Tot. No. of Pat. Referred	Diagnosis	
1974	$\frac{7}{479}$ (1.4 %)	Glutethimide	5
		Imipramine	1
		Barbiturate/ Salicylate	1
1975	$\frac{5}{449}$ (0.9 %)	Barbiturate	3
		Barbiturate/ alcohol	1
		Paraquat	1
1976	$\frac{8}{344}$ (2.3 %)	Glutethimide	4
		Amitriptyline	1
		Imipramine	1
		Paracetamol	1
		Methaqualone	1
1977	$\frac{1}{?}$	Tuinal	1

Glutethimide and barbiturates have been most frequently
encountered in the severe cases. The incidence of
poisoning by tricyclic antdepressants is increasing
overall although fortunately very few are severe. In
1976 it amounted to about 6 % of all cases.

Table 3
Acute Drug Intoxication - Cases Treated by Cellulose
Coated Carbon Hemoperfusion

Toxin	No. of cases	Mean Blood Level (mg/ltr)		Toxin Clearance (ml/min)
		Pre	Post	
Glutethimide	4	61	46	103 - 151
Amylobarbitone	3	34	19	10 - 43
Tuinal	1	40	19	108
Tricyclic Antidepressants	2	3.03	2.1	33
Methaqualone	1	31	20	49 - 190
Paracetamol	1	76	48	186 - 237
Paraquat	1	Treated by combined Hemoperfusion and Hemodialysis		

Q_B 120 - 280 ml/min; T 2 - 4 hrs

Table 3 shows the cases treated by cellulose coated
carbon hemoperfusion. The duration of treatments
ranged from 2 to 4 hours with blood flow rates of
120 to 280 ml/min. The paracetamol case presented with
a blood level of 76 mg/ltr, 52 hours after ingestion
and was in hepato-renal failure. No adverse reactions
to the hemoperfusion procedure have been observed.
There has been no fall in blood pressure recorded but
it is important to try and normalise the central venous
pressure in these cases before any extracorporeal
circulation is undertaken.

Table 4
Platelet Changes before and after Hemoperfusion in Acute
Drug Intoxication (mean)

		Pre	Post (x 10^9/ltr)
Glutethimide	(4)	185	125
Amylobarbitone	(3)	190	190
Tuinal	(1)	170	150
Tricyclic Antidepressants	(2)	170	120
Methaqualone	(1)	300	57

In all but the one case of methaqualone poisoning the platelet change as a result of perfusion has been minimal. In this case the platelet count was normal within 12 hours (Table 4).

The mortality in drug intoxication and ultimate diagnosis is reviewed and ranges from 0.4 to 1.4 %.

Table 5
Mortality in Acute Drug Intoxication

Year	Number	Diagnosis
1974	$\frac{3}{479}$ (0.6%)	Salicylate - Gastric coating - Cardio-Resp. arrest Glutethimide - brain infarction Imipramine - brain infarction (perfused)
1975	$\frac{2}{449}$ (0.4%)	Salicylate - Gastric coating - Cardio-Resp. arrest Barbiturate/Tricyclic - Bronchopneumonia
1976	$\frac{5}{344}$ (1.4%)	Barbiturate (bronchopneumonia) Glutethimide - brain infarction (perfused) Glutethimide - brain infarction (perfused) Amitriptyline- brain infarction (perfused) Paraquat - GI, Haemorrhage, Resp. arrest

Two cases of salicylate poisoning died, (neither of whom had perfusion or dialysis) and at post mortem the gastric mucosa was found to be coated with solid aspirin which had defied gastric lavage and at no time had the blood level exceeded 800 mg/ltr). Cerebral infarction was the post mortem finding in the 2 cases of tricyclic and 2 cases of glutethimide poisoning. Both tricyclic cases developed severe diabetes insipidus terminally and the cerebral substance virtually flowed out of the cranial cavity at necropsy. There was complete pituitary infarction. The 2 cases of glutethimide poisoning who died despite perfusion were admitted moribund 24 - 36 hours after ingestion.

SHORT TERM STUDIES IN URAEMIA

There may be a role for hemoperfusion in the
management of uraemia, but this will depend on the
demonstration of some superiority in performance as
compared with dialysis. Ideally this would amount to
developing a selective adsorbant system. For the
present we, the clinicians, concentrate on characterise-
ing the patient reactions and the adsorptive spectrum
of existing materials while the bioengineers, chemists
and manufacturers explore new materials. Cellulose
coated carbon hemoperfusion was undertaken on 19
occasions in 4 end stage uraemics who were on regular
dialysis. No adverse reactions to the procedure were
observed.

Table 6
Cellulose Coated Carbon Hemoperfusion in Uremia
(Blood Chemistry and Platelets)

	Concentration		Clearance (ml/min)
	Pre	Post	
Serum Creatinine (mMol/ltr)	1114	625	101 - 179
Serum Uric Acid (mMol/ltr)	0,48	0,25	105 - 127
Platelets (x 10^9/ltr)	279	274	

(Q_B 240 - 280 ml/min; T 2 - 3 1/2 hrs)

Perfusion time ranged from 2 to 3 1/2 hours with blood
flow rates of 240 to 280 ml/min. There was no significant
platelet change as a result of these perfusions. The
creatinine clearance ranged from 101 to 179 ml/min.,
uric acid clearance 105 to 127 ml/min. The fall in blood
levels amounting to about 50 % of the pre perfusion
concentration in most cases.

Phenols have been suspected as contributing to the
clinical features of uraemia for many years, although
views have been conflicting, 3,4,5,6,7. It has been
suggested that a combination of acidosis and phenol

retention is responsible for red cell metabolic defects.
Phenols can inhibit cerebral enzymes and cause
uncoupling of oxidative phosphorylation. Phenol
inhalation by chemical workers results in definite
neurological disturbances. Standard dietary and dialysis
treatment in renal failure does decrease the concentration of phenols in parallel with urea[8]. The phenolic
compounds include volatile phenols (phenol and cresol
isomers) and a number of phenolic acids. They are
mainly protein bound but also lipid soluble being
mainly unionized. The mean molecular weight is about
150 but the conjugates can be much larger molecules.
The normal blood level is around 2 mg/ltr, levels 6
times higher being commonly found in renal failure.

        A comparison of phenol removal by hemodialysis and
carbon hemoperfusion was made. Total free phenols were
measured colorimetrically. Plasma is first deproteinised,
treated with sulphuric acid and ether, then the ether
layer separated and mixed with sodium hydroxide.
Evaporation of the ether leaves a solution of the phenols
in alkali, acetate and diazotised nitro aniline is
added followed by sodium carbonate and colorimetric
measurement. The method gives a colour with all phenolic
compounds but excludes phenolic compounds which have a
basic group present.

        The figures on Figure 1 demonstrate the effect of
dialysis and perfusion on blood phenol levels. The broken
lines indicate the corresponding serum creatinine change.
There was a 50 % reduction in plasma phenol levels in
3 hours hemodialysis using a 1 square metre gambro, blood
flow 250 ml/min, dialysate flow 500 ml/min. There was
a linear fall in concentration with time and rebound
after dialysis was minimal similar in magnitude to
creatinine rebound. The fall in serum creatinine is
plotted with a broken line. The effect of hemoperfusion
has been variable in the limited number of studies undertaken. Blood flow rates were constant at 250 ml/min.
Within the first hour the fall in phenol levels ranged
from 30 to 60 %. During the second hour the drop
continued in 2 cases but a rise in concentration was
observed in one patient. This continued into the 3rd hour
and a 2nd patients plasma levels started to rise. This
rise continued after the end of perfusion in one patient.
The rise in concentration was observed despite continuing
clearance across the column, in other words saturation
had not occurred. Although the study is limited it would
suggest that adsorption of phenols results in a rapid

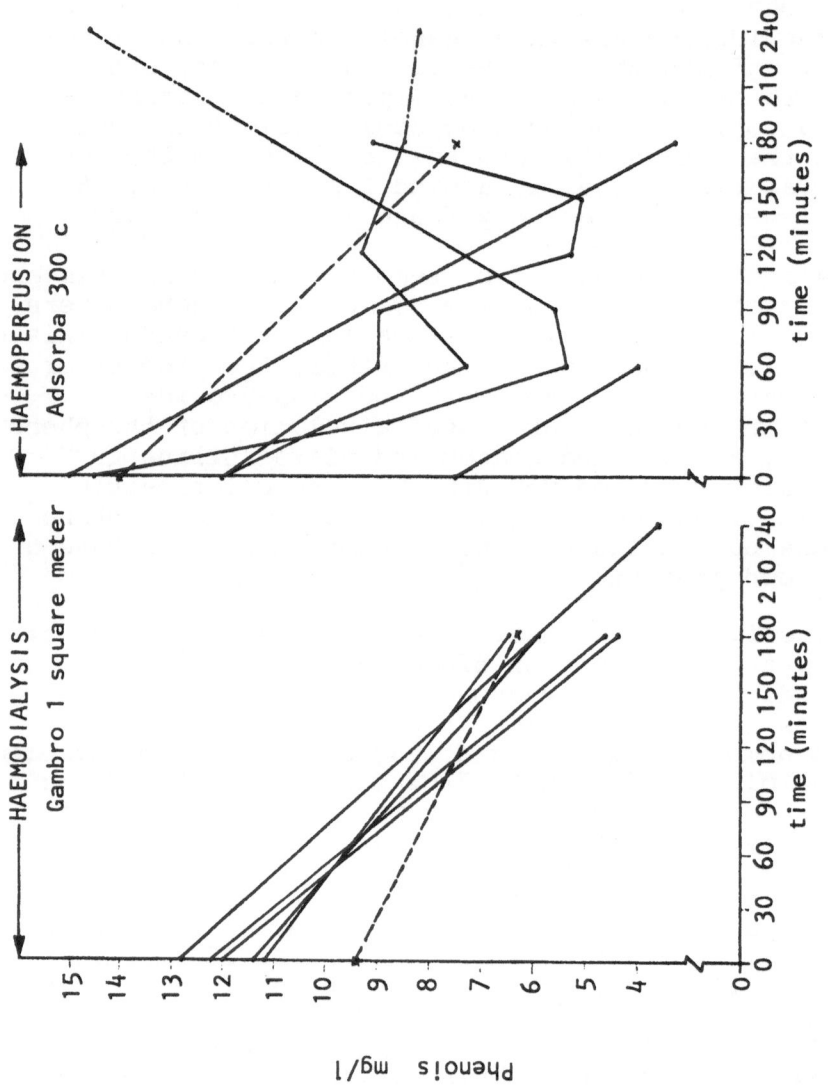

Figure 1

release of free phenols from protein receptor sites or tissues stores. We have undertaken desorption studies on the used columns and defined a mean of 800 mg of phenols from a column used for 3 hours. The change in serum creatinin levels is indicated by the broken line and represents a mean value. No significant variation in adsorption similar to the phenol behaviour was observed.

Conclusions

1. Hemoperfusion with the Adsorba 300 C column is an effective means of drug and chemical removal in patients with severe intoxication.

2. No adverse reactions to its use have been observed in short term studies on drug intoxication and uraemia.

3. Over a 3 hour treatment period creatinine and uric acid clearance is superior to hemodialysis.

4. Phenol adsorption has been demonstrated.

References

1. Thysell, H., Lindholm, T., Heinegard, D., Jonsson, E., Bylen U., Svensson, T., Bergkvist, G., Gullberg, C-A., (1975) Proceedings European Society for Artificial Organs.

2. Schreiner, G.E., Techan, B.P., Dialysis of Poisons and Drugs ASAIO Transaction.

3. Becker, E., (1933) Ergebnisse der Gesamten Medizin, 18, 51 - 59.

4. Schmidt E.G., McElvain, N.F., Bowens, J.J., (1950) Am. J. Clin. Path. 20, 253.

5. Muting, D. (1965) Clinica Chimica Acta, 12, 551-554.

6. Dunn, I., Weinstein, M., Maxwell, H., Kleeman, C.R. (1958) Proc. Soc. Exp. Bid and Med. 99, 86 - 88.

7. Wardle, E.N., Wilkinson, K., (1976) Clinical Nephrology 6, 2, 361 - 364

8. Wengle, B., Hellström, K. (1972) Clinical Science 43, 493 - 498.

HEMOPERFUSION AND REMOVAL OF

ENDOGENOUS UREMIC MIDDLE MOLECULES

R. Oulès[*], H. Asaba, M. Neuhäuser[**], V. Yahiel[†],
S. Bæhrendtz[††], B. Gunnarsson[†††], J. Bergström,
and P. Fürst

From the Metabolic Research Laboratory and the
Dept of Nephrology, St. Eriks sjukhus, Stockholm,
Sweden

INTRODUCTION

According to the middle molecule hypothesis (1), uremic solutes in the molecular weight range of 350 to 2,000 daltons are assumed to be toxic and evidence has been brought forward that uremic patients accumulate these substances in their body fluids (2–6). Serum middle molecule levels determined by gel filtration were reported by Chang et al. (7) to be more reduced following 2 hours of hemoperfusion than after hemodialysis for 6 to 10 hours as found by Dzúrik et al. (8).

It was therefore suggested that middle molecule removal by hemoperfusion is more effective than by hemodialysis.

Using new analytical methods it is now possible to obtain quantitative data on individual middle molecule fractions (9).

This technique was used in the study of endogenous middle molecule removal by hemoperfusion, which was compared with results obtained in hemodialysis.

Present addresses: * Dept of Nephrology, Centre Hospitalier Régional, Nîmes, France; ** Justus Liebig University, Giessen, West Germany; † University of Marseille, France; †† Dept of Medicine I, Södersjukhuset, Stockholm, Sweden; ††† Hospital Pharmacy, Södersjukhuset, Stockholm, Sweden.

This work was supported by NIAMDD (contract no. NO1-AM-2-2215), Bethesda, Md, U.S.A., the Swedish Medical Research Council (project no. B77-19X-1002-12C), Stockholm, and Gambro AB, Lund, Sweden.

Table I. Clinical data

Patient	Age, year	Sex	Diagnosis	Residual creatinine clearance, ml/min	Body weight, kg
1	34	F	Glomerulonephritis	0	50
2	44	M	Pyelonephritis	Binephrectomized	53
3	64	M	Cancer of the kidney pelvis	Binephrectomized	68
4	66	F	Pyelonephritis	2.24	59

MATERIAL AND METHODS

Four patients on regular dialysis treatment were studied. Clinical data are presented in Table I. One single hemoperfusion was performed on each patient for a period of 3 hours, using a Gambro hemoperfusion column (Adsorba 300 C) containing 300 g activated charcoal encapsulated with cellulose. The patients had arteriovenous fistulas for blood access and the extracorporeal circuit was prepared with standard hemodialysis blood lines. The column was rinsed with 1000 ml of 0.9 % saline and 500 ml of 5.5 % glucose followed by 2,000 ml of 0.9 % saline containing 2,000 I.U. of heparin. The patients were connected to the column without wasting the priming fluid.

At the start of the perfusion, a priming dose of heparin, 5,000 I.U., was given, and followed by a continuous infusion to the arterial line by a heparin pump with a rate about 1,000 I.U. per hour.

We aimed at keeping a constant blood flow at 200 ml/min during the perfusion by presetting the blood pump. The blood flow was measured by the air bubble method in a 1 M 'race-track' at the time of blood sampling. Using this method, no significant changes in blood flow rate were recorded.

Heparinized blood samples were drawn simultaneously from the inlet and outlet blood lines. The first inlet sample was drawn at the start of the perfusion, while the corresponding outlet sample was taken after 5 min. Subsequent samples from inlet and outlet lines were obtained at 30, 60, 120, and 180 minutes, respectively, after the start of hemoperfusion.

Plasma creatinine and middle molecules were determined. Plasma creatinine was measured by a kinetic method using an I L automatic analyser. Plasma middle molecules were determined by the combined HSGF–GEC method using a newly developed automatic middle molecule analyser, basically similar to the analytical system described earlier (9). The analytical procedures are schematically illustrated in Fig. 1. The plasma samples were ultrafiltrated through a millipore membrane with a cut-off at 50,000 daltons. This ultrafiltrate was separated by high speed gel filtration (HSGF) on Sephadex G15. The solutes were detected by ultraviolet absorption at 254 and 206 nm. The middle molecule fraction, namely peak 7, is prominent in uremic patients but not detectable in non-uremic subjects. The molecular weight range of this fraction was assessed against standards of known mo-

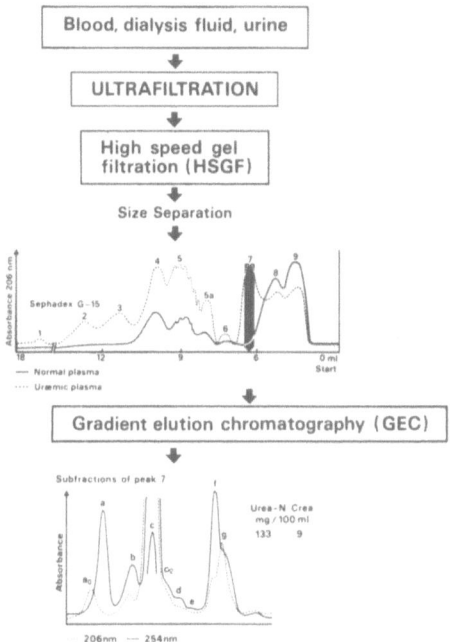

Fig. 1. Schematic illustration of the combined HSGF–GEC method.

lecular weight and estimated to be between 1,000 and 2,000 daltons as recorded in Fig. 2. This peak 7 is overlapping the decapeptide Angiotensin I,
of which the molecular weight is about 1,200 daltons. Using gradient elution
chromatography, on gel Sephadex DEAE 25, the material in this peak was
separated into 6 to 8 UV absorbing subfractions, peaks 7a, 7b, 7c, 7d, 7e,
7f, and 7g. Peaks 7a, b, c, and d were quantitated by integration of the
peak areas at 254 nm on the chromatograms and are presented in this communication. Peak 7e was less frequent and peaks 7f and 7g were unsuitable
for integration because of heterogeneity of the peak material.

RESULTS

The mean inlet concentrations for creatinine and the estimated clearance
over the column are given in Fig. 3. The clearance over the column was
estimated according to the formula: $(C_i - C_o)/C_i \times Q_B$, where C_i was the
concentration at the inlet, C_o was the concentration of the outlet, and Q_B
was the blood flow. The inlet concentrations for peaks 7a, 7b, 7c, and 7d
were expressed as percentage of the initial values and are presented in
Figures 4–7 as well as the estimated middle molecule clearances over the
column.

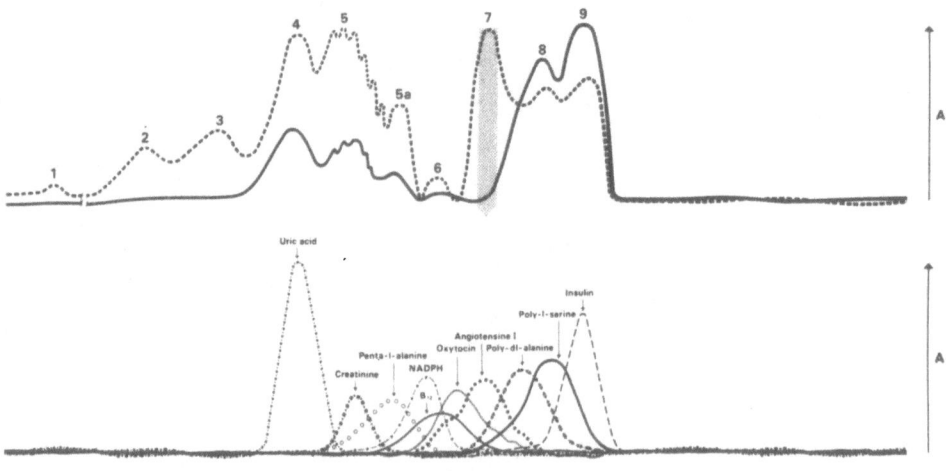

Fig. 2. High speed gel chromatograms of normal (——) and uremic (- - -)
plasma (above) and, for comparison, of various reference substances
(below). The molecular weights of the reference substances are as follows: creatinine 113, uric acid 168, penta-L-alanine 373, NADPH 765,
oxytocin 1,080, angiotensine I 1,129, B$_{12}$ 1,354, poly-DL-alanine 3,400,
poly-L-serine 5,200, and insulin 24,430.

   The inlet concentration of peak 7a decreased gradually to about 53% of
the initial values. The extraction (calculated from the inlet-outlet concentration differences and expressed as percentage of the inlet concentrations)
which was primarily high (61%) decreased throughout the hemoperfusion
and there was even evidence of some release (−24.8%) at the end of the
procedure. The clearance, initially 118.0 ml/min, fell to 25.3 ml/min
after 3 hours of perfusion.

   Peak 7b showed the same profile. The inlet concentration dropped to
61% of the initial values at the end of the perfusion. The initial extraction
(71%) and the clearance (137 ml/min) decreased rapidly with some release
at the end of the perfusion.

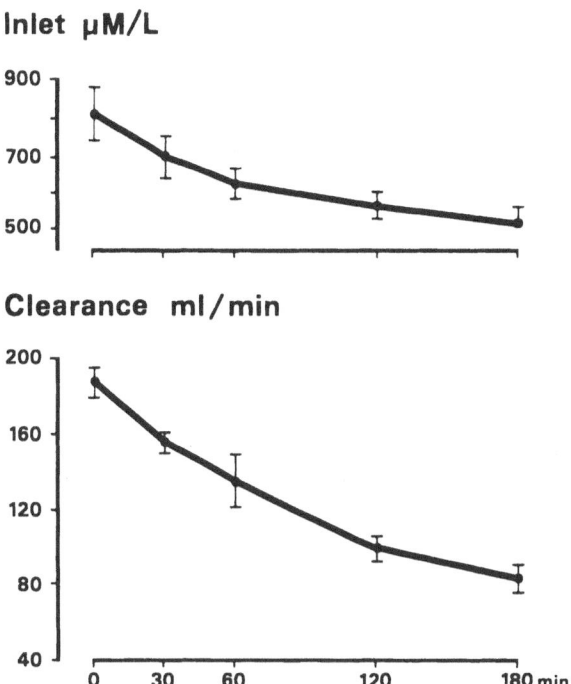

Fig. 3. Mean inlet creatinine concentrations and the estimated clearances over the hemoperfusion column in 5 uremic patients (10) (mean
± S. E.).

The inlet concentration of peak 7c exhibited a steady decrease throughout the study. The extraction percentage (initially 61 %) fell gradually to
10.6 % after 3 hours of hemoperfusion. Peak 7c clearance was 118 ml/min
after 5 min and fell to 25 ml/min at the end of the perfusion. Thus, an uptake still occurred at the end of hemoperfusion.

In contrast to the other peak concentrations the inlet concentrations of
peak 7d did not decrease more than 81 % of the initial values after 3 hours
of hemoperfusion. The extraction rate, on the other hand, fell to 20–30 %
within 30 min and then remained stable. Peak 7d clearance was estimated
to 125 ml/min at the start of the perfusion which value fell to 25 ml/min
at the end of the study.

A rough determination of the mean clearance of each peak could be based
upon their total uptake and first and last inlet concentrations. By this way,
the mean clearance can be estimated to be 41.2 ± 5.08 ml/min (mean ± S. E.)
for peak 7a, 50.0 ± 4.72 ml/min for peak 7b, 61.8 ± 7.75 ml/min for peak
7c, and 49.3 ± 6.02 ml/min for peak 7d.

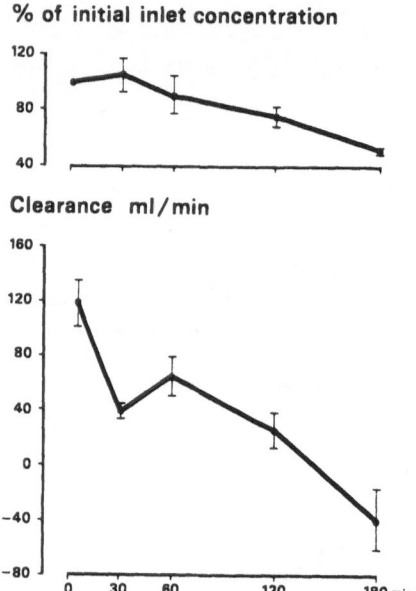

Fig. 4. Mean percentage of initial inlet concentrations for peak 7a and the estimated clearances over the hemoperfusion column in 4 uremic patients (mean ± S. E.).

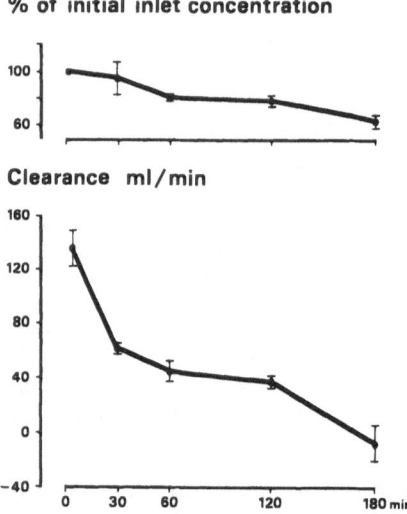

Fig. 5. Mean percentage of initial inlet concentrations for peak 7b and the estimated clearances over the hemoperfusion column in 4 uremic patients (mean ± S. E.).

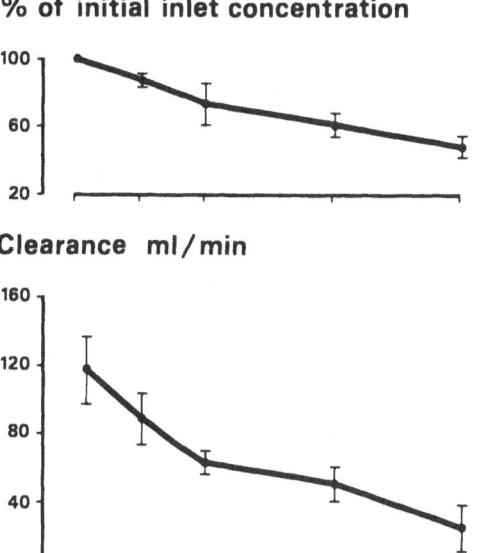

Fig. 6. Mean percentage of initial inlet concentrations for peak 7c and the estimated clearances over the hemoperfusion column in 4 uremic patients (mean ± S.E.).

DISCUSSION

The therapeutic potential of activated charcoal in uremia has been investigated in several applications (11). It was demonstrated that activated charcoal adsorbs creatinine, uric acid, guanidines, amino acids, and other organic compounds (12–14). In good agreement with these studies we found that a single hemoperfusion, using a column with cellulose encapsulated activated charcoal adsorbs uric acid, creatinine, and amino acids during a 3-hour hemoperfusion (10). Winchester et al. (15) reported clearance values for creatinine using Smith and Nephew Column 151 ml/min after 15 min perfusion and 110 ml/min after 2-hour perfusion. In the present investigation we found similarly 170 ml/min and 98 ml/min for the corresponding perfusion times. We observed somewhat higher initial creatinine clearance (190 ml/min) than that found by Chang using ACAC column (16), who reported initial creatinine clearance of about 160 ml/min. As a result of a higher initial removal of creatinine we were able to show an uptake of 9.8 mmol creatinine after 2 hours and 12.3 mmol after 3 hours of hemoperfusion. These removal values were higher than found by Winchester et al. (15) who observed an uptake of creatinine of 6.7 mmol after 2 hours. Chang and co-workers (7) reported that a crude UV-absorbing middle molecule fraction isolated by gel filtration decreased in plasma following 2 hours of hemoperfusion using a microcapsule artificial kidney containing albumin coated activated carbon. In contrast Winchester et al. (15) were not able to demonstrate a large removal of middle molecules following

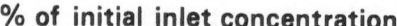

% of initial inlet concentration

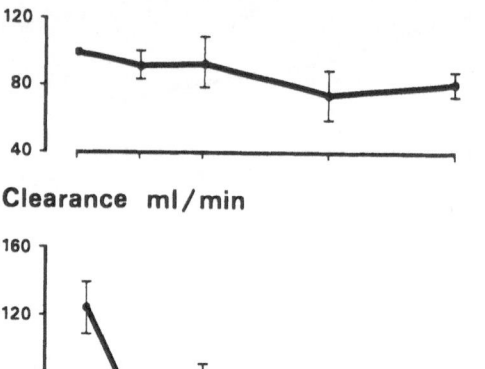

Clearance ml / min

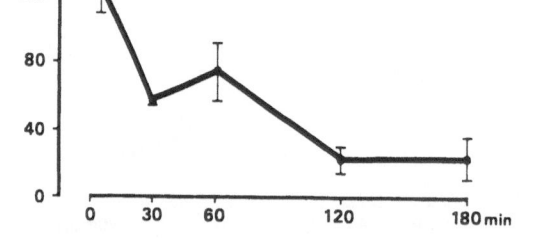

Fig. 7.   Mean percentage of initial inlet concentrations for peak 7d and
the estimated clearances over the hemoperfusion column in 4 uremic patients (mean ± S. E.).

hemoperfusion with the analytical techniques used (2). However, they found
that middle molecules were reduced with standard hemodialysis and with
combined hemoperfusion–hemodialysis treatment. M. Neuhäuser (17) has
also estimated the total amount of remaining middle molecules following
hemoperfusion and hemodialysis by using gel filtration techniques on Sephadex G15 (18). Compared with hemodialysis the reduction of plasma middle
molecules was significantly less following hemoperfusion. However, one of
the middle molecule fractions, considered to inhibit the activity of α-amino
levulinic dehydrase, was found to be removed more effectively by hemocol-
perfusion than by using RP 6 high flux membrane dialyser.

In the present study the removal of 4 different middle molecule fractions
are reported. The initial clearances for all fractions determined were
about 120 ml/min. These values are in good agreement with that reported
by Chang et al. in 1974 (7), who found a crude middle molecule clearance
of 120 ml/min at a blood flow of 300 ml/min. On the other hand after 2 hours
of hemoperfusion the estimated middle molecule clearances varied between
50 and 20 ml/min and after 3 hours between 25 and −40 ml/min. These findings indicate that the removal of the different middle molecule solutes may
vary independently of each other due to variations in production and elimination rates probably depending on the physico-chemical properties. By using
a crude determination of middle molecule substances in the molecular weight
range of 1,500–300 Chang et al. reported a lowering of serum middle molecules to 45 % following 2 hours of hemoperfusion (7). We found that 3 hours
of hemoperfusion resulted in a lowering of the middle molecule concentra-

BEFORE HEMOPERFUSION

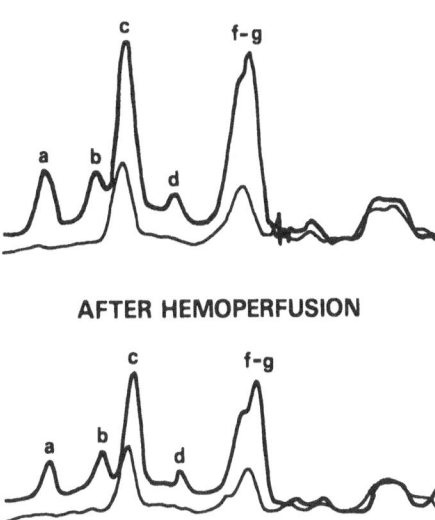

AFTER HEMOPERFUSION

Fig. 8. Typical chromatograms in patient 1 before and after 3 hours of hemoperfusion.

tions by about 50 % of the initial values except for peak 7d material, which was only reduced by about 20 %. However, after 2 hours of hemoperfusion peak 7c concentration exhibited a 45 % reduction, whereas the remaining peaks were only decreased by about 20 % of the initial values. In Fig. 8 the effect of hemoperfusion is illustrated by chromatograms in one patient before and after 3 hours of hemoperfusion.

Peak 7c was often found to be prominent in patients with severe uremic symptoms (19). It cannot be ruled out whether the results reported by Chang et al. (7) were related to this peak 7c material only, not considering that the crude peak material consists of a mixture of different polypeptides and other middle molecule solutes.

It was proposed (20) that hemoperfusion time of two hours is sufficient for maintenance therapy in uremia. The presented data support this and suggest that prolongation of the perfusion time beyond 2 hours appears to be of little benefit, if the aim of the treatment is to eliminate middle molecules.

We also compared the effects on middle molecule plasma concentrations of 3 hours of hemoperfusion with 3 hours of single pass dialysis on Gambro Major 1.5 m^2 and 3 hours of dialysis with the RP 6 high flux membrane dialyser in a 75 litre recirculating system on the plasma middle molecule concentration. The remaining solute concentration expressed as per cent of the initial values, is presented in Fig. 9. No significant differences were found except for peak 7d which was less reduced after hemoperfusion. We also observed in one patient with a very high peak 7c (case 2) that approxi-

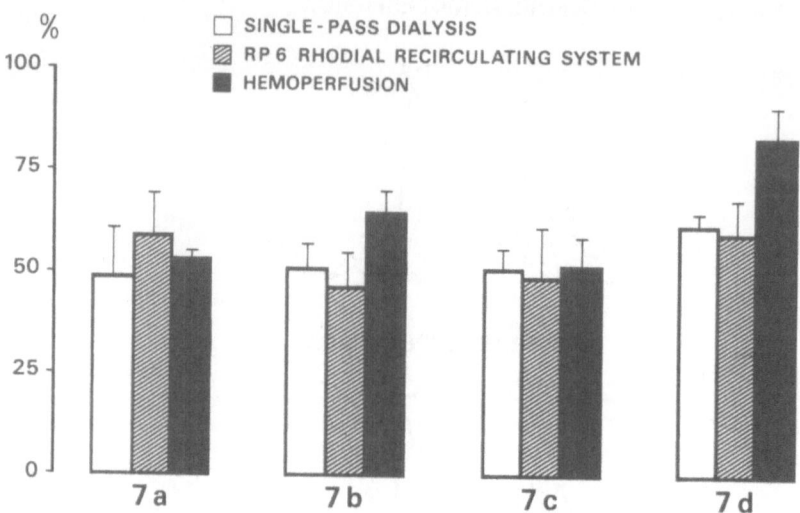

Fig. 9. Plasma middle molecule fractions after hemodialysis and after hemoperfusion. Per cent of the initial values are recorded (mean ± S.E.).

mately the same amount of 7c material was recovered in the circulating dialysate following dialysis with RP 6 (991 · 10³ cm²) as was taken up by the column during hemoperfusion (921 · 10³ cm²).

In conclusion, hemoperfusion during 3 hours on cellulose coated activated charcoal appears not to afford any advantage over dialysis with a large surface dialyser or a high flux membrane existing today as far as middle molecule removal is concerned.

REFERENCES

1. Babb, A.L., Farrell, P.D., Uvelli, D.A., and Scribner, B.H., Hemodialyzer evaluation by examination of solute molecular spectra. Trans. Am. Soc. Artif. Intern. Organs 18, 98, 1972.

2. Dall'Aglio, P., Buzio, C., Cambi, V., Arisi, L., and Migone, L., La retention de moyennes molecules dans le serum uremique. Proc. Eur. Dialysis Transplant Ass. 9, 408, 1972.

3. Gajdos, M., and Dzúrik, R., Erythrocyte glycolysis in uraemia; dynamic balance caused by the opposite action of various factors. Int. Urol. Nephrol. 5, 331, 1973.

4. Man, N.K., Terlain, B., Paris, J., Werner, G., Sausse, A., and Funck-Brentano, J.-L., An approach to "middle molecules" identification in artificial kidney dialysate, with reference to neuropathy prevention. Trans. Am. Soc. Artif. Intern. Organs 19, 320, 1973.

5. Migone, L., Dall'Aglio, P., and Buzio, C., Middle molecules in uremic serum, urine and dialysis fluid. Clin. Nephrol. 3, 82, 1975.

6. Funck-Brentano, J.L., Man, N.K., Sausse, A., Zingraff, J., Boudet, J., Becker, A., and Cueille, G.F., Characterization of a 1100–1300 MW uremic neurotoxin. Trans. Am. Soc. Artif. Intern. Organs 22, 163, 1976.

7. Chang, T.M.S., Migchelsen, M., Coffey, J.F., and Stark, A., Serum middle molecule levels in uremia during long term intermittent hemoperfusions with the ACAC (coated charcoal) microcapsule artificial kidney. Trans. Am. Soc. Artif. Intern. Organs 20, 364, 1974.

8. Dzúrik, R., Bozek, P., Reznicek, J., and Obornikova, A., Blood level of middle molecular substances during uraemia and haemodialysis. Proc. Eur. Dialysis Transplant Ass. 10, 263, 1973.

9. Fürst, P., Zimmerman, L., and Bergström, J., Determination of endogenous middle molecules in normal and uremic body fluids. Clin. Nephrol. 5, 178, 1976.

10. Oulès, R., Asaba, H., Neuhäuser, M., Yahiel, V., Gunnarsson, B., Bergström, J., and Fürst, P., The removal of uremic small and middle molecules and free amino acids by carbon hemoperfusion. Trans. Am. Soc. Artif. Intern. Organs, in press.

11. 'Sorbents', Kidney Int. 10, Suppl. 7, S-209, 1976.

12. Yatzidis, H., A convenient haemoperfusion micro-apparatus over charcoal for the treatment of endogenous and exogenous intoxication. Proc. Eur. Dialysis Transplant Ass., 1, 83, 1965.

13. Gazzard, B.G., Portmann, B.A., Weston, M.J., Langley, P.G., Murray-Lyon, I.M., Dunlop, E.H., Flax, H., Mellon, P.J., Record, C.O., Ward, M.B., and Williams, R., Charcoal haemoperfusion in the treatment of fulminant hepatic failure. Lancet 1, 1301, 1974.

14. Vale, J.A., Rees, A.J., Widdop, B., and Goulding, R., Use of charcoal haemoperfusion in the management of severely poisoned patients. Br. Med. J. 1, 5, 1975.

15. Winchester, J.F., Apiliga, M.T., and Kennedy, A.C., Short-term evaluation of charcoal hemoperfusion combined with dialysis in uremic patients. Kidney Int. 10, S-315, 1976.

16. Chang, T.M.S., Hemoperfusion alone and in series with ultrafiltration or dialysis for uremia, poisoning and liver failure. Kidney Int. 10, S-305, 1976.

17. Neuhäuser, M., Untersuchungen zur Elimination von Endprodukten des Proteinstoffwechsels durch Hämodialyse oder Hämoperfusion bei Patienten mit chronischer Niereninsuffizienz. Thesis, Justus-Liebig-Universität, Giessen, West-Germany, 1976.

18. Goubeaud, G., and Schott, H.H., Aufrennung von "Mittelmolekülen" im Urämikerserum durch Molekularsiebchromatographie. Klin. Wochenschr., in press.

19. Bergström, J., and Fürst, P., Uremic middle molecules. Clin. Nephrol. 5, 143, 1976.

20. Chang, T.M.S., Chirito, E., Barre, B., Cole, C., and Hewish, M., Clinical performance-characteristics of a new combined system for simultaneous hemoperfusion–hemodialysis-ultrafiltration in series. Trans. Am. Soc. Artif. Int. Organs 21, 502, 1975.

CHARCOAL HEMOPERFUSION IN MUSHROOM POISONING: AMANITA PHALLOIDES

E.DENTI°, R.TRIOLO*, V.GRIVET* AND A.RAMELLO*

°SORIN BIOMEDICA, 13040 SALUGGIA, ITALY

*OSPEDALE MARTINI, Iˆ DIV. MEDICINA, VIA TOFA-
NE 71, 10141 TORINO, ITALY

Of the many genera and species of poisonous mushrooms the most dangerous are some species of Amanita
especially Amanita phalloides, A. verna, A. virosa and
A. bisporigera. Amanita phalloides is the most common
mushroom in Europe and is also present in North America
but Amanita bisporigera and Amanita virosa appear to be
more abundant. During rainy summers poisoning due to
eating Amanita phalloides is relatively common in Europe
but far less common in North America where wild mushroom
picking is less common. Fig. 1 shows the general appearance of some typical varieties of poisonous
Amanita sp. mushrooms. The cap size varies from two to
five inches, and the shape from conical to broad and
flat. The color ranges from white (A. verna, A. virosa,
A. bisporigera) to yellow, brown and especially to green.
The stem is generally three to seven inches tall and
coloured with a bulbous base. A. virosa, bisporigera and
verna are white in colour and contain the same family of
toxins of the phalloides variety. Although a little work
has been done since the end of 19th century to elucidate
the chemical nature of A. phalloides poisons, it was only
from 1907 to 1959 that the isolation and identification
of Amanita toxins was performed (1, 2, 3, 4, 5). The
toxic components that can be extracted from A. phalloides

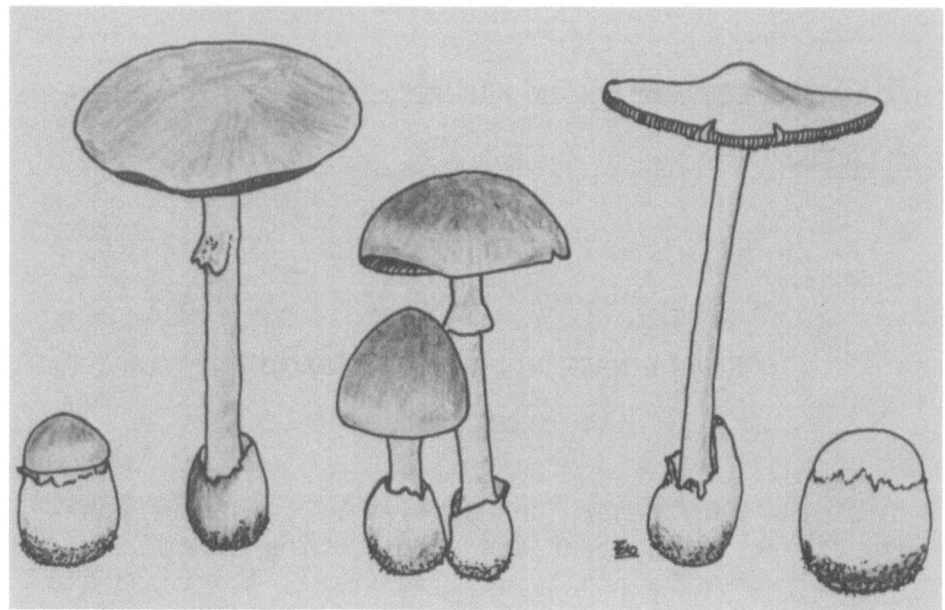

Figure 1

α –Amanitin

Figure 2

mushrooms can be divided into two group:
1. the amanitines, slow acting and more poisonous
2. the phalloidines, fast acting but less toxic.
All A. phalloides toxins have a cyclopeptide structure,
their molecular weight ranging from 730 to 1072. The
cyclopeptides may associate together and/or with a poly-
saccaride molecule to form large and relatively unstable
macromolecules ranging from 10.000 to 50.000 m.w. The
toxins are water soluble, stable in the gastrointestinal
tract and are able to be easily adsorbed in the gut.
The toxins are also stable in the temperature range used
in cooking.

Figure 2 shows the structure of α -Amanitin. This
toxin , like all the other amanitines contains eight
aminoacids while the phalloidines contain seven aminoacids. The mode of action of those toxins is not completely clear. Nevertheless, it appears evident from various experiments that the poisons are easily adsorbed
in the gut. REHBINDER and coworkers (6) have studied the
distribution of the toxins two hours after injection in
rats. The toxins appear to be concentrated particularly
in the liver as shown in table I. The mechanism of the
action of the amanitines seems to be related to a specific inhibitory action on the endonuclear RNA - polymera-
sis (7, 8). The phalloidines appear to affect the cellular membrane. It is generally accepted that death from
Amanita poisoning is due mainly to the amanitines than
to the phalloidines.

Clinical and laboratory findings

The principal symptoms of acute A. phalloides poisoning are summarized in table II. The latent interval
after the early gastrointestinal manifestations of poisoning (nausea, vomiting, abdominal pain) is about 12 - 24
hours. During this period of time the patient's well-
being is relatively good and in some instances actually
seems to improve. The following phase is characterized
by severe nausea, diarrhea, bloody vomitus and stools,
painful tenderness and enlargement of the liver.
Confusional status followed by coma, jaundice and all
symptoms of acute liver failure are present in heavily

TABLE I

Distribution of Amanita toxins two
hours after injection in rats (6).

LIVER	57%
SKELETAL MUSCLE	10%
BLOOD	6%
KIDNEYS	3%

TABLE II

AMANITA PHALLOIDES POISONING

1. 3-8 hours after ingestion : ABDOMINAL PAIN,NAUSEA

2. 12-24 hours after ingestions : APPARENT RECOVERY

3. After 24 hours : CONFUSION, HALLUCINATIONS, NAUSEA
   CONVULSION

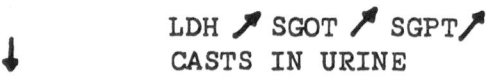
LDH ↗ SGOT ↗ SGPT↗
CASTS IN URINE

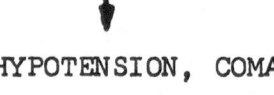

OLIGURIA OR ANURIA

↓

HYPOTENSION, COMA

↓

RECOVERY OR DEATH

poisoned patients. Pulmonary oedema, anuria and acute
failure quite often follows. Laboratory findings show
impairment of liver function tests, a rise in LDH, SGOT,
SGPT, bilirubinemia, fall in glucose and serum proteins.
The urine examination could show red cells and protein-
aceous cast. Unfortunately the identification of the
Amanita toxins is not easy; only a qualitative method
based on a chromatographic technique is normally available (9, 10). This makes a laboratory diagnosis very
difficult and limits the possibility of an early and
agressive therapeutic treatment. The best method of diagnosis is often the identification of the mushrooms by
a microscopic examination and spore determination of the
residues left in the kitchen of the patient. Very recently Fiume and Busi (11) of University of Bologna, Istitu-
to di Patologia Generale,have developed a radioimmunoassay technique to quantitate the amanitine in plasma.
We hope to take advantage in the near future of this
useful analysis. It has been reported that in severe
intoxications 50-70% of the patients will die. In our
experience, based on seven cases of severe intoxications
in over four years, we have had only two deaths.

Treatment of poisoned patients

A number of studies have been made with the aim of
finding a specific antidote for the amanita toxins.
The use of antisera, silimarine, antiamanide, thioctic
acid have been proposed. The low molecular weight of the
amanitins make it practically impossible to obtain specific antisera simply by sublethal injections of toxins
in animals. The use of other "antidote" molecules requires, to be effective,a very early diagnosis and treatment.
For those reasons the clinical treatment is symptomatic
and based on the following:
1. GASTRIC LAVAGE (within 6-7 hours from ingestion)
2. CORRECTION OF THE HYDROELECTROLITIC DISEQUILIBRIUM
   (Vomiting, diarrhea and profuse sweating cause a
   marked disequilibrium that should be corrected by
   careful control of fluid and electrolyte balance).
3. ANTISHOCK AND CARDIOCIRCULATORY THERAPY (Idrocorti-
   sol, ACTH, Dopamine, Adrenaline etc. may be indicated in some particular situation).

A complete review of the supportive treatment in A. phalloides poisoning, based on 74 cases was recently published by Ciocatto and coworkers (12). Other measures include the use of thioctic acid (200-600 mg/day), UDPG (70 mg/day), use of high doses of penicillin to compete with α-amanitin in binding with albumin (0.5 - 1 million of Units/Kg of body weight/day). The pain could be controlled by codeine or morphine if necessary.
The use of hemodialysis may be useful for the correction of anuria and electrolyte unbalance. Thölen and coworkers (13) have proposed early and in some instances prolonged (8-16 hours) hemodialysis treatment as a therapeutic measure probably effective to some extent.
Recently Seeger and Barteles (14) pointed out in vitro experiments using α-Amanitin in a aqueous and plasma solutions, the ability of activated carbon to quickly remove the toxins by adsorption. Encouraged by those findings and by the single case succesfully treated by Williams and coworkers (15) using activated carbon hemoperfusion, we treated in Autumn, 1976 three heavily poisoned patients by hemoperfusion with DETOXYL 1 (coated carbon columns manufactured by SORIN BIOMEDICA, 13040 Saluggia, Italy).

S.F., 35 years old male, S.R. 8 years old girl and G.I., 67 years old male were treated by a full range of supportive measures:
- Fluid infusion therapy for electrolyte balance correction,
- Dextrose infusion,
- Tioctic acid (500 mg/day),
- Penicillin (1 million of Units/Kg/day).

All patients were severely ill in comatous state showing very high transaminases level. In particular G.I., transferred from Sardinia six days after the ingestion of the mushrooms was in deep coma and anuric with symptoms of acute liver and kidney failure.

A plasmapheresis treatment was immediately started on the three patients until the total protein fell down to 4 g% ml of serum. A total of five hemoperfusion with DETOXYL columns was done. S.F. and S.R. made on evident improvement of the clinical conditions after the hemoperfusions. Both patients recovered completely and were

dismissed by the hospital three weeks later. The clinical conditions of G.I. do not improve until the exitus
seven days after the ingestion.

Discussion

The difficulty to quantitate and to follow the removal of the Amanita toxins by a reliable and simple
analytical method has made it extremely difficult to
draw conclusions on the effectiveness of such types of
treatments. We think that from our limited clinical
experience it is useful to point out the following:

1. The use of hemoperfusion in Amanita sp. poisoned patients is possible but requires particular care to
   prevent and dominate hypotensive fenomena during the
   extracorporeal circulation (100 mg dopamin and 1 g
   hydrocortisol i.v.).
2. The platelet drop after the hemoperfusion as well
   after hemodialysis and plasmapheresis was particularly severe although spontaneous bleeding was never observed.
3. The recovery of the two patients treated early by hemoperfusion was particularly fast conpared with our
   previous experience.

In conclusion we think that the early treatment of Amanita sp. poisoned patients by activated carbon hemoperfusion is worth consideration as a therapeutic measure
for the affinity showed by α -Amanitine for activated
carbon. More extensive clinical studies are required
to confirm the real effectiveness of this treatment.

ACKNOWLEDGEMENTS

The authors would like to express their sincere
appreciation to Dr. Francesco GORGERINO, M.D., Ph. D.,
Director of the intensive care unit where the patients
were treated.

BIBLIOGRAPHY

1. WIELAND, TH. Pure Appl. Chem. $\underline{9}$, 145, (1964).

2. LYNEN, F., WIELAND, U., Ann. $\underline{533}$, 93, (1937).

3. WIELAND, TH., GEBERT, U., Ann. $\underline{700}$, 157, (1966).

4. WIELAND, TH., WIELAND, O., Pharmacol. Rev. $\underline{II}$, 87, (1959).

5. ARIETTI and TOMASI "I funghi velenosi" Ed. Edagricole, Bologna, Italy (1975).

6. REHBINDER, D. et al., Z. physiol. Chem. $\underline{331}$, 132, (1963).

7. STIRPE, F., FIUME, L., Biochem. J. $\underline{105}$, 779, (1967).

8. NOVELLO, F. et al., Biochem. J. $\underline{116}$, 177 (1970)

9. DHEW PUBLICATION N°. (NIH) 76-725, Fogarty International Center Proceedings N° 22 "Diseases of the liver and Biliary tract" (1976).

10. FAULSTICH, H. et al, Jour. of chromatography $\underline{79}$, 257, (1973).

11. FIUME, L., personal comunication.

12. DELFINO, U., CIOCATTO, E., BUFFA, I. - Min. Anest. $\underline{41}$, 426, (1975).

13. THÖLEN, H. et al. German. Med. Monthly $\underline{11}$, 89, (1966).

14. SEEGER, R., BARTELES, O., Stsch. Med. Wschr. $\underline{101}$, 1456, (1976).

15. WILLIAMS, R. et al., LANCET, June 29, 130, (1974).

BIOCOMPATIBILITY STUDIES OF HEMOPERFUSION SYSTEMS FOR LIVER AND KIDNEY SUPPORT

S.Sideman*,E.Hoffer,L.Mor,J.M.Brandes,I.Rousseau,
O.Better,D.Ben-Arie and S.Lupovitch

Department of Chemical Engineering and School of Medicine
Technion-Israel Institute of Technology
Haifa,Israel

ABSTRACT

The biocompatibility of liver and kidney support hemoperfusion systems operating in-vitro with blood taken from a number of donors was investigated. The liver support system, aimed at the specific removal of Bilirubin, consisted of a column of Dowex 1X2 beads coated with an Acrylic polymer and a crosslinked Albumin. The kidney support system, aimed at the specific removal of phosphate ions, consisted of a packed-bed of alumina particles coated with a modified collodion. Comparison tests with empty columns show that the adsorbents do not significantly affect the depletion of erythrocytes leukocytes and thrombocytes.

LIVER SUPPORT HEMOPERFUSION SYSTEM

The study relates to high risk pregnancy. Premature babies represent 10% of the newborns, exhibiting a high prenatal mortality and a much higher morbidity rate. One of the crucial problems is neurological and 'minimal' brain damage. Jaundice, which appears in about half of the prematures, is one of the major factors which contributes to these sequelae. The serum bilirubin (BIL) concentration in hemolytic diseases may reach toxic levels, penetrating cerebral tissues and impairing cellular function by blocking the oxidative phosphorylation, inhibiting respiration and resulting in the development of brain damage, kernicterus and death.

---

* Presently on sabbatical leave, Dept. of Chemical Engineering, The City College of New York, 10031

Currently, systems of mild hyperbilirubinaemia are treated by phototherapy or by the administration of human serum albumin (HSA) solution. In cases of severe hyperbilirubinaemia an incremental exchange transfusion is necessary. In some clinics the administration of drugs is used to induce hepatic activity of bilirubin UDP glucoronyl transferase [1]. Our objective is to develop a small cartridge capable of removing BIL from whole bilirubinaemic blood of newborn babies in a closed hemoperfusion cycle, thus replacing exchange transfusion and reducing the dependency on the application of phototherapy, of which the long-term effects are still undetermined.

Anion exchanger - Dowex 1X2 - coated with biocompatible polymers including poly-HEMA, acrylic polymer and human albumin, removed between 50 to 75% of the initial Bilirubin from blood in 2-3 hours of in-vitro hemoperfusion [2]. Here, we report on the biocompatibility of the hemoperfusion system which includes the coated Dowex 1X2 beads. Citrated fresh human blood was chosen for this purpose. The advantages of citrate as an anticoagulant in in-vitro tests were recently demonstrated [3] and its careful use was suggested for in-vivo hemoperfusion [4].

Materials and Methods

The hemoperfusion system, which consists of a small two-facet conical Perspex column [2], and a peristaltic pump, had a volume of 28 ml. The system, including the tubing, was siliconized with Dow Medical Fluid No.360 [5]. The Dowex 1X2 beads 50-100 mesh (SERVA, fein biochemica Heidelberg, P.A.) were coated with Acrylic AG-1039 polymer (Hydrophilics Ltd.,Haifa) and then with human albumin crosslinked with glutaraldehyde [2]. Prior to each run, the resin was equilibrated with a 15% solution in PBS (0.14 M NaCl, 0.01 M phosphate buffer, pH 7.4) of Acid Citrate Dextrose (ACD) or buffered citrate.

Fresh human blood (from the Maccabi Hematological Laboratory) was used throughout. 15% ACD (or buffered citrate) was used as anticoagulant. Soluble BIL in PBS (7.5 mg BIL in 5 ml PBS for 50 ml blood) was added, in some runs, to the fresh blood sample. The blood volume in each run was 50 ml.

Control tests, in which the blood was circulated through an identical but empty column, were run in parallel. Blood flow rate in both columns was 12 ml/min. Platelet, erythrocyte and leukocyte counts were taken during the various runs, utilizing a Coulter Counter model Z-B, with a 50μ orifice. Size distribution before and after perfusion were obtained with Size Distribution Analyzer Model P 64.

Results

Erythrocytes, thrombocytes and leukocytes were counted in both empty and packed-column experiments. In order to try and establish the time dependence of these counts, measurements were taken every 30 minutes, up to 3 hours. The erythrocyte and thrombocyte counts showed no significant change after the first measuring period. Hence, later measurements were regarded as repetitious. As such, they were averaged, giving the results in table I. The leukocytes were found to be time dependent. The values in table I represent counts after 3 hrs of perfusion.

Table I indicates that there is, on the average, practically no difference in the erythrocyte and thrombocyte depletion in the packed bed and the empty control system. On the other hand, the leukocytes are unaffected by the empty system but, are affected by the presence of the coated Dowex beads; some 10-20% adhere to the packed bed, which possibly acts as a mechanical filter for these relatively large blood cells.

An analysis of the size distribution of the platelets before and after the hemoperfusion test may be helpful in explaining the different behavior noted with blood taken from different individuals. Fig.1 represents the size distribution of the platelets in the blood used in Exp. Nos. 2 and 5. The area under the graph is proportional to the total number of platelets. The scale is so normalized, that this area is unity for blood before perfusion. Inspection of these figures shows that (a) the average platelet size decreases during hemoperfusion [6] and (b) larger platelets seem to adhere to the foreign surfaces more than smaller ones. In fact, some 30% of the larger platelets (Exp.2), remain, whereas practically none of the smaller ones are depleted from the blood. It is possible that some of the originally larger platelets shrink

Exp.No.	Thrombocytes		Leukocytes		Erythrocytes	
	Empty	Packed	Empty	Packed	Empty	Packed
1	85.1	83.9	79	62	97.3	95.9
2	52.4	48.6	92	80	92.5	88.2
3	89	85.6	102	90	97.4	100
4	78	92.4	106	99	89.9	93.8
5	104.3	93.8	83	65	95.2	95.2

Table I:% Blood cells remaining in blood after 3 hrs circulation

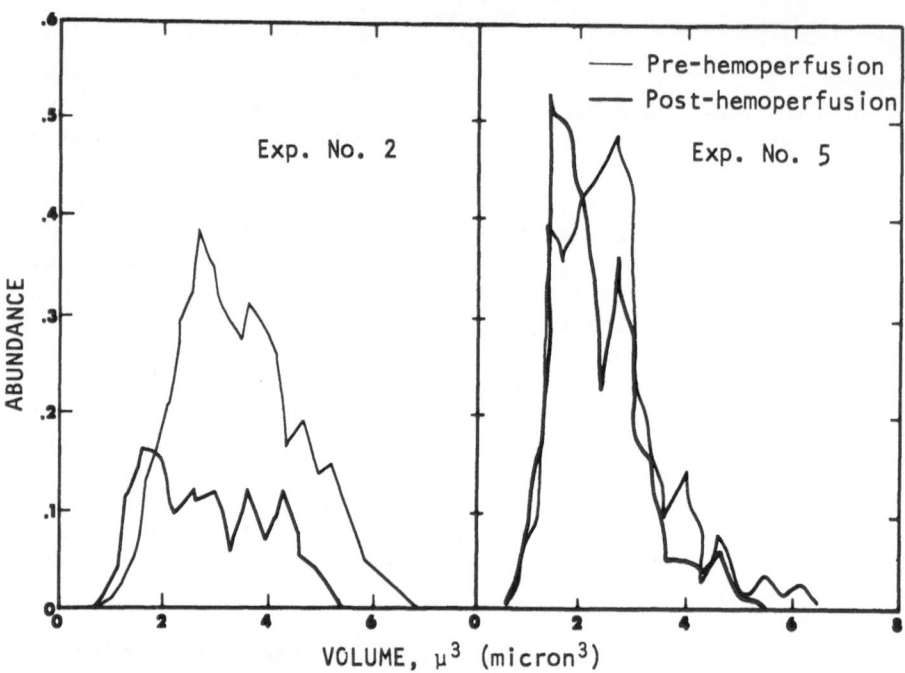

Fig. 1: Normalized size distribution of platelets
before and after hemoperfusion

Element		Empty column	Packed column
K	meq/ℓ	4.6 ± 1.5	5.1 ± 1.5
Cl	meq/ℓ	93 ± 22	87.4 ± 21.3
Na	meq/ℓ	159.7 ± 16.5	158 ± 15.7
Cholesterol	mg%	139 ± 13.4	135.6 ± 16.9
Tot.protein	gr%	6.9 ± 0.9	6.7 ± 1.1
Albumin	gr%	4.0 ± 0.7	4.2 ± 1.3
Globulin	gr%	2.7 ± 0.8	2.3 ± 0.6
Uric acid	mg%	5.4 ± 2.3	3.6 ± 1.0
Urea	mg%	13.9 ± 1.8	15.7 ± 3.3
P	mg%	5.8 ± 0.4	4.1 ± 1.4
Ca	mg%	4.1 ± 2.0	6.3 ± 1.5

Table II: Blood chemistry after 3 hrs hemoperfusion

in size during the in-vitro operation. It is, however, quite reason-
able to assume that the different adhesion characteristics of
different blood is due to their differing size distributions.

Table II represents the average values of some of the blood
components after perfusion through an empty and a packed column,
in the five individuals' blood. These preliminary results do not
indicate any significant effect of the resin bed on the blood
chemistry, and the evident differences between the columns are
within the spread of the experimental error. The low amount of
calcium is due to the presence of citrate as an anticoagulant.

KIDNEY SUPPORT HEMOPERFUSION SYSTEM

The blood level of inorganic phosphate ions in patients
suffering from acute or chronic renal failure is, in many cases,
excessively high. The high concentration of phosphate ions disturbs
the delicate calcium phosphate balance in the blood and may
ultimately lead to osteodistrophy or calcification of soft tissue.
Neither hemodialysis nor the activated carbon hemoperfusion systems
are effective in controlling excess phosphate ions in the blood
stream. Extracorporeal hemoperfusion with alumina packed bed columns
was recently suggested for the controlled removal of inorganic
phosphate from the blood of uremic patients, [7,8]. Column size,
duration and frequency of the alumina hemoperfusion required to meet
specific needs of the patients, are under study (9,10].

As shown in Ref.[8], 5 grms of 14-28 mesh alumina practically
remove all the phosphate (15 mg %P) from a 100 ml buffered saline
solution after two hours, while collodion coated alumina particles
remove 80% of that amount. These results are quite encouraging,
since one wishes to reduce the phosphate concentration in the blood
to a normal level rather than remove it completely. Furthermore,
coating of alumina particles eliminated the release of fine particles from the bed to the blood stream [8]. Preliminary blood
compatibility experiments [8] indicated the lack of interaction
between the alumina granules and the blood components. Here we
report additional blood compatibility experiments carried out with
fresh human blood under standardized experimental conditions.

Materials and Methods

The experimental hemoperfusion system consisted of a Pharmacia
column (K9, 15 cm length) packed with 5 gr alumina. The priming
volume of the alumina filled cell is 4.5 ml. The system was
siliconized with Dow Medical Fluid No.360. The alumina granules of
14-28 mesh size were coated with either collodion or modified

collodion. The latter was obtained by a chemical reaction between
the collodion layer and a dichlorotriazine reactive dye.

The fresh blood volume in each run was 50 ml. 15% ACD was used
as anticoagulant. A flow rate of 3 ml/min was maintained with a
peristaltic pump. Prior to each run, the system was washed with
saline for a couple of hours. Control tests with an identical, but
alumina free, system were also carried out. It is perhaps noteworthy
that this flow rate corresponds to the residence time realized in
clinical carbon hemoperfusion with the Smith & Nephew commercial
columns.

Platelets and leukocytes were counted from samples taken from
the blood reservoir at various time intervals, utilizing a Coulter
Counter model Z-B with a 50μ orifice. A sample of each donor's blood
was subjected to a platelet adhesiveness test [11] whereby 2 ml
blood were passed, within 40 seconds, by a syringe pump through a
small column filled with 2 gr glass beads. The ratio of the platelet
count in the effluent blood to that in the influent blood is used
as a measure of platelet adhesiveness.

Results and Discussion

The adherence of platelets to foreign surfaces may vary
considerably from one donor's blood to another. (Even with the same
donors, a state of stress, or drugs taken, may have a strong
influence on platelet adherence). The platelet adhesiveness test was
therefore utilized to ascertain that there were no exceedingly large
variations in the blood samples received for the perfusion experiments. As seen in Table III the platelets' adhesiveness varied
between 70% and 90% in the various blood samples tested.

The percent of blood cells remaining in circulation in the
perfusion experiments with the various columns is summarized in
Table III. The particle bed reduces the leukocyte count by some 30%
relative to the empty column. The average drop in platelet concentration is 40% in the uncoated alumina columns, 50% in collodion
coated alumina and only 35% of the initial count in the column with
the modified collodion, coated alumina. The finding that the
modified collodion coated alumina is somewhat more thromboresistent
than the collodion coated alumina is consistent with the work of
Nishizawa et al [12], who found that platelet adherence to polymeric
surfaces was inhibited by coating these surfaces with Chicago acid.
It is possible that the negatively charged surface may decrease the
adherence of the platelets which carry an overall negative charge.

The platelet depletion noted in the empty column is close to
that obtained in the packed bed, in agreement with the results shown

Column	Time	Platelet adhesiveness	Leukocytes x10^3/μl	%	Platelets x10^5/μl	%	Platelet adhesiveness	Leukocytes x10^3/μl	%	Platelets x10^5/μl	%
Empty cell	0		4.35	100	5.10	100		4.06	100	2.83	100
	30				3.09	60				2.12	75
	60				3.21	63				2.15	76
	90		3.99	92	3.32	65		3.90	96	2.09	74
	120				2.39	47				1.95	69
Uncoated Alumina	0	73	3.83	100	1.44	100	90	0.94	100	1.49	100
	30				0.69	48				1.14	76
	60				0.73	51				0.99	67
	90				0.91	63				0.92	62
	120		2.05	53	0.92	63		0.73	77	0.94	63
Collodion Coated Alumina	0	80	4.51	100	1.42	100	89	6.68	100	2.80	100
	30				0.59	42				2.25	80
	60				0.49	35				1.60	57
	90				0.62	44				1.61	57
	120		2.58	57				4.23	63	1.60	57
Modified Collodion Coated Alumina	0	73	3.67	100	1.41	100		3.75	100	2.88	100
	30				0.68	49				2.15	75
	60				0.95	67				2.22	77
	90				1.11	83				1.84	64
	120		2.14	58	1.02	72		2.22	59	1.87	65

Table III: Blood compatibility of various columns. % remaining.

in Table I for the liver support system. This is substantiated by
the relative high drop in platelet concentration noted in in-vivo
experiments with animals [13] when blood was circulated through a
by-pass, before the extracorporeal device was inserted. Evidently,
comparison of platelets depletion in different hemoperfusion systems
requires better specification of the operating conditions and,
ideally, an identical reference state.

It is rather surprising to note that the contact of the blood
with the uncoated alumina particles does not induce a more
appreciable change in the platelet and leukocyte counts. Evidently,
the alumina surface is relatively biocompatible, and one may assume
that the coating is superfluous. However, as shown earlier [8], the
uncoated alumina releases fines into the blood stream. Thus, the
coating is required to prevent this undesired physical phenomena,
as well as to slightly improve the biocompatibility characteristics
of the system.

In general, the measured fall of the platelet concentration in
the alumina column is of the same order of magnitude as that
reported in hemoperfusion with coated activated carbon (38%) [14]
and in hemodialysis [15].

The analysis of some of the common chemical elements in the
plasma, before and after the alumina perfusion with fresh whole
blood, was undertaken in order to check the specificity of the
system. As can be seen in Table IV, there is no significant
depletion of any of the main chemical elements in the plasma. The
decrease of calcium concentration during perfusion is probably due

Element	Initial Concentration	Final Concentration	
		Collodion Coated Alumina	Modified Collodion Coated Alumina
Total protein gr%	7	7.2	6.9
Urea (mg%)	18	20.5	24
Uric acid (mg%)	7	6.6	6.8
Na (meq/ℓ)	160	156	160
K (meq/ℓ)	7.9	8.5	8.1
Cl (meq/ℓ)	88	98	
Ca (mg%)	9		5

Table IV: Blood chemistry before and after hemoperfusion

to the deposition of calcium citrate on the alumina column. Thus, for phosphate removal experiments with whole blood, another anticoagulant must be used.

CONCLUSIONS

The liver and kidney hemoperfusion support systems tested here did not show adverse effects on blood composition and cellular count, thus encouraging further work towards the clinical application of these support systems.

Comparison of platelets depletion in empty and packed bed systems indicates the important role played by the supporting equipment. On the other hand, the particle bed accounts for an additional decrease in the leukocyte counts, but the overall loss is in the acceptable practice.

Different blood samples exhibit different platelet adhesion characteristics. In general, larger platelets tend to deplete more than smaller ones.

Acknowledgement

This work was supported in part by a grant from the B.DeRothschild Foundation for the advancement of science in Israel and in part by a special grant from Mr.H.Grunfeld of the Herbert Grunfeld and Ernest Grunfeld Trust, N.Y.

Thanks are due to Dr.I.Blank for supplying the Acrylic AG-1039 polymer and to Dr.D.Frenkel, Chairman, Life International for facilitating the write-up of this report.

References

1. Radzialowski,F.M.,"Effect of Spironolactone and Pregnenolone-16α Carbonil on BIL Metabolism and Plasma Levels in Male and Female Rats",Biochem.Pharma.22,1607 (1973).

2. Sideman,S.,Mor,L.,Rousseau,I.,Brandes,J.M.and Ben-Arie,D., "Removal of Bilirubin from the Blood of Jaundiced Infants",Proc. 2nd Strathclyde Bioengineering Seminar - "Artificial organs", (1976),Kenedi,Courtney,Gaylor and Gilchrist,eds.,MacMillan Press, London 1977.

3. Winchester,J.F.,MacKay,J.M.,Forbes,C.D.Blakely,E., Prentice,C.R.M. and Kennedy,A.C. "Haemostatic Changes Induced in-vitro by Activated Charcoal Haemoperfusion",Thromb.Diath.,34(2), 587, (1975).

4. Scharschmidt,B.F.,Martin,J.F.,Shapiro,L.J.,Plotz,P.H. and Berk,P.D.,"Use of calcium chelating agents and prostaglandin $E_1(PGE_1)$ to eliminate platelet losses during hemoperfusion through various adsorbents", Gastroentr. 69 (3), 864, (1975).

5. Plotz,P.H.,Berk,P.D.,and Scharschmidt,B.F.,"Removing substances from blood by affinity chromatography. I.Removing bilirubin and other albumin-bound substances from plasma and blood with albumin-conjugated agarose beads",J.Clin.Invest.,53,778 (1974).

6. Williams,R.,"Approaches to the development of artificial liver support", Proc.2nd Strathclyde Bioengineering Seminar - "Artificial organs",(1976),Kenedi,Courtney,Gaylor and Gilchrist,eds., MacMillan Press,London,1977.

7. Hoffer,E.,Rousseau,I.,Sideman,S.,Better,O. and Raziel,A,"Selective removal of waste metabolites from human serum",Proc.XXIV International Symposium on macromolecules;Jerusalem,July 1975.

8. Sideman,S.,Hoffer,E.,Better,O.and Lupovitch,S,"Selective removal of phosphate ions from the blood of uremic patients",Proc. 2nd Strathclyde Bioengineering Seminar - "Artificial Organs",(1976), Kenedi,Courtney,Gaylor & Gilchrist,eds.,MacMillan Press,London, 1977.

9. Yaniv,A,"Removal of waste metabolites from the blood serum - inorganic phosphate",M.Sc.Thesis (in Hebrew) Technion,Haifa, August,1976.

10. Ramon,O, "Selective removal of metabolites from the blood serum by hemoperfusion",M.Sc.Thesis (in Hebrew),Technion,Haifa,Aug.1976.

11. Salzman,E.W. "Measurement of platelet adhesiveness - A simple in-vitro technique demonstrating an abnormality in Von Willebrand's disease",J.Lab.Clin.Med.,62, 724 (1963).

12. Nishizawa,E.E.,Wynalda,D.J. and Lednicer,D,"Non-thrombogenic surface with Evan's blue","Platelets,Thrombosis and Inhibitors", P.Didisheim,T.Shimamoto and H.Yamazaki,eds.,p.135,F.K.Shattauer Verlag,1974.

13. de Leval,M.R.,Hill,J.D.,Mielke,C.H.,Macur,M.F. and Gerbode,F. "Blood platelets and extracorporeal circulation",J.Thor.Cardiovas. Surg.,69, 144 (1975).

14 Vale,J.A.,Rees,A.J.,Widdop,B.and Goulding,R."The use of charcoal hemoperfusion in the management of severely poisoned patients",in "Artif.Liver Support",p.352,R.Williams and I.M. Murray Lyon,eds.,Pitman Medical Publishing Co.,1975.

15. Lindsay,R.M.,Prentice,C.R.M.,Davidson,J.F.,Burton,J.A. and McNicol,G.P.,"Haemostatic changes during dialysis associated with thrombus formation on dialysis membranes",Brit.Med.J. 11,454 (1972).

OTHER ADSORBENT HEMOPERFUSION APPROACHES

THE USE OF MEMBRANES AND SORBENTS FOR BLOOD DETOXIFICATION:

CUPROPHAN SORBENT MEMBRANES

P.S. Malchesky and Y. Nose

Cleveland Clinic, Department of Artificial Organs

9500 Euclid Avenue, Cleveland, Ohio 44106

INTRODUCTION

The use of membranes and sorbents for blood detoxification are well published topics in the field of artificial organs. The advantage of the membrane process is that it exhibits low trauma in contact with blood, no particulate is generated, and the removal of large molecular weight substances or cells can be prevented from passage due to the porosity or permeability of the membrane's wall. Herein lies also a disadvantage in that transport is a function of solute size and discriminate solute removal patterns are thus not possible. The advantage of sorbents is that their physical and chemical characteristics can be matched with those of the solute to be removed. Thereby, specific solute removal patterns different than that of membrane separations and not really as dependent as molecular size can be achieved. Disadvantages in the use of sorbents, however, have been the blood trauma related to damage of blood components or the removal of the cellular elements and particular generation with carryover into the vascular system. As a practical consideration in the use of sorbents for blood detoxification in the treatment of most disease states in which the range of solutes to be removed is broad and generally no one sorbent is totally effective, multiple sorbents must be employed. Past studies have concentrated primarily on the use of a single sorbent.

In order to employ the advantages of sorbents and to employ multiple sorbent systems, specialized sorbent-membrane systems are being studied for blood detoxification as related to hepatic and renal failure. Two specific systems are plasma filtration hemoperfusion and the employment of sorbent membranes.

PLASMA FILTRATION HEMOPERFUSION

In the removal of large molecular weight substances in blood, such as protein or protein-bound substances, high porosity membranes are needed. Our principle of plasma filtration hemoperfusion [1,2] involves the perfusion of blood over high porosity membranes (less than one micron pore diameter with a sieving coefficient of albumin of about one). Under a pressure gradient, plasma is filtered through the membrane and enters the reactor compartment. In the reactor compartment the sorbents interact with the plasma to remove those select solutes, and the plasma is allowed to be returned to the mainstream blood flow after passage through a second porous membrane which prevents the passage of the reactor. Thus, the disadvantages of the sorbents can be overcome by the proper choice of membrane. This system is also amendable to the incorporation of biologically active systems such as enzymes, cells, or tissue in the reactor compartment to provide metabolic support. At the present, the Nuclepore 040 and 060 membranes (Nuclepore Corp., Pleasanton, Calif.) have the most acceptable plasma flux rates of the membranes studied with high sieving coefficients for albumin and protein-bound substances. Using surgically created hepatic failure dog models, three appropriate sorbents have been selected to date for studies in the support of hepatic insufficiency. Recently, Maini et al also showed the feasibility of this plasma filtration hemoperfusion system for hepatic assist [3]. This concept has been applied clinically in the treatment of hepatic failure by Yamazaki et al [4]. They used cellulose acetate hollow fiber membranes of $0.2 \mu m$ and activated charcoal as the sorbent.

SORBENT MEMBRANES

While the problem of hepatic assist is quite complex, and the degree to which detoxification alone can be helpful still requires further work, the past history on renal support and drug or chemical overdose has indicated that select sorbents can be employed. Past studies in these applications have indicated their advantages [5-7]. The necessity of making such systems practical and safe is of paramount importance.

Recently, Cuprophan membranes containing sorbents have been made available (Enka Glanzstoff, Wuppertal-Barmen, West Germany). Three general types have been made available for our studies, as shown schematically in Figure 1. The sorbent (S) fiber is essentially a Cuprophan hollow fiber filled with sorbents in a matrix of Cuprophan. The membrane wall is between 3 and 15 microns thick

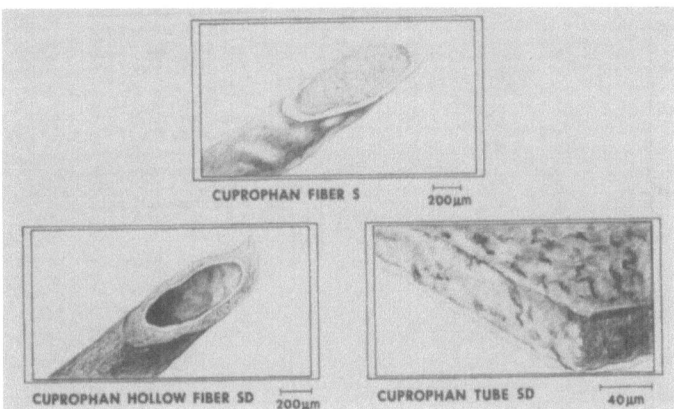

Figure 1. Schematic representation of the Cuprophan membranes containing sorbents (a) sorbent (S) fiber, (b) sorbent dialyzing (SD) hollow fiber, and (c) SD tube.

and overall fiber diameter between 300 and 330 microns, depending on the fiber style. Overall sorbent content is between 40 and 65%. To date, two types of sorbents have been incorporated in these fibers, activated charcoal and aluminum oxide. The sorbent dialyzing fiber is a hollow fiber with a bilayer of about 300 micron internal diameter and 400 micron outer diameter. The wall consists of a 5 to 10 micron inner wall of Cuprophan with an outer wall of about 40 micron thick of the sorbent in a matrix of Cuprophan. Overall sorbent content of the fiber is about 50%. Presently, only activated charcoal fibers have been made available. The sorbent dialyzing tubular membrane is similar in wall structure to the sorbent dialyzing fiber. The pure Cuprophan layer is on the inside of the tube. Tubes with activated charcoal have been made available with a width of 15 cm and overall charcoal content of about 40%. The tubes can be employed in parallel plate or coil type devices. For more technical information concerning the composition and general characteristics of these Cuprophan membranes containing sorbents, one is referred to published literature from the manufacturer [8].

The advantages of Cuprophan as a carrier for sorbents are quite obvious. Its history of use in the treatment of chronic renal failure has shown it to be biocompatible. It is acceptably permeable to low molecular weight solutes desired to be removed, yet impermeable to the large molecular weight species as proteins and blood cells and to the finest of sorbent particles. Based upon the manufacturing techniques employed for these sorbent membranes, particulate release is prevented, and multiple sorbents have been employed.

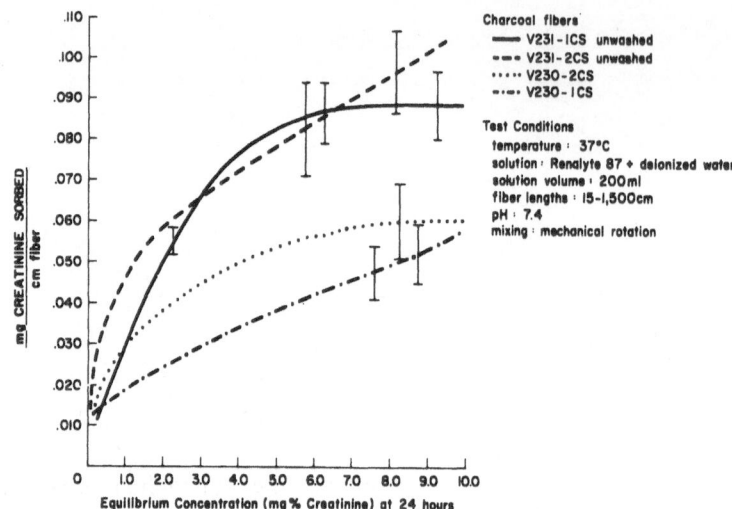

Figure 2.   Sorption isotherms for various activated charcoal
            fibers.

       Studies on these materials have been reported by the authors
elsewhere [9,10]; therefore, a brief summary only will be given here.
To evaluate the solute capacity of the sorbent, membrane sorption
isotherms are run in dialysate solution to which the solutes under
study are added at 37°C, pH 7.4, for contact times of 24 hours.
Figure 2 shows a plot of mg creatinine sorbed per cm fiber length
for various charcoal fibers versus the equilibrium concentration
of creatinine. Differences among the fibers are readily discern-
able but at an equilibrium concentration of close to zero; while
sorption is significantly greater than zero, it is comparable for
all fibers. Very similar is the plot of mg of creatinine sorbed
per gm of activated charcoal versus the equilibrium concentration.
The isotherms are best described as the Langmuir type sorption
which fit the Freundlich equation expressed as: $x/m = KC^{1/n}$ where
x/m is the amount of solute sorbed per unit weight of sorbent. C
is the equilibrium concentration taken to be at 24 hours and K and
n are constants for the sorbent membrane. K is the value of x/m
at C=1 and n is the value taken from the slope (=1/n) of the plot
of ln x/m versus lnC. Table 1 shows data generated on some activated charcoal fibers. Particularly noteworthy is the high K values for these fibers. For a given fiber, uric acid was removed
better than creatinine and creatinine better than salicylate. No
significant urea removal was noted.

       Various types of units have been constructed using the sor-
bent membranes. Figure 3 shows a canister type unit utilizing a
coil of the sorbent fiber. Figure 4 shows a rectangular design

Table 1. Activated Charcoal Fiber Isotherm Data

Fiber	Solute	n	K mg/gm
V-67	Creatinine	3.7	82.46
	Salicylate	8.33	52.46
V-124	Creatinine	3.33	68.49
	Uric Acid	4.87	81.28
	Salicylate	2.90	33.88
V-230-1CS	Creatinine	2.94	57.84
V-230-2CS	Creatinine	2.92	74.35
V-231-1CS	Creatinine	1.30	90.90
	Uric Acid	2.11	143.86
V-231-2CS	Creatinine	2.21	160.32

unit employing the charcoal and aluminum oxide sorbent fibers.
The blood porting is perpendicular to the flow in the device. Devices similar in shape have also been made with the sorbent dialyzing fibers incorporating the necessary lumen porting. Figure 5
shows a coil dialyzer constructed with the charcoal dialyzing tube.
All devices are tested under stabilized conditions [10]. For the
sorbent fiber devices, removal rates per gram weight of sorbent is
sufficiently high in four hour studies that practical device designs are feasible. Creatinine and uric acid removal by the activated charcoal sorbent fibers ranged between 15 and 35 mg/gm and
for phosphorous removal by the aluminum oxide fiber 20-40 mg/gm.

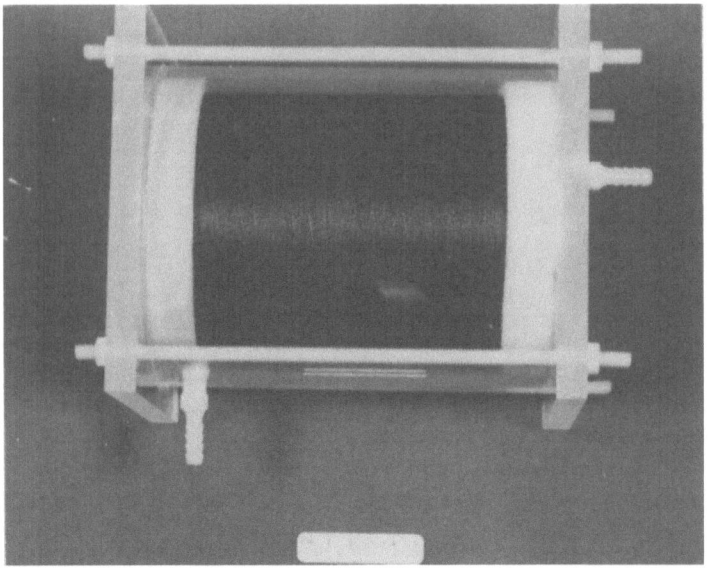

Figure 3. Canister activated charcoal sorbent fiber device.
Blood porting is from the front and side.

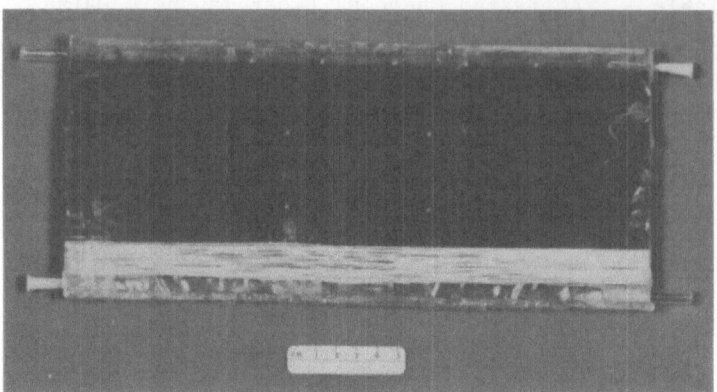

Figure 4. Rectangular plate design employing activated charcoal and aluminum oxide sorbent fibers. Blood enters and exits the device axially with the fibers and flows across the fibers.

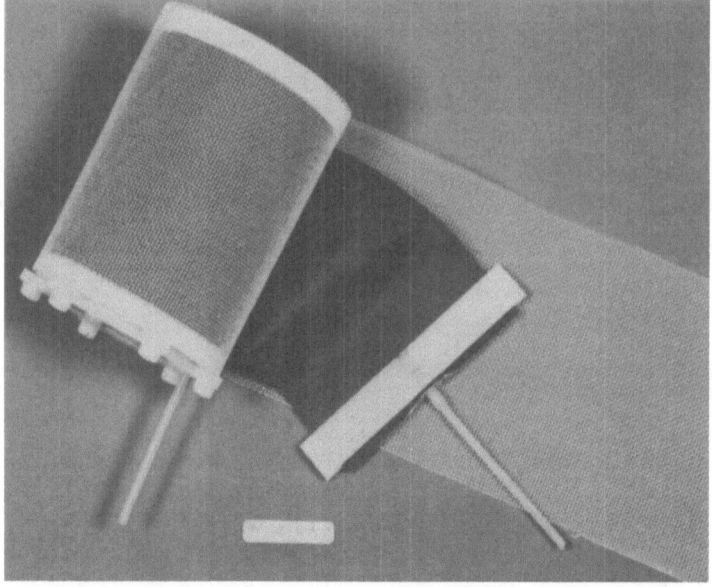

Figure 5. Activated charcoal sorbent dialyzing tube used in construction of a coil dialyzer by techniques employed in the construction of the Coiled Envelope Kidney.

No significant removal of urea was noted. Note that the removal rates for the charcoal fibers are less than the K values for the given fibers. Therefore, high concentration gradients can be maintained between solution and sorbent fiber even up to the four hours studied. Uric acid is removed better than creatinine which is just the opposite to be expected by dialysis alone. For the small molecules studied, the fibers appear to act more like sorbents than membranes in their transport characteristics. The transport of molecules more easily sorbed by the sorbents appear to be facilitated. In the studies with the aluminum oxide fiber, the phosphorous removal was limited by the quantity of sorbent employed. Variations in removal among the various devices is related to differences in fluid dynamics. These studies indicate that construction parameters which affect the flow dynamics are critical for the solutes studied as is the case in dialyzer design. No electrolyte variations were noted in the use of these fibers and no particulate generation was observed [10]. Acute animal studies carried out to date do not indicate any problems related to the use of these sorbent membranes in vivo. Heparin levels have been comparable to those used in extracorporeal circuits with standard dialyzers.

In the evaluation of the sorbent membranes and device designs incorporating them, testing has been standardized. A major difficulty has arisen in the literature in that standardized reporting of sorbent properties and device results has not been made, particularly making comparisons difficult. Sorption is a function of the sorbent, solution, and transfer properties of the device. Present analysis (in press) relating all these parameters has indicated that device designs tested to date have overall efficiencies of 50-95% calculated based upon the fiber characteristics. It is believed that efforts in the future should be made in this direction to relate device design characteristics in order to optimize designs for clinical application.

SUMMARY

With a design goal of removal of known low molecular weight solutes, biocompatibility, ability to employ multiple sorbents, as is required in the disease state, with no particle releases is required for chronic applications, the Cuprophan sorbent membranes offer great potential in the design of novel treatment modalities. It is believed that the appropriate combination of membranes and sorbents, as outlined in the plasma filtration hemoperfusion system, and sorbent membrane configurations, can be useful in meeting the needs of blood detoxification in various disease states.

1. Nose, Y., Malchesky, P.S., Castino, F., Koshino, I., Scheucher, K. and Nokoff, R.: Improved hemoperfusion systems for renal-hepatic support. Kidney International, 10:S244, 1976.

2. Castino, F., Scheucher, K., Malchesky, P.S., Koshino, I. and Nose, Y.: Microemboli-free blood detoxification utilizing plasma filtration. Trans. Amer. Soc. Artif. Int. Organs, 22:637, 1976.

3. Maini, R. and Baillie, H.: Detoxification system utilizing microporous membranes and sorbents. Program, Conference on Fulminant Hepatic Failure, February 29, 1977, NIH, Bethesda, Maryland.

4. Yamazaki, Z., Fujimori, Y., Sanjo, K., Sugiura, M., Wada, T., Inoue, N., Oda, T., Kominami, N., Fujisaki, U. and Hayano, F.: New artificial liver support system (plasma perfusion detoxification) for hepatic coma. Abstracts Amer. Soc. Artif. Int. Organs, 6:99, 1977.

5. Chang, T.M.S., Gonda, A., Dirks, J.H., Coffey, J.F. and Lee-Burns, T.: ACAC microcapsule artificial kidney for the long-term and short term management of eleven patients with chronic renal failure. Trans. Amer. Soc. Artif. Int. Organs, 18:465, 1972.

6. Rosenbaum, J.L., Kramer, M.S., Raja, R. and Boreyko, C.: Resin hemoperfusion: A new treatment for acute drug intoxication. New Eng. J. Med., 284:874, 1971.

7. Gordon, A., Better, O.S., Greenbaum, M.A., Marantz, L.B., Gral, L., Maxwell, M.H.: Clinical maintenance hemodialysis with a sorbent based low volume dialysate regeneration system. Trans. Amer. Soc. Artif. Int. Organs, 17:253, 1971.

8. Enka Glanzstoff, Cuprophan Technical Information Bulletin No. 12, 1976, 'Wuppertal-Barmen, West Germany.

9. Malchesky, P.S., Varnes, W., Nokoff, R. and Nose, Y.: The charcoal capillary hemoperfusion system. Proc. EDTA, 13: 242, 1976.

10. Malchesky, P.S., Varnes, W., Piatkiewicz, W. and Nose, Y.: Membranes containing sorbents for blood detoxification. Trans. Amer. Soc. Artif. Int. Organs, 23: 659, 1977.

COMBINATION OF HEMODIALYSIS AND HEMOPERFUSION IN A SINGLE

HOLLOW-FIBER UNIT FOR TREATMENT OF UREMIA

L.A. Castro, G. Hampel, R. Gebhardt, A. Fateh
and H.J. Gurland

Med. Klinik I Grosshadern, Munich University
Fed. Rep. of Germany

In the past, various researchers have attempted to obtain improved permeability in the middle molecular range by the development of new dialysis membranes. As a consequence of this, it is clearly indicated that an improvement in this area can only be achieved at the expense of an increased hydrodynamic permeability. This additionally requires new techniques to regulate ultra-filtration. Therefore, it was intended to avoid this high ultra-filtration side-effect by combining diffusion and adsorption in a single membrane. The result was a new double-layer cuprophane-membrane of hollow-fiber type consisting on the inner (blood compartment) side of a thin layer of pure cuprophane-cellulose and on the outer (dialysate compartment) side of a second layer, containing about 40 to 50 % activated charcoal. The total thickness of the charcoal containing hollow-fiber therefore increased by three as compared to the conventional hollow-fiber (Figures 1 and 2).

Materials and Methods

In-vitro investigations of the double-layer hollow-fiber* with and without the use of dialysate were compared with the conventional cuprophane hollow-fiber*.

Two manufacturers of hollow-fiber dialyzers presently in clinical use made test dialyzers available in identical configurations as their commercially available models. The surface area of the charcoal hollow-fiber differed from the conventional cuprophane units by 0.1 and 0.3 m^2. The clearance values given in Figure 3 have been recalculated to 1.0 m^2 for comparison purposes.

*ENKA Glanzstoff AG, Wuppertal-Barmen, Fed. Rep. of Germany

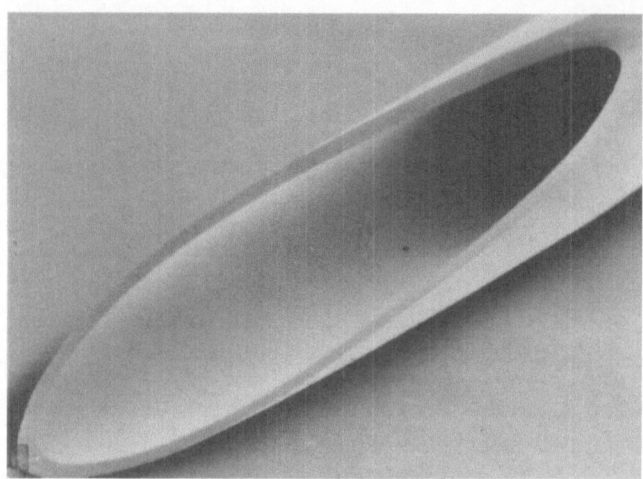

Figure 1
Conventional Cuprophan Hollow-Fiber B4 IM
Wall thickness   19 μm
Inside diameter 300 μm

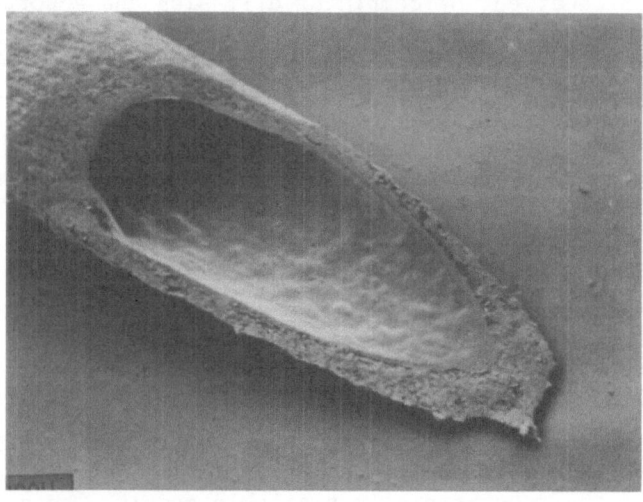

Figure 2
Double-layer Cuprophan Hollow-Fiber SD-M 50/9/290
Wall thickness inner layer   9 μm
Wall thickness outer layer   50 μm
Inside diameter   290 μm

For all clearance evaluations, the Cobe Centry 2 single-pass proportioning system (Cobe Laboratories, Inc.) was used. Dialysate flow rate was 500 ml/min.

The simulated blood was a solution corresponding to normal dialysate and to which the following test substances were added. The blood flow rate was measured by electro-magnetic flow meters. In order to alleviate ultrafiltration effects, the transmembrane pressure was held at 0 mmHg.

Clearance determinations were made for the following radio-isotope-marked substances: Urea, creatinine, phenobarbital, carbromal, digoxin, vitamin B_{12} and inulin with molecular weights of 62, 150, 233, 237, 781, 1355, 5175 respectively.

The ultrafiltration was measured as the reduction in volume in the "blood" reservoir after recirculation of the simulated blood. A regression curve was drawn from the experimentally determined values ($y = a + bx$).

Results

As may be expected, a comparison of the hollow-fiber containing activated charcoal with and without the use of dialysate resulted in a remarkable difference in the clearance of urea. For all other test substances higher clearance values were obtained using the charcoal fiber even without dialysate.

With the use of dialysate the hollow-fiber containing charcoal achieved the highest clearance values for all substances, with the exception of urea. This improvement of clearance was significant in all test substances with the exception of inulin (Figure 3).

Comparing the conventional with the double-layer membrane the ultrafiltration rates were 2.6 ml/h/mmHg and 3.3 ml/h/mmHg respectively.

Until now we performed clinical trials with three patients in chronic hemodialysis using 18 dialyzers with double-layer membranes. Side-effects, such as changes in blood pressure or blood cell count, have not been recognized. The gel chromatographic evaluations before and after dialysis clearly showed an improved elimination of middle molecular substances with the charcoal fiber dialyzer over the conventional type. As yet we have not sufficient in-vivo data available to enable us to present a final comment concerning clinical applications. More detailed studies of clinical aspects will be the subject of future investigations.

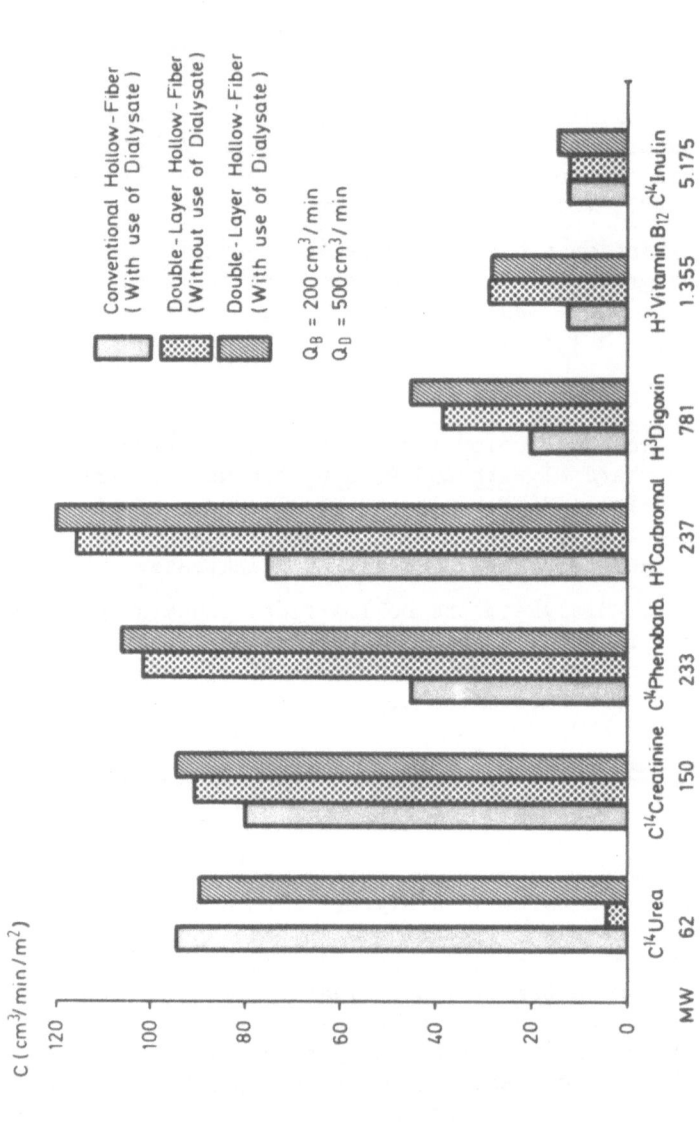

Figure 3. Clearances obtained from in-vitro tests with conventional and double-layer Cuprophan hollow-fiber dialyzers.

Conclusion and Summary

Our preliminary in-vitro results show that an improvement of clearances in the middle molecular range between 150 and 1,350 can be achieved with the use of a new double-layer hollow-fiber. These new technological considerations indicate that a combination of dialysis and adsorption in a single membrane for treatment of uremia is not only possible but highly advantageous as well.

The following presents a summary of our results as obtained until today:

1. Double-layer charcoal fibers gave significantly higher in-vitro clearances for all test substances with the exception of urea.

2. Ultrafiltration rates were comparable despite differences in membrane thickness.

3. Negligible effect on clearance with and without dialysate offered the possibility of reduction or elimination of dialysate.

4. Preliminary clinical trials indicated feasible application for treatment of uremia.

THE B-D HEMODETOXIFIER: PARTICULATE RELEASE AND ITS SIGNIFICANCE

John B. Hill and C. Russell Horres

Becton, Dickinson and Company Research Center

P. O. Box 12016, Research Triangle Park, N. C. 27709

When a clinician considers the use of an extracorporeal blood circuit in treating a patient, in addition to the therapeutic value of the procedure, he should know what exogenous material the circuit adds to the blood flowing through it and what is the significance of this addition to the patient. The data presented in this communication represent preliminary attempts to address these questions in regard to the Becton, Dickinson HEMODETOXIFIER, an adsorption device containing activated charcoal immobilized to produce a minimum of particulate release with a maximum of adsorptive surface in direct contact with the bloodstream (1). Of primary interest was quantification of particulate release from the device under simulated use conditions and the evaluation of possible untoward biological effects of intravenous administration of such particulate material. A gravimetric technique was developed using Nuclepore® filters to trap and weigh microgram amounts of material released during perfusion of the devices. To monitor biological effects of intravenous charcoal particulates, single injections of pulverized charcoal in a saline-DEXTRAN vehicle were given to Sprague-Dawley rats.

MATERIALS AND METHODS

Particulate Release Tests. A diagram of the circuit used in the experiments may be seen in Figure 1. A hemodialysis roller pump and an arterial bloodline with the bubble trap removed were used with luer adapters to complete the circuit (HEMODETOXIFIER, Blood Pump N-4504 and hemodialysis tubing #8851, B-D Drake Willock, Portland, Or.). Nuclepore® filters - .8μ (N080CPR04700) and filter holders (FH04700108) were obtained from the Nuclepore

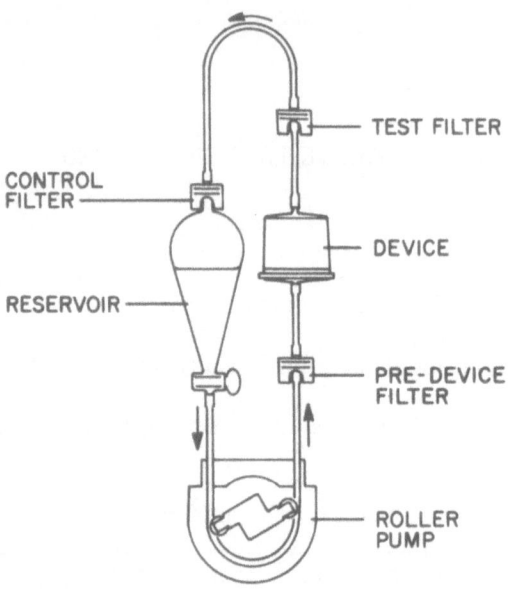

Figure 1. Circuit used to evaluate particulate release by B-D
    HEMODETOXIFIERS. Positions of the Nuclepore® filter holders
    containing 0.8µ filters are shown.

Corporation, Pleasanton, Ca. Both the filters and the holders
were washed with distilled water which was previously filtered
through 0.45µ Millipore® filters (Millipore Millex® 0.45µ Disposable Filter Unit, Millipore Corporation, Bedford, Mass.). In
addition, the filter holders were pre-washed in an ultrasonic
cleaner. A pre-weighed Nuclepore® filter in a holder assembly was
attached to the outlet of the HEMODETOXIFIER and three liters of
distilled water were pumped through the pre-HEMODETOXIFIER filter,
the device and test filter at 200 ml/min. This water was discarded
and the test filter was removed, dried and weighed as described
below. A fresh pre-weighed test Nuclepore® filter was placed on
the outlet of the device and the entire circuit connected for the
re-circulation experiments. The total volume of water in the
circuit was approximately seven hundred milliliters and it was
circulated at two hundred milliliters per minute for the time
period noted in the text. Two types of control experiments were
done. In the first there was no device in the circuit and the pre-
filter and test filter were separated by approximately six inches
of plastic tubing. Water was circulated for four hours, and the
test filter dried and weighed. In other experiments the control
consisted of a third Nuclepore® filter and holder in the circuit

following the test filter on the device outlet. The test filter
was weighed for particulates and the additional filter was weighed
as a control for the drying and weighing procedures. The
hemodetoxifiers evaluated were obtained from several production
lots. Filter weight changes are reported in the text. No attempt
was made to subtract the control data from the experimental data
changes.

Gravimetric Analysis of Filters. The Nuclepore® filter, in
the filter holder, was connected to a vacuum flask and 0.45 Millex®
filtered air pulled through it to remove excess water. The
Nuclepore® filters were removed from the holders with smooth tipped
forceps and placed in covered plastic containers (RODAC® Plate
#1034, Falcon, Oxnard, Ca.) on a coiled stainless steel wire which
prevented the filter from sticking to the bottom of the plastic
container and thus facilitated handling. The seal on the plastic
containers was not air tight but did keep airborne particulates
off the filter. The filters in the plastic containers were dried
in a 55°C oven for at least twelve hours and transferred directly
to a glove box (Fisher isolator/lab chamber, Fisher Scientific Co.,
Raleigh, N. C.) containing a balance (Cahn Model 4700 Electro
Balance, Cahn Instruments, Cerritos, Ca.), ionizing units for
removing static electricity (Nuclear Products Co., El Monte, Ca.)
and a humidity monitor (Bacharach Instrument Co., Pittsburgh, Pa.).
The filters in the plastic containers were allowed to equilibrate
in the chamber for one hour prior to weighing the filters. Relative
humidity was carefully controlled in the glove box by means of dry
nitrogen so that weighings with and without particulates for a
given filter were made at a similar relative humidity ($\pm$ 5% RH).
The filters were passed over the ionizing unit just prior to each
weighing.

A stainless steel wire loop was used as an aid to transfer
the filter from the plastic container to the weighing stirrup.
The filters were weighed at least three times at intervals never
less than thirty minutes. The filter was discarded if the range
of three consecutive weighings was more than 4 µg. Filters were
tared in the same manner.

Rat Injection Studies. Coconut shell charcoal (Type PCB,
Pittsburgh Activated Carbon, Division of Calgon Corporation,
Pittsburgh, Pa.) was ground with a porcelain mortar and pestle.
The resulting dry powder was screened through a monofilament
polyester screen with 43µ openings (DAFAB, D-120, Wire Cloth
Enterprises Inc., Pittsburgh, Pa.). The screened particles were
suspended in physiological saline in 6% DEXTRAN solution and were
injected intravenously into the tail veins of Sprague-Dawley strain
rats (ARS, Madison, Wi.) ranging from 120 gm to 250 gm in weight.
One hundred each of male and female rats were used. The single
injections were made to include a vehicle control and three doses

of charcoal particles (0, 0.2, 2.0 and 20 mg/Kg). Twenty-five
animals of each sex received each treatment. The particulates
were kept suspended by means of magnetic stirring bars until
aspirated into the injection syringe. The rats were caged
individually, fed and watered ad libitum, and were weighed
periodically. Surviving animals were sacrificed after two years.
The size distributions of the charcoal particles for injection and
those found in washes of the HEMODETOXIFIER as determined by sizing
with a scanning electron microscope were comparable.

RESULTS

The mean increase in weight of the Nuclepore® filters through
which the three liter rinse from the twenty devices studied had
passed was 15 µg. The smallest increase was 1 µg and the largest
was 32 µg. These devices had been shipped in their regular
packaging some 700 miles by truck. Since each of the devices was
washed to minimize particulate release prior to packaging and
sterilization, these data suggest that relatively little particulate matter was generated during sterilization and shipment.

Figure 2 shows the results of the twenty re-circulation
experiments; ten for four hours and five each at one and two hours.
The eleven control data points are plotted at the zero time point
on the graph. Though there is variance at each point, the values
for the means give a reasonably straight line which passes very
close to the mean for the control values. This latter finding
could be interpreted as indicating that there was an increase in
weight of these filters (6.6 µg) unassociated with device perfusion.
In any case, if the control values are ignored, particulates were
released at approximately 7.5 µg per device-hour. This figure is
similar to that reported by Temple, Walker and Done (2).

Figure 3 shows the body weight gains for the rats given the
various doses of intravenous charcoal. No differences are apparent.
A plot of survival of each of the four treatment groups may be seen
in Figure 4. An analysis of variance, based on survival days up
to the sacrifice day some two years after the injection, showed no
significant differences between the dose levels (0, 0.2, 2.0 and
20 mg/Kg). These injection experiments have not been completed in
that postmortem evaluation of tissue sections is still in progress.
The data so far, however, strongly suggest that these doses of
charcoal did not effect the growth or survival of the rats.

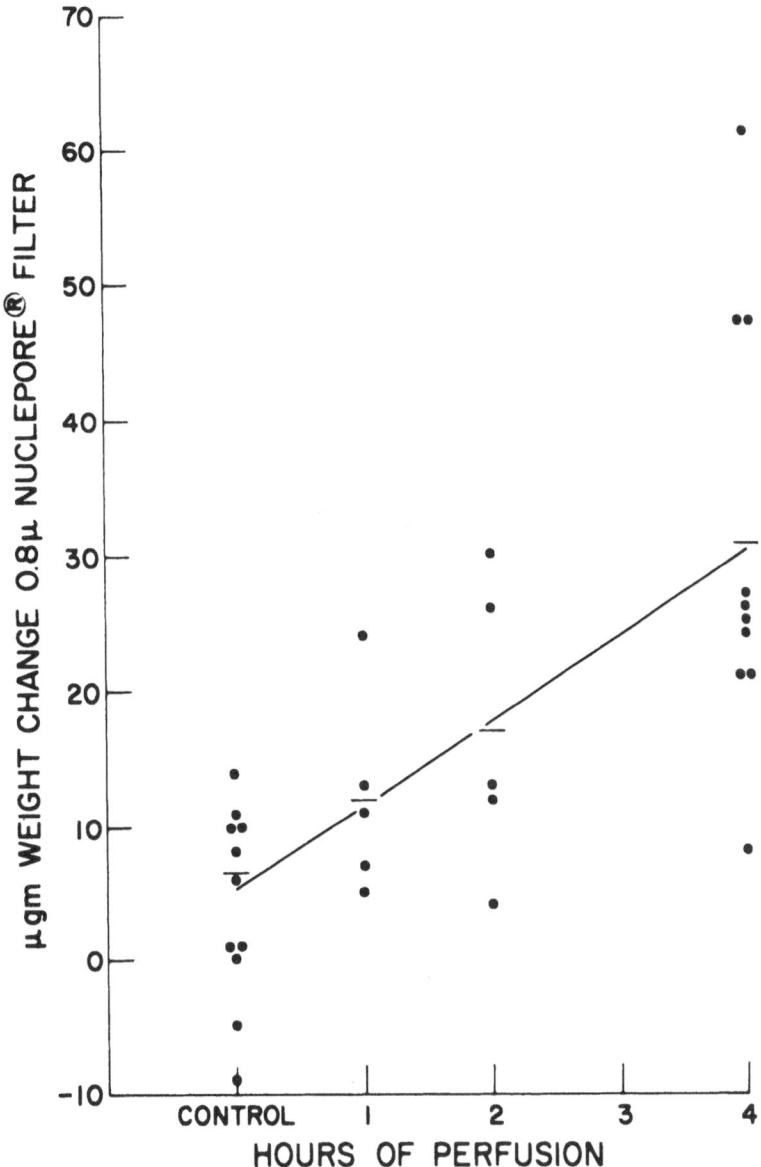

Figure 2. Particulate release by B-D HEMODETOXIFIERS during
    200 ml/min water perfusions. (-) represents the mean value.

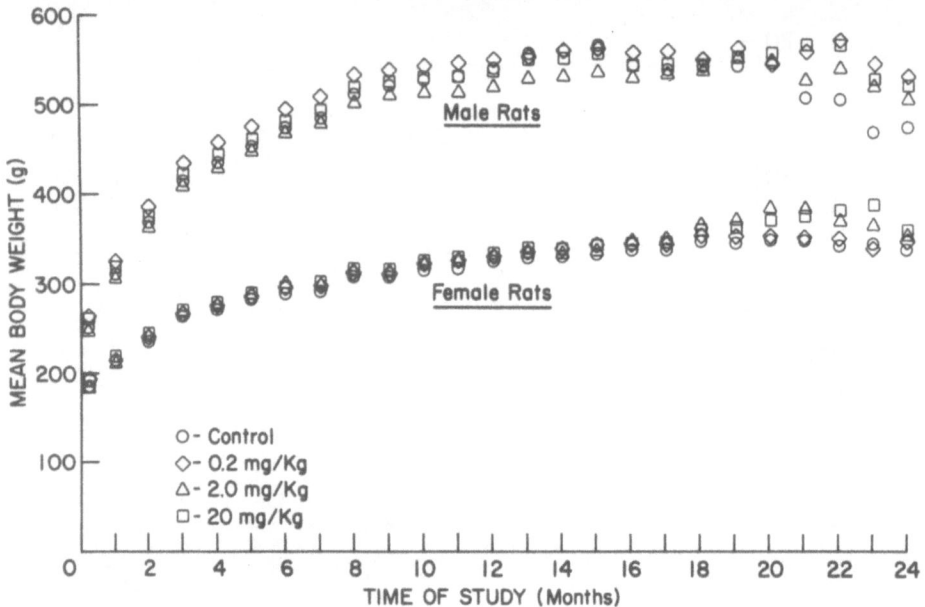

Figure 3.   Body weight changes of rats injected intravenously with charcoal particulates.

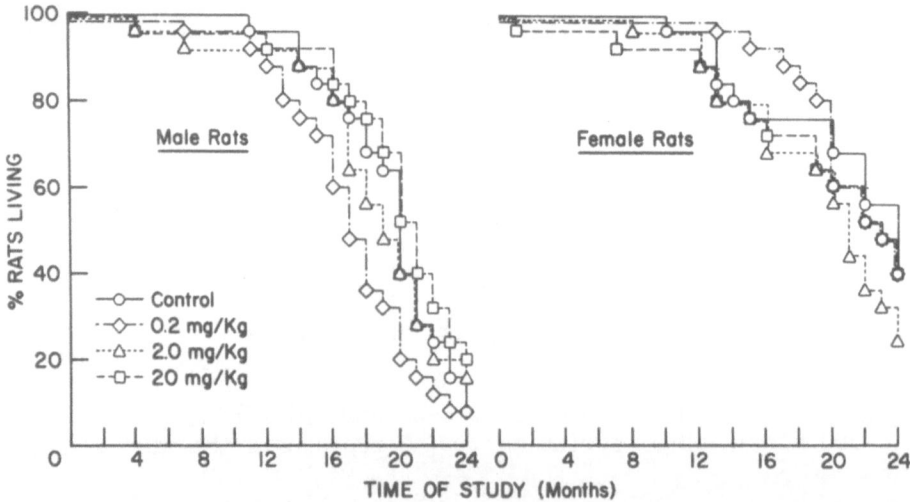

Figure 4.   Survival in rats injected with charcoal particulates.

DISCUSSION

The measurement of particulates in whole blood is a challenging task. Since blood contains endogenous particles, red cells, white cells and platelets, the measuring technique would have to be capable of detecting charcoal particles among some five billion other particles per milliliter of blood. As yet, no such technique has been described. The use of a radioactive label on the charcoal may appear to be a solution to evaluating particulate release in vivo. The label, however, must be uniformly distributed throughout the charcoal on a molecular level and must not separate from it. Short of growing coconuts in an atmosphere of $C^{14}O_2$ such a label does not appear to exist.

An alternative approach might be to relate tissue levels to particulate release. Van Wagenen, Coleman and Andrade (3) injected charcoal particulates intravenously into mice. A dose of 10 mg/Kg body weight was required before particles could readily be found in tissue sections. Similar results were seen in the rat studies described here. It is clear, therefore, that histological techniques are not a sensitive measure of particulate infusion.

In view of these difficulties studies of particulate release to date have been limited to those in which aqueous solutions were pumped through devices and analyzed. It is recognized that distilled water does not approximate the viscosity or surface tension properties of blood. Attempts to use saline and DEXTRAN solutions, however, were unsuccessful because of high control filters weights (no device present in circuit) which were possibly related to infusion of the test solution under the seal areas of the filter housing over the course of the experiment thereby preventing adequate wash out.

The gravimetric procedure described here is lengthy and requires careful technique. The Nuclepore®filters weigh approximately 15 mg and the particulates weigh only micrograms, thus requiring a high degree of precision in the weighing as well as the constant avoidance of airborne particulate contamination. Previously reported studies (1), utilizing a simpler visual comparison technique and 150 ml/min flows, estimated 2 µg of particulates in a ten liter effluent from one device. The studies reported here averaged 7.5 µg in twelve liters of effluent from twenty devices with a flow of two hundred ml/min. In spite of the fact that visual estimates of particulate weight did not take into consideration the size distribution of the charcoal particulates, the estimates were of the same order of magnitude as the gravimetric results. The visual technique would be more practical for high volume quality control procedures.

Observation of postmortem tissues so far studied has revealed no foreign body reaction to the charcoal. Indeed, the length of time between the charcoal infusion and the death of the animal cannot be ascertained by looking at the charcoal in the tissue. Minimal tissue reaction to charcoal has been reported previously (4).

The experiments reported here were done with uncoated coconut shell charcoal. What effects the infusion into the bloodstream of other types of charcoal or the polymer coating used to encapsulate charcoal cannot be answered from these data. Such answers can come only from experiments in which the specific type of charcoal or polymer or combinations thereof are infused into animals. It should be emphasized that the re-circulation system used in this study isolates the test device from particulates generated by pump operation which would have to be considered along with residual particulates in blood tubing and particulates created from needle punctures of the injection ports during an extracorporeal procedure.

The results of the intravenous injection studies have not demonstrated untoward effects over the life span of the test animal. By way of comparison assuming a 50 Kg patient, with a 10 µg/device-hour release rate, some 1000 to 100,000 hours of perfusion would be required to accumulate the particulate load on a per kilogram body weight basis used in these rat studies. Since no signs of toxicity have yet been noticed, a sufficient margin of safety seems to exist for this procedure, even on a repeated basis.

CONCLUSIONS

Particulates are released by the Becton, Dickinson HEMODETOX-IFIER at approximately 7.5 µg/device-hour at a flow rate of 200 ml/min distilled water. These relatively small amounts of material and the apparent lack of toxic response from much larger amounts suggest that particulate release from the HEMODETOXIFIER should not be of significance in the use of this device in an extracorporeal procedure.

ACKNOWLEDGMENT

The authors wish to acknowledge the assistance of J. L. McAdams, S. M. Maret and C. C. Ramaley in this work.

REFERENCES

1. Hill, J. B.; F. L. Palaia; J. L. McAdams; P. J. Palmer;
    J. T. Skinner; and S. M. Maret, The Rationale for Fixed-
    Bed Charcoal in Hemoperfusion, Kidney International 10
    (1976), S-328.

2. Temple, A. R.; J. Walker; and G. A. Done, "A Comparative
    Evaluation of Activated Charcoal Hemoperfusion Devices,"
    presented at a joint meeting of the American Academy of
    Clinical Toxicology, The American Association of Poison
    Control Centers and the Canadian Academy of Clinical
    Toxicology, Seattle, Washington, 5 August 1976.

3. Van Wagenen, R.; D. L. Coleman; and J. D. Andrade, Adsorbent
    Hemoperfusion: Non-biological Particulate Matter, Kidney
    International 7 (1975), S-397.

4. Hagstam, K. E.; L. E. Larsson; and H. Thysell, Experimental
    Studies on Charcoal Haemoperfusion in Phenobarbital
    Intoxication and Uraemia, Including Histopathologic
    Findings, Acta Medica Scandinavica 180 (1966), p. 593.

FIXED-BED CHARCOAL HEMOPERFUSION IN THE TREATMENT OF DRUG OVERDOSE AND CHRONIC RENAL FAILURE

Benjamin H. Barbour, M.D.

White Memorial Medical Center and University of Southern

California, Los Angeles, California

INTRODUCTION

The fixed bed charcoal hemoperfusion system has now been applied extensively in animals and humans for evaluation of safety and efficacy in a variety of disorders.[1,2] It is clearly appropriate that all of the methods which have been applied to treating intoxication by hemoperfusion be considered together although it is doubtful that an agreement will be reached on the superiority of one technique over any other at this time. The classic loose-bed arrangement of clean charcoal packed loosely in a column with blood perculating through its matrix was initially evaluated by Yatzidis and it was found to have some intolerable side effects, particularly on formed blood elements.[3] Furthermore, charcoal particulate emboli was a definite threat to the safty of such a device. Chang in his pioneering studies of the artifical cell attempted to overcome both problems of emboli as well as the platelet depression by placing a thin coat over the charcoal.[4] A still unsettled issue using Chang's approach is the probability that the coat will decrease charcoal's absorability and therefore its efficiency, partially offseting the advantage of charcoal as a therapeutic agent to remove noxious substances. Hill devised an arrangement of the charcoal being glued to a plastic sheet and rolled in a coil, thus minimizing the possibility of charcoal emboli while retaining its native uncoated absorbing qualities.[1] In the preceding paper Hill describes some aspects of this system. The contents of this paper describes solely the author's experience using the fixed-bed approach designed by Hill.

METHODS AND MATERIALS

The initial evaluation of the fixed-bed approach was designed out of skeptism that charcoal glued to a surface would not give up embolic particles and that other side effects might just as well arise from charcoal fixed to a sheet of plastic as a loose bed packed in a column. Consequently, the original studies were done in dogs.

Five dogs were operated on to have an arterial-venous shunt established from the internal carotid to the external jugular vein so that each could be studied over a two- to eight-week period. The shunt is placed across the dorsal of the neck so the animal cannot use his paws to traumatize it. The dogs were kept alive for as long as eight weeks following charcoal hemoperfusion and they all appeared generally healthy. Evidence that renal function, liver function, pulmonary and cardiac functions were impared was sought after but no significant changes could be ascertained. Prior to the use of the device a rinse test was performed and effluent solution was passed through 0.8 mm filters. The filters were examined under 30 power optical magnification and compared to filters with known weights of charcoal. It was estimated that less than five micrograms of particular matter might be infussed per hour during fixed-bed charcoal hemoperfusion. Data accumulated by Dr. Hill indicated that the LD 50 in rats was somewhere between 40 and 100 mg per kilo, so the possible delivery of only 5 micrograms helped to delay a great deal of anxiety about significant charcoal microemboli.[5] The dogs were all killed and the tissue examined. No evidence of charcoal microemboli was seen in the lungs, heart, liver, kidney, spleen or sketetal muscle. The platelet counts fell rapidly during hemoperfusion in all animals, but none of the animals showed evidence of bleeding and they had no evidence of leukopenia.

PATIENT MATERIAL

In August, 1974, all of the dog data had been accumulated and it was decided that if a patient who was in a life-threatening situation from drug overdose appeared, it would be an acceptable risk to try charcoal hemoperfusion as a means of eliminating the offending drug. Furthermore, it was known that when dogs given 175 grams a kilo of phenobarbital were treated by charcoal hemoperfusion and compared to an untreated perfused group through an empty extracoporeal circuit, 13% of the dogs died whereas all of the dogs died that were untreated.[1]

The first patient treated was an 18 year-old girl who had ingested 7 grams of phenobarbital. It was striking that within 3 hours of beginning treatment she was responsive to her name and attempted to answer questions. The patient is still alive and well, having no physical abnormalities at the date of this publication.

Since the first patient was treated, over 70 patients have under-gone therapy for a variety of drug intoxications. There has been a rather consistent decrease in paltelet count when the fixed-bed device is used. In Figure la the changes in the platelet count are shown. The parentheses enclose the number of patients. Figure lb shows an insignificant difference in platelet count across the device. All patients underwent perfusion for 3 hours and had an average fall in platelet count of approximately 30 percent. If the platelet count was followed for several days, it usually required longer than 48 hours to return to normal. There may be a further decrease in plate-let count after perfusion is discontinued and this finding, in addi-to the lack of a difference in platelet count across the device, has led to the speculation that the cause for the low platelet count is probably destruction within the body. Perhaps hemoperfusion damages platelets so that their life span is shortened. Bone marrow examina-tion on a few patients shows no abnormalities or megakaryocytes. Another finding is a decrease in the hematocrit after hemoperfusion. This has been attributed to a combination of blood loss due to blood testing and hemodilution during therapy although the amount of fluid administered was invariably less than one liter. No signs of hemo-dialysis were seen in any of the treatments.

The question remains as to the value of charcoal hemoperfusion as a means of drug overdose therapy when other conservative measures

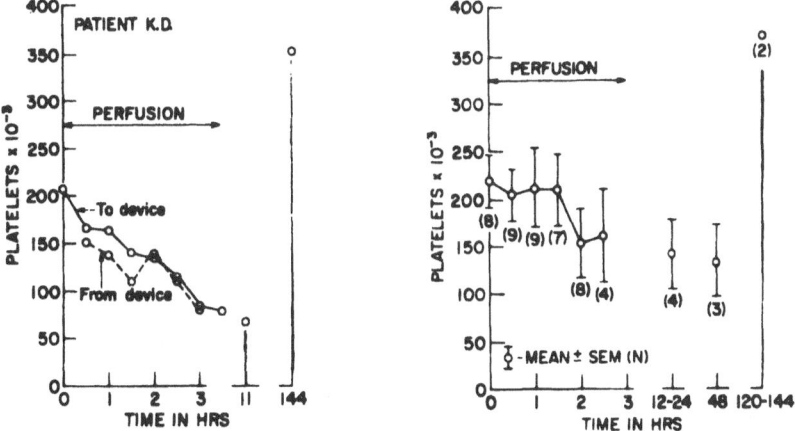

FIG. la & b. Platelet changes after fixed-bed charcoal hemoperfusion.

are considered as alternatives. The same question arises in the consideration of hemodialysis as therapy for drug overdose cases and the
questions are difficult if not impossible to answer. Many will point
to the very low mortality found in barbituate intoxication if the
patients are simply given good nursing care.[6] There is currently no
objective evidence available that would support the merits of one
approach over the other. The evidence gained clinically from the use
of charcoal hemoperfusion with a fixed bed of charcoal is that it
shortens the coma period at the risk of thrombocytopenia and perhaps
anemia.

In order to further evaluate the problem of relative efficacy, a
group of patients intoxicated with barbituates were accumulated and
their outcome was examined. The findings are shown in Table I. The
amount of heparin used was about equal, considerably less IV fluid

TABLE I

	Phenobarbital Intoxication	
	Hemodialysis (N = 7)	Hemoperfusion (N = 6)
Treatment Hours	4.7	2.7
Blood Level % Drop	36%	46%
mg/100 ml/hr Drop	1.33	3.25
Coma Level Change	3.0 - 1.8	2.8 - 1.0
Days between Admission to Treatment	1.5	1.1
Hospital Days	10.9	10.7
I.C.U. Days	6.2	5.5
Days of Intubation	5.3	2.8
Incidence of Tracheotomy	36%	33%
Incidence of Pneumonia	73%	44%
Mortality	18%	0

was administered and blood pressure appeared more stable in the group treated by hemoperfusion. The number of hours of treatment was less, the percent drop in blood level was greater and the coma changed quicker in the hemoperfusion group. If one looks at other parameters such as the number of hours intubated, the incidence of pneumonia and the mortality rate, the differences were not statistically significant but the number of cases was small. The changes in the blood components seen between the two groups are generally in the same direction; however, the platelets were not measured in the hemodialysis group.

There is no doubt that charcoal hemoperfusion is technically easier than hemodialysis. Hemoperfusion shortens coma level but is associated with a drop in platelet count. The data still does not answer the question as to the importance of hemoperfusion in the overall management of drug intoxication and once again there are no objective data to establish an unasailable position on this question. The clinical impression is gained that in a deeply comatose patient with high barbituate blood level, charcoal hemoperfusion using a fixed-bed device is of value and is clearly superior to hemodialysis.

OTHER DRUGS

A variety of other drug intoxications with measurable blood levels have been treated but far fewer cases have been accumulated. However, there is a consistent fall in the barbituate blood levels following the use of charcoal hemoperfusion in all cases of barbituate intoxication treated thus far, both short and long acting. In addition, salicylate and glutethimide blood levels are reduced by hemoperfusion. It is impossible to reach a conclusion regarding the overall value of hemoperfusion in the treatment of intoxication with these other drugs but it clearly lowers their blood concentration.

OTHER APPLICATIONS

Another obvious potential of charcoal hemoperfusion is in uremia. Once again, although there have been several reports of the use of charcoal hemoperfusion to treat uremia, there is no body of data to support its importance. Hemoperfusion in a fixed-bed device has been used in these patients for variable periods of time. Each patient had chronic renal failure and required maintainence hemodialysis to sustain life. A total of 34 treatments were administered in conjunction with dialysis for 4 hours each treatment. The major problem encountered was a fall in arterial pressure and a fall in platelet count. The platelet count fell approximately 30 percent but was back to the prior level by the next dialysis treatment. Arterial pressure fell during hemoperfusion in 33% of the cases. The cause of the fall in arterial pressures was not clear but may be related to the removal of circulating catecholamines.

The charcoal cartridge is placed after the dialyzer and the values of commonly measured metabolites are shown in Table II. The prevalues are from blood samples taken from patients while the PD and PC values are from simultaneously obtained blood samples taken from the venous side of the dialyzer and the charcoal, respectively. The lack of the removal of urea by charcoal is well known. Uric acid and creatinine are removed by the device and it is continuously removed up to 4 hours. Although charcoal is known to absorb glucose, this has not been a clinical problem.

The present status of charcoal hemoperfusion as a means of treating renal failure remains unclear. Ultrafiltration is obviously a problem when one considers charcoal alone. The need to remove urea could be a problem as well as the need to remove potassium and phosphorus. A combination of charcoal and dialysis as proposed by Chang could provide an alternative approach to uremia.[7] The major problems when charcoal and dialysis were used together were a frequent drop in arterial blood pressure. This device is associated with platelet loss and the clinical significance of this in chronic renal failure is unclear. Further evaluation is clearly indicated.

CONCLUSION

Charcoal hemoperfusion using a fixed-bed device is a reasonably safe method to treat drug overdose patients. It decreases coma time more rapidly than hemodialysis in phenobarbital intoxication. Other barbituates and miscellaneous drugs with a measurable blood level are removed from the blood by charcoal hemoperfusion. A drop in

TABLE II

	DIALYSIS THEN CHARCOAL		
	PRE	P_D	P_C
BUN	89	32	33
Cr	7.2	3.0	0.8
K	6.1	3.5	3.3
Ca	7.5	8.2	7.2
P	6.3	3.8	3.8
Uric Ac	4.8	2.7	0.8

platelet count of approximately 30 percent consistently occurs but has not posed a clinical problem. The fixed-bed device has been used to treat uremia but its role is not yet defined. Hypotension and thrombocytomia were seen when used in patients with chronic renal failure.

REFERENCES

1. Hill, J. B., Palaia, F. L., McAdams, J. L., Palmer, P. J., and Maret, S. M.: Etticacy of Activated Charcoal Hemoperfusion in Removing Lethal Doses of Barbiturates and Salicylates from the Blood of Rats and Dogs. Clinical Chemistry 22:754-760, 1976.

2. Barbour, B. H., LaSette, A. M., Koffler, A.: Fixed-bed Charcoal Hemoperfusion for the Treatment of Drug Overdose. Kidney International 10:S333-337, 1976.

3. Yatzidis, H., Oreopoulos, D., Triantaphylidis, D., Voudiclari, S., Tsaparas, N., Gavras, C., Stravroulaki, A.: Treatment of Severe Barbiturate Poisoning. Lancet 2:216-217, 1965.

4. Chang, T. M. S.: Artificial Cells. Springfield, ILL., Charles C. Thomas, 1972, p. 207.

5. Hill, J. B.: Unpublished Observations.

6. Matthew, H. and Lawson, A. A. H.: Treatment of Common Acute Poisonings. New York, Churchill Livingston, 1975, p. 202.

7. Chang, T. M. S., Gonda, A., Dirks, J. H., and Malave, N.: Clinical Evaluation of Chronic Intermittent and Short Term Hemoperfusion in Patients with Chronic Renal Failure using Semipermeable Microcapsules (artifical cells) formed from Membrane Coated Activated Charcoal. Trans. Amer. Society for Artifical Internal Organs 17:246-252, 1971.

EXPERIENCE WITH RESIN HEMOPERFUSION

Jerry L. Rosenbaum, M.D.

Albert Einstein Medical Center, Northern Division

York and Tabor Roads, Philadelphia, Pennsylvania 19141

In 1948 Muirhead and Reid introduced the concept of a "resin artificial kidney" using anion (Deacidite) and cation (Amberlite IR-100H) exchange resins to remove urea from the blood of uremic dogs by hemoperfusion (1). The resin capacity for urea and creatinine was quite limited and more effective adsorptive spectra are offered by charcoal adsorbents for uremic retention products.

More recently, the technique of hemoperfusion through uncoated resin columns has been applied clinically to patients with life-threatening, acute drug overdose. Amberlite XAD-2 is an uncoated and uncharged macroreticular, styrene, divinylbenzene copolymer with particular adsorptive attraction for lipid-soluble molecules. In 1970, hemoperfusion with a column containing 312 Gms (dry weight) of Amberlite XAD-2 resin was shown to be more effective than hemodialysis by treating 5 patients with drug overdose using the two systems in parallel (2). During treatment the intoxicated patients had a dramatic improvement in the depth of their coma and became responsive to verbal command within a few hours. There was an average reduction in circulating platelet concentration of 40% with no evidence of clinical toxicity. Further studies with Amberlite XAD-2 column hemoperfusion in patients with profound overdose continued to demonstrate dramatic lessening of coma time and improvement in vital functions in patients intoxicated with overdoses of glutethimide, ethchlorvynol, methaqualone and a variety of barbiturates (3).

Amberlite XAD-4 is chemically identical to XAD-2 but differs in physical properties with a larger surface area of 750 M^2/Gm compared to 330 M^2/Gm. This difference in adsorptive capacity was measured in-vitro by circulating a dialysate solution containing

217

approximately 20 mg/dl of phenobarbital through 312 Gm resin
columns of Amberlite XAD-2 and XAD-4 in parallel (4). The Amberlite
XAD-4 column removed over 13 Gms of phenobarbital and the clearance rate was still over 150 ml/min after 6 hours of perfusion.
The result of hemoperfusion with the 312 Gm Amberlite XAD-4 column
was reported initially in 8 patients with severe intoxication with
a variety of drugs including glutethimide and various barbiturates
(5). Hemoperfusion extended from 2½ to 10 hours with a blood flow
rate of 300 ml/min. No clinical toxicity was noted. The average
platelet concentration decreased by 50% during the procedure and
returned to 80% of the pre-perfusion levels 18 hours later. Seven
of the 8 patients had an immediate dramatic clinical response usually with spontaneous stabilization of the blood pressure and the
respiratory rate by 30 to 45 minutes, response to painful stimuli
within 45 minutes and response to verbal command by the end of
hemoperfusion. All of the patients had a complete clinical recovery. Two patients with glutethimide intoxication had a modest
clinical rebound after hemoperfusion, but not enough to require
repeat therapy. Another patient ingested 75 Gms of glutethimide
then received 3 daily hemoperfusions for 9, 10 and 8 hours respectively. She recovered after the columns removed over 30 Gms of
drug. The column drug clearance from the blood ranged from 222 to
300 ml/min in the 5 patients with glutethimide intoxication and
from 207 to 300 ml/min in the 3 patients with barbiturate intoxication. It was common for the column clearance of drug to equal or
closely approximate the blood flow rate. Moreover, there was no
evidence of saturation of the column in any of the procedures.

    Occasional patients demonstrated persistent coma for several
days following effective removal of the intoxicant drug by hemoperfusion with either the Amberlite XAD-2 or the Amberlite XAD-4
column (3,5). However, the coma was followed by complete clinical
recovery within a few days. It appears that rapid removal of glutethimide and barbiturates by hemoperfusion allows the identification of the more common rapid responder in whom the coma is likely
due to the drug excess itself, and a less common slow responder in
whom associated ischemia or drug toxicity to the central nervous
system may be important contributing factors to the coma. Release
of resin particles from the Amberlite XAD-4 column into the systemic circulation may be effectively controlled by inserting a
loosely packed dacron-wool filter into the column outflow blood
line (6).

    Hemoperfusion and hemodialysis clearance data generally are
assumed to represent whole blood passing through the column or
dialyzer although the drug concentrations are usually calculated
from plasma. However, the plasma may not necessarily reflect erythrocyte concentration of a solute being rapidly removed by an artificial device (7). Drug concentrations in both the plasma and
erythrocyte compartments were determined in 5 patients with acute

drug intoxication treated with the Amberlite XAD-4 resin hemoperfusion column (6,8). Three patients with glutethimide intoxication
had a higher concentration of drug in the erythrocyte compartment,
whereas 2 patients with barbiturate concentration had a considerably higher concentration of drug in the plasma compartment of the
column inflow blood samples. All 5 patients had a marked reduction in both the erythrocyte and plasma concentrations of the drugs
in the outflow blood samples. Due to these variations in blood
compartments for different drugs, it is advisable to determine
either whole blood or separate erythrocyte and plasma compartment
concentrations for precise calculations of column removal rates of
drugs during hemoperfusion.

    Clinical hemoperfusion with the Amberlite XAD-4 resin column
has consistently demonstrated exceptionally high clearance rates
for barbiturates, glutethimide, ethchlorvynol, methaqualone and
tricyclic antidepressant drugs (5,6,8,9,10). The clearance data
during hemoperfusion with the Amberlite XAD-4 resin column are
represented for 13 previously reported patients with glutethimide
or barbiturate overdose in Figure #1 (5,6,8). The blood flow rates
through the column were 300 ml/min. In 8 patients the clearances
were calculated from whole blood flow rates and plasma drug concentrations (5). This may introduce a small error with overestimation

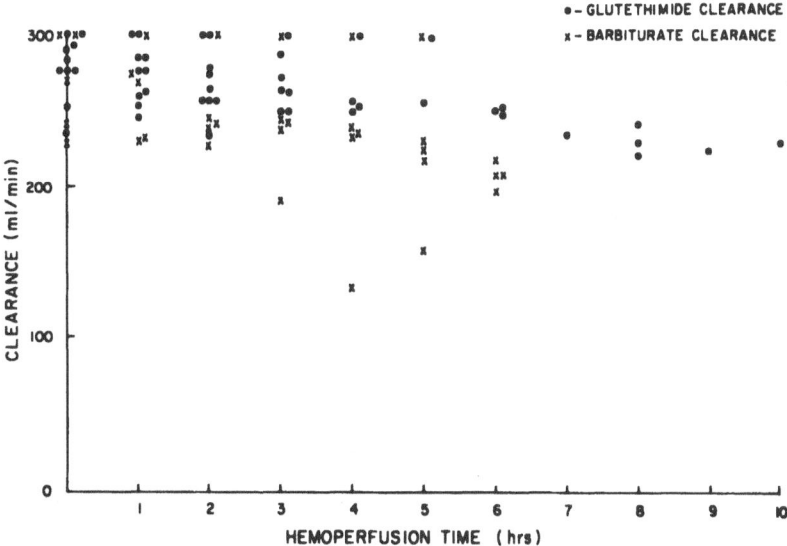

Figure #1: Blood clearance rates during 15 hemoperfusions in 13
patients with glutethimide or barbiturate overdose using a 312 Gm
column of Amberlite XAD-4 resin. The barbiturate overdoses include 1 phenobarbital, 1 pentobarbital, 1 secobarbital and 2 combined pentobarbital-amobarbital.

of barbiturate and underestimation of glutethimide clearance (6).
Amberlite hemoperfusion has resulted in dramatic clinical responses
with no appreciable clinical toxicity. The resin does not require
any protective coating, thereby allowing a highly effective adsorptive surface that usually surpasses the coated carbons for many
of the common drug intoxicants. Since hemoperfusion with various
adsorbent columns markedly shortens coma time with improvement of
hypotension and respiratory depression, we should anticipate that
it will result in a reduction in morbidity and mortality for patients with severe, life-threatening drug intoxication.

In contrast to its high efficiency for the treatment of acute
drug intoxication, uncoated Amberlite XAD-4 resin is not effective
in adsorbing the retention products commonly associated with renal
failure. Activated charcoal does offer such an adsorptive spectrum
but requires a protective semipermeable coating to reduce platelet
adsorption and to reduce embolization of charcoal particles into

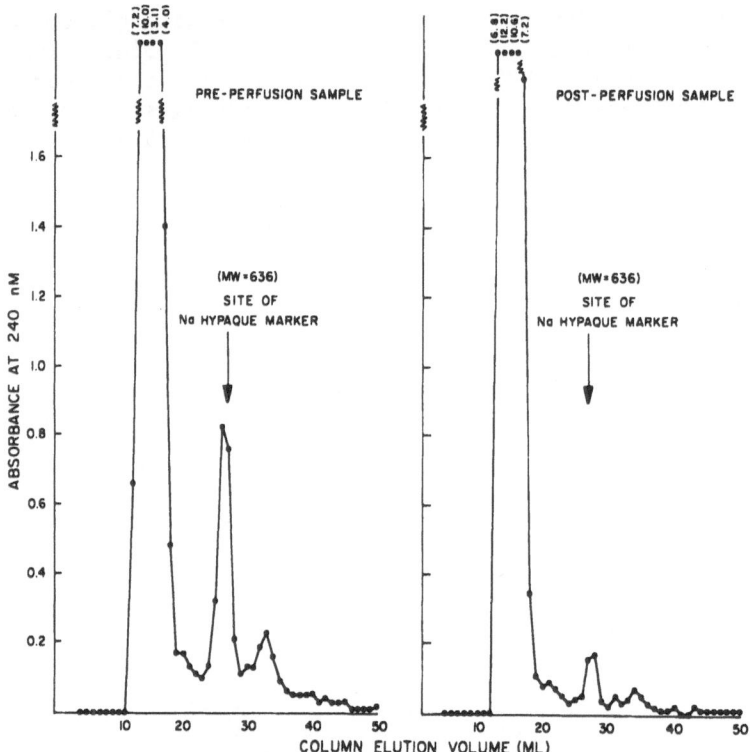

Figure #2: Chromatograms obtained by gel filtration chromatography
using a 160 Gm column of Sephadex G-15 (particle size 40 to 120
microns). The column inflow and outflow blood samples were obtained
simultaneously after ½ hour of hemoperfusion with a 400 Gm Amberlite XE-336 column at a blood flow rate of 300 ml/min in a uremic
dog.

the systemic circulation (11). The feasibility of charcoal coating
and its application to the treatment of drug and uremic intoxication has been introduced by Chang (12,13). Recently, a new synthetic and uncoated resin, Amberlite XE-336[1], has been developed
with a broad adsorptive spectrum similar to charcoal. The adsorbent is an uncharged, uncoated macroreticular polystyrene resin
which is pyrolized to form a carbonaceous surface. The resin beads
are 20 to 50 mesh in diameter with a pore size of 100 Angstroms
and a surface area of 400 to 500 M^2/Gm.

Five normal (Group I) and five uremic (Group II) dogs with
bilateral ureteral ligations 3 days prior to study were
hemoperfused for 6 hours with a 400 Gm column of Amberlite XE-336
resin[2]. The blood flow rate was 300 ml/min. The column was
primed with 350 ml and the blood lines with 150 ml of 6% dextran in
isotonic saline containing 1,500 units of heparin. The blood was
circulated from the femoral artery back to the femoral vein using
a Sarns roller pump. Exogenous clearances were performed for
bromsulphalein (BSP) in Group I and for inulin in Group II. The
plasma middle molecules were measured by gel filtration through a
Sephadex G-15 column. The concentration of the first and major
peak, primarily consisting of large molecular proteins, was not
appreciably affected by hemoperfusion. Therefore, the second peak,
consisting of middle molecules, was quantitated as a percent of the
first peak (Figure 2). During hemoperfusion both the normal and
uremic dogs had transient hypotension, hypocalcemia, leukopenia
and thrombocytopenia. After one hour of hemoperfusion the platelet
concentration maximally decreased from 180,000±61,000 to 60,000±
18,000/ml in Group I and from 198,000±79,000 to 67,000±30,000/ml
in Group II. It was unlikely that resin emboli had any physiologic
significance in this study. Two of the uremic dogs in Group II
had a dacron-wool filter inserted in the outflow line without any
change in the pattern of response to hemoperfusion. In-vitro
analysis was performed on three 200 Gm Amberlite XE-336 resin
columns with a dacron-wool filter inserted in the outflow line.
They were perfused with isotonic saline for 6 hours at a flow rate
of 300 ml/min through a 0.22 micron milipore filter. There was
minimal release of particulate matter. The total mean particulate
count for the three columns was 9 particles over 75 microns, 18
particles from 50 to 75 microns, 165 particles from 25 to 49 microns and 1,500 particles from 5 to 24 microns in diameter[3]. In the
uremic dogs the plasma clearance of creatinine was initially quite
high then decreased almost linearly during hemoperfusion from 273,

---

[1] Supplied by Rohm and Haas Chemical Company, Philadelphia, PA.,
    U.S.A.
[2] Prepared through the courtesy of Extracorporeal Medical Special-
    ties, King of Prussia, PA., U.S.A.
[3] Studies performed at the Quality Control Laboratories Division,
    Industrial Highway, South Hampton, PA., 18966, U.S.A.

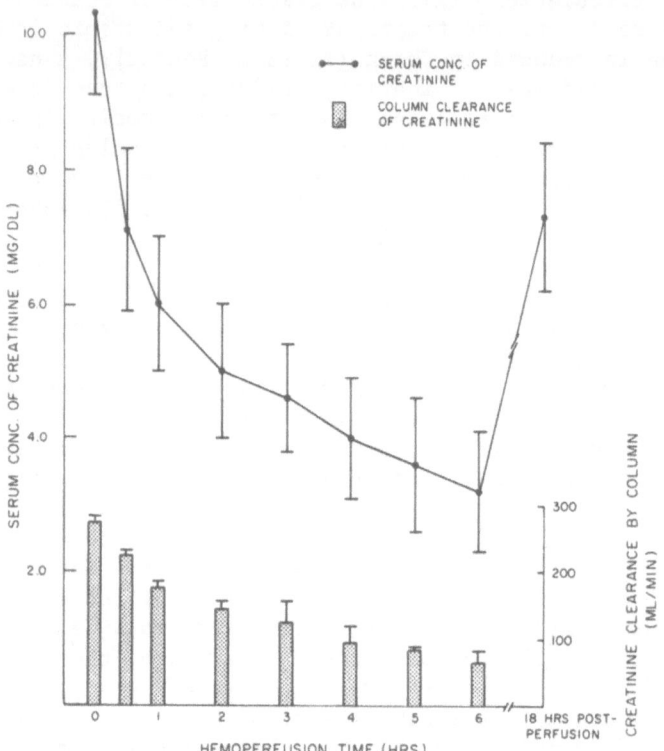

Figure #3: The effect on plasma creatinine concentration of hemoperfusion with a 400 Gm Amberlite XE-336 resin column at a blood
flow rate of 300 ml/min in 5 uremic dogs. Plasma clearances of
creatinine by the column are also recorded. The data represent
the mean ±1 SD.

±10 to 64±17 ml/min. The plasma creatinine concentration decreased
from 10.4±1.3 to 3.2±0.9 mg/dl (Figure 3). In Group I the BSP
clearance ranged from 53±14 to 107±34 ml/min; in Group II the inulin
clearance ranged from 42±25 to 13±36 ml/min. After ½ hour of hemoperfusion the mean column clearance of middle molecules in the
uremic dogs was 241±18 ml/min. In one of the uremic dogs serial
middle molecule clearances were recorded during the 6 hour hemoperfusion (Figure 4). The plasma concentration of the middle
molecules (percent of the area of the middle molecular weight peak
to the area of the large molecular weight peak) ranged from 10.2
to 4.1%.

Since Amberlite XE-336 is uncoated, there is no inhibition of

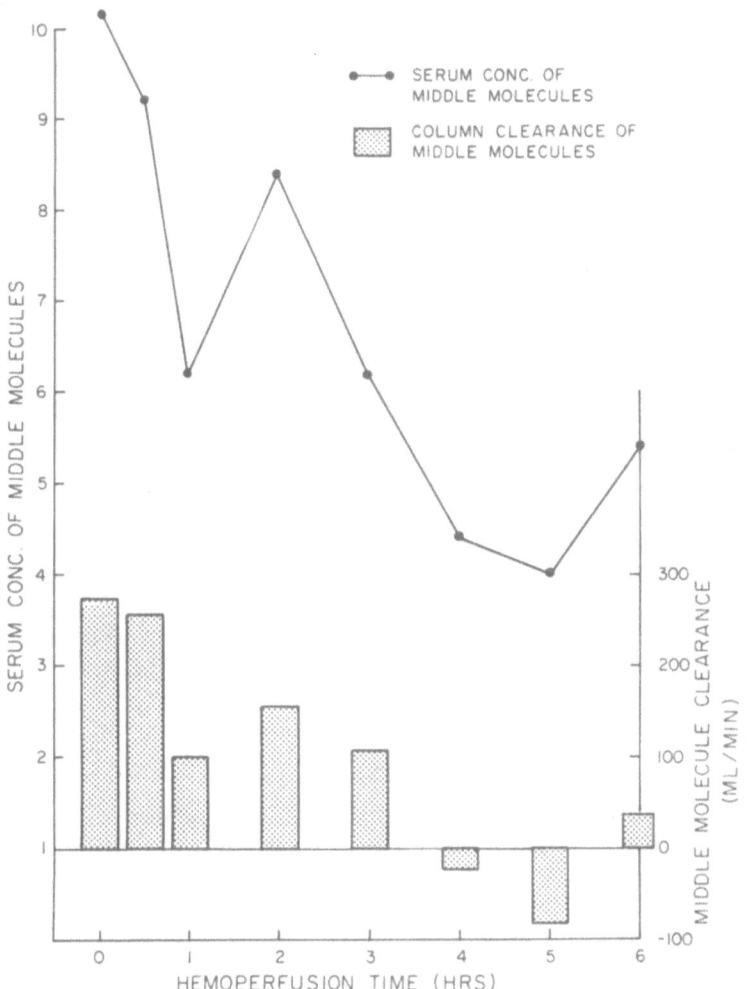

Figure #4: The effect of hemoperfusion with a 400 Gm Amberlite
XE-336 resin column at a blood flow rate of 300 ml/min on plasma
middle molecules in a uremic dog 3 days following bilateral ureteral ligation. The plasma concentration of middle molecules was
derived from the ratio of the area of the second or middle molecular weight protein peak to the area of the first or large molecular weight protein peak miltiplied by 100.

adsorption rate as compared to coated activated carbons. This may
explain the high initial clearance rates of middle molecules and
creatinine. If hypotension and adsorption of formed blood elements
can be resolved in uremic man, hemoperfusion through Amberlite

XE-336 should provide an efficient method of clearing many of the small and middle molecules from uremic blood.

REFERENCES

1. Muirhead, E.E., and Reid, A.F.: A resin artificial kidney. J. Lab. Clin. Med. 33:841-844, 1948.
2. Rosenbaum, J.L., Winsten, D., Kramer, M.S., Moros, J., and Raja, R.: Resin hemoperfusion in the treatment of drug intoxication. Trans. Am. Soc. Artif. Int. Organs 16:134-140, 1970.
3. Rosenbaum, J.L., Kramer, M.S., Raja, R., and Boreyko, C.: Resin hemoperfusion : A new treatment for acute drug intoxication. New Eng. J. Med. 284:874-877, 1971.
4. Rosenbaum, J.L.: Resin hemoperfusion in the treatment of acute drug intoxication. I & EC Products Res. and Devel. 14:99-101, 1975.
5. Rosenbaum, J.L., Kramer, M.S., and Raja, R.: Resin hemoperfusion for acute drug intoxication. Arch. Int. Med. 136:263-266, 1976.
6. Rosenbaum, J.L.: Hemoperfusion in the treatment of acute poisoning. Biomedical Engineering Approaches to Artif. Lung, Kidney and Liver, Glasgow. To be published by Messrs. Macmillan, 1976.
7. Nolph, K.D., Bass, O.E., and Maher, J.F.: Acute effects of hemodialysis on removal of intracellular solutes. Trans. Amer. Soc. Artif. Organs 20:622-627, 1974.
8. Rosenbaum, J.L., Kramer, M.S., Raja, R., Winsten, S., and Dalal, F.: Hemoperfusion for acute drug intoxication. Kidney Intern. 10:S341-S342, 1976.
9. Trafford, J.A.P., Jones, R., and Evans, R.: Haemoperfusion with DX-60 hemoperfusion cartridge (Rosenbaum design) in acute poisoning. Abstr. Am. Soc. Artif. Int. Organs 5:81, 1976.
10. Leber, H.W.: Hemoperfusion and hemodialysis in carbromal intoxication. Intern. Cong. of Europ. Assoc. of Poison Control Centers, Oslo, 1976 (In press).
11. Andrade, J.D., Coleman, D.L., Kim, S.W., and Lentz, D.J.: The coating of activated carbons for optimal blood compatibility. Artif. Liver Support, R. Williams and I.M. Murray-Lyon, editors. Pitman Med. Publ. Co. Ltd., London:84-92, 1974.
12. Chang, T.M.S., Johnson, L.J., and Ransome, O.J.: Semipermeable aqueous microcapsules. Canad. J. Physiol. and Pharmacol. 45:705-715, 1967.
13. Chang, T.M.S.: Microencapsulated adsorbent hemoperfusion for uremia, intoxication and hepatic failure. Kid Intern. 7:S387-S392, 1975.

STRATHCLYDE APPROACH TOWARDS ARTIFICIAL KIDNEY, ARTIFICIAL LIVER AND DETOXIFICATION

J.M. Courtney, J.D.S. Gaylor, R. Maini, G.B. Park and E.M. Smith

Bioengineering Unit, University of Strathclyde
106 Rottenrow, Glasgow G4 0NW, U.K.

INTRODUCTION

The Bioengineering Unit at the University of Strathclyde has been engaged in research relating to the use of adsorbents in medicine since 1972. The decision to undertake research in this area was influenced by the work of Chang on artificial cells (Chang, 1972) and a Unit involvement in the development of synthetic polymer membranes for haemodialysis (Courtney, 1969; Muir et al, 1971, 1973). The initial effort concerned activated carbon granules and was directed towards the selection of a suitable grade of carbon, development of a method of coating the granules with polymer and the design of a polymer coating.

The grade of carbon was selected as a result of a joint evaluation programme between the Bioengineering Unit and Norit-Clydesdale Co. Ltd. (Cameron et al, 1974; Walker, 1974). The carbon is a peat-based, extruded material, now designated Norit RBX1, Haemoperfusion Grade. The coating method which was developed (Courtney et al, 1976a) involves rotating the carbon granules in an inclined glass vessel, utilising electrostatic repulsion to minimise contact between the granules during rotation and applying the polymer in the form of a solution in an organic solvent.

With the grade of carbon and the coating procedure established, emphasis has been placed on the preparation and evaluation of suitable polymer coatings. Consideration has also been given to the evaluation of alternative forms of carbon and, in particular, an activated carbon cloth with a high adsorption capacity.

The evaluation of our polymer-coated granules in hepatic support
(Abouna et al, 1975) increased our interest in the artificial liver area.
The current approach (Maini et al, 1977) is that of a system utilising
microporous membranes and sorbents.

The polymer-coated carbon granules have been investigated for the
removal of paracetamol and glutethimide (Edwards, 1975).   However, the
recent effort in the area of detoxification has been to consider the application
of ion exchange resins (Maini, 1975).   This is exemplified by the use of a
cation exchange resin to achieve removal of the herbicide paraquat (Maini
et al, 1976).

ARTIFICIAL KIDNEY

Our selection of polymer coatings was influenced by a previous evaluation of haemodialysis membranes (Courtney, 1969).   This evaluation
demonstrated the advantages of selecting a copolymer system, where one
monomer contributes to copolymer mechanical strength and the other to
copolymer sensitivity or reactivity.   Various copolymer systems have been
considered (Courtney et al, 1976b) but the work has been concentrated on
copolymers of dimethylaminoethyl methacrylate (DMAEMA), a water-soluble
aminoester of methacrylic acid.

The patent literature suggests the application of DMAEMA copolymers in
pharmaceutical coatings (Volker and Wenzel, 1962; Tuji, 1969) and medical
adhesives (Gander, 1967).   Advantage has been taken of the fact that
DMAEMA renders copolymers cationic in procedures for the ionic attachment
of the anticoagulant heparin (Falb et al, 1966; Idezuki et al, 1975;
Courtney et al, 1976c; Lindsay et al, 1976).

Our original choice of comonomer for DMAEMA was acrylonitrile (AN)
and AN-DMAEMA coated granules have been evaluated for solute removal
and blood compatibility (Edwards, 1975; Gilchrist et al, 1975; Winchester,
1977).   While interest in the AN-DMAEMA copolymer system has been maintained, our preferred choice of comonomer for DMAEMA is, at present,
methyl methacrylate.   Polymers of methyl methacrylate have been widely
used as bone cements (Charnley, 1970).   Copolymers of MMA have been
proposed for coating both organic and inorganic substances generally (Gusman,
1960) and for coating medicaments (Utsumi et al, 1963).

MMA-DMAEMA copolymers are produced by solution or emulsion polymerisation.   Solution polymerisation is carried out in acetone and the
emulsion polymerisation procedure makes use of the nonionic surfactant

Pluronic F68 (Courtney et al, 1977a).   In a blood compatibility assessment
based on modified recalcification times, both the solution and emulsion
copolymers demonstrated enhanced compatibility following contact with
heparin (Courtney et al, 1977b).

The carbon granules are coated by the Rotacoat procedure of Hood
(Courtney et al, 1976) using solutions of the MMA-DMAEMA copolymers
in acetone/ethanol.   The coated granules have been assessed for solute
removal by passing creatinine solution, concentration 20mg/100ml, from a
reservoir at 37°C, through a column containing 130g of granules.   The
solution flow rate was 200ml/min.

Figure 1 shows the relationship between creatinine clearance after 60 min
and DMAEMA content in the copolymer for various solution and emulsion
copolymers.   In each case, the coating weight was 1%.   The general trend
is that creatinine clearance increases with increasing DMAEMA level for
both solution and emulsion polymerisation.   The extent to which the DMAEMA
content can be increased is limited by the need to maintain a satisfactory
balance between copolymer strength and copolymer sensitivity.   On the
basis of the clearance results, the blood compatibility assessment (Courtney
et al, 1977b) and animal studies (Park et al, 1977), we have chosen a
particular copolymer.

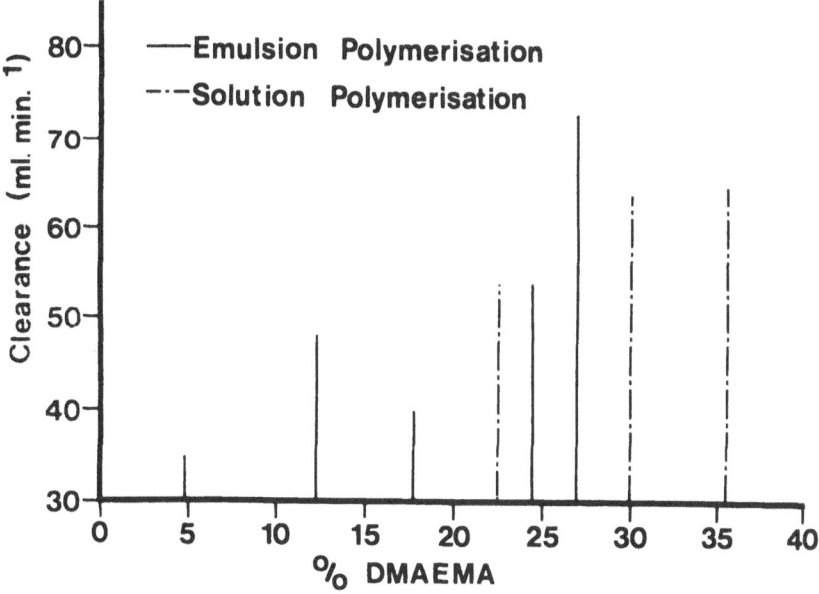

Figure 1:-   MMA-DMAEMA coated carbon granules, coating weight of 1%:
creatinine cleara ice after 60 min against DMAEMA content.

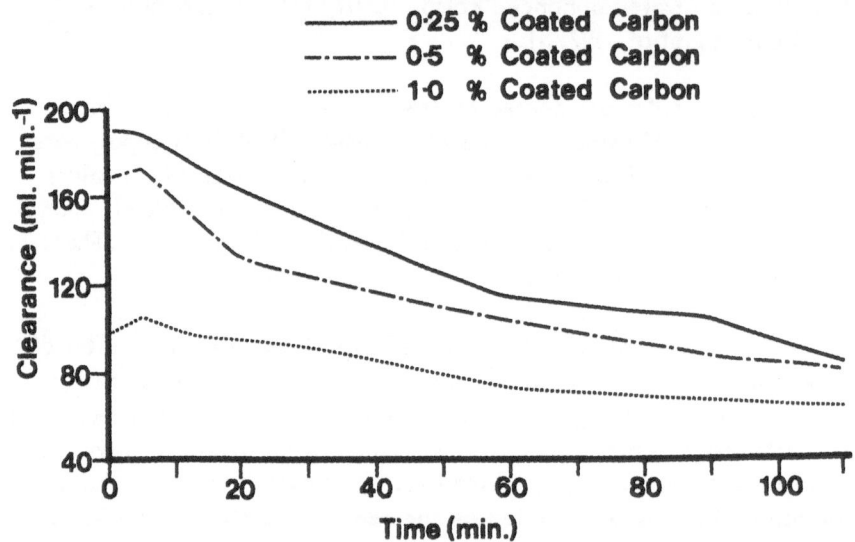

Figure 2:- MMA-DMAEMA coated carbon granules: creatinine clearance
against time for coating weights of 0.25, 0.5 and 1.0%.

This copolymer is prepared by emulsion polymerisation from a
monomer weight ratio MMA:DMAEMA of 50:50.   This corresponds to a
DMAEMA level in the copolymer of about 27%.

Plots of creatinine clearance against time for 3 different coating weights
of the preferred copolymer are shown in Figure 2.   As expected, the best
solute removal is obtained with the lowest coating weight.   Our approach
(Courtney et al, 1977a) is that of applying the minimum amount of polymer
commensurate with achieving satisfactory levels of blood compatibility and
fine carbon particle generation.   We have, therefore, selected a coating
weight of MMA-DMAEMA copolymer of 0.25%.

An alternative to the use of activated carbon granules is solute removal
by passage over activated carbon in fibre or cloth form.   Our interest lies
in a particular carbon cloth (Bailey et al, 1973), which is produced from a
rayon precursor.   The performance of this cloth has been compared with that
of the Norit RBX1 granules (Gaylor et al, 1976).   Results obtained from
batch stirring tests are demonstrated in Figure 3.   These tests involved the use
or 2g carbon in 300 ml creatinine solution, initial concentration 10mg/100 ml,
and were carried out at 37° C.

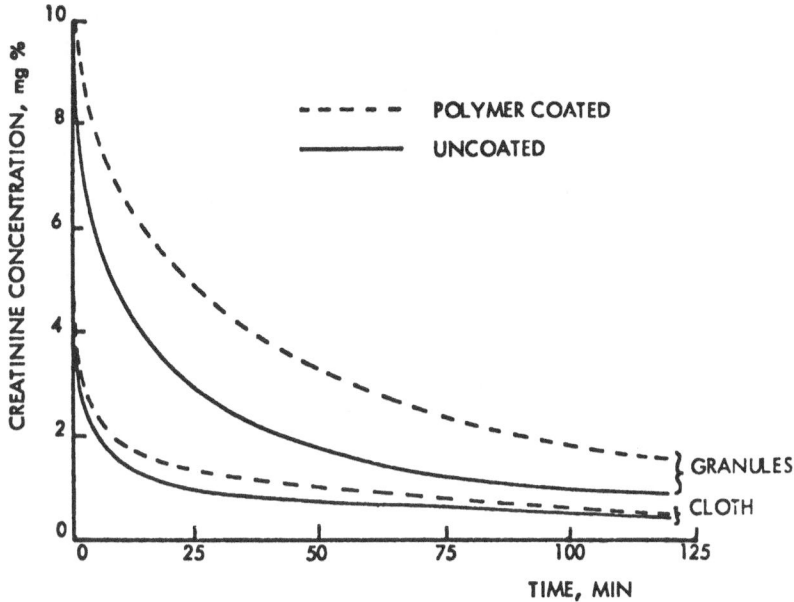

Figure 3: – Comparison between carbon cloth and Norit RBX1 carbon granules: creatinine removal for materials uncoated and coated with 0.25% by weight MMA–DMAEMA copolymer.

The carbon cloth and the Norit RBX1 granules were evaluated uncoated and coated with 0.25% by weight of MMA–DMAEMA copolymer. Figure 3 indicates the superiority of the cloth in both the uncoated and coated states.

It is our view (Hood et al, 1975) that the carbon cloth offers potential advantages in solute removal and in device preparation. It could prove particularly useful in the design of devices incorporating adsorption and membrane separation processes such as dialysis and ultrafiltration. Preliminary animal studies have been conducted and emphasis is now being placed on the preparation of fabric precursors which will ensure the best cloth geometry after carbonisation.

ARTIFICIAL LIVER

It is believed (Maini et al, 1977) that a system suitable for artificial liver support should be capable of removing a wide range of substances, both free and protein bound. The system should also have the ability to operate for long periods. The Strathclyde approach is based on a haemodialyser containing microporous membranes, permeable to serum proteins but impermeable to cellular blood components.   Dialysate composed of banked plasma is recirculated in a closed loop through a mixture of sorbents. Toxins of small and middle molecular weight diffuse rapidly across the membrane. The transport of high molecular weight, protein bound toxins is increased by convective flux provided by ultrafiltration.   The toxins are removed by the sorbents and the excess ultrafiltered plasma is recombined with the blood circuit.   The proposed system is shown in schematic form in Figure 4.

This system permits the use of large quantities of uncoated sorbent of small particle size.   The proposed sorbents are activated carbon for amino acids, fatty acids, mercaptans and phenols; anion exchange resin for the removal of bilirubin and other protein bound anions; cation exchange resin for the removal of ammonia and uncharged polymeric adsorbents for the removal of bile acids.

Work has been carried out using a Kiil haemodialyser, area 1 m^2, containing 50 μm thick Goretex expanded polytetrafluoroethylene membrane, 1 μm x 0.2 μm pore size.   This has produced a sustained ultrafiltrate flow rate of 40 ml/min for bovine blood in vitro at a blood flow rate of 200 ml/min.

DETOXIFICATION

The poison paraquat is a widely used herbicide, which exists as a cation at normal blood pH.   The Strathclyde approach to the removal of paraquat (Maini et al, 1976) is that of haemoperfusion over a cation exchange resin. The approach is based on the views that the effect of paraquat depends not only on the quantity ingested but also on the rate of removal and that the toxic effects of paraquat appear to result from selective accumulation of the poison from blood into lung tissue over an extended period of time.   The approach aims at achieving the rapid removal of paraquat from blood to a concentration which does not permit accumulation to dangerous levels.

The cation exchange resin used is Zerolit 225 SRC21 (Z225/21) supplied by Permutit Co. Ltd., London.   This resin is a strong acid cation exchanger based upon sulphonated polystyrene – divinylbenzene matrix of high cross-linkage (20% divinylbenzene).

In vivo studies have been conducted with beagle dogs (Maini and Winchester, 1975; Maini et al, 1976).   Paraquat dichloride was administered to 9 dogs.   After 2 h, 3 dogs were treated by haemoperfusion over Z225/21 resin, 3 dogs were treated by haemoperfusion over uncoated Norit RBX1 and 3 dogs remained untreated.

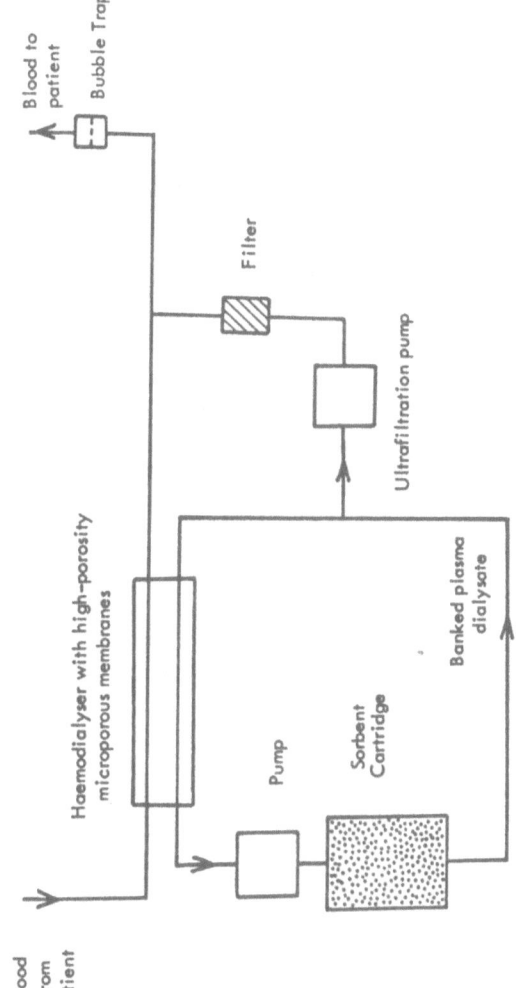

Figure 4: Proposed artificial liver support system utilising microporous membranes and sorbents.

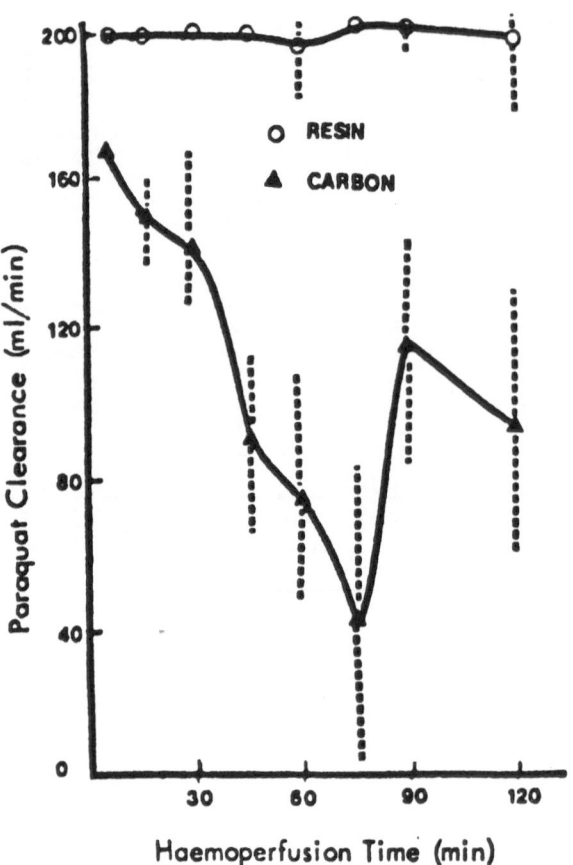

Figure 5:- Paraquat clearances for Z225/2l cation exchange resin and Norit RBX1 carbon granules: means and ranges of 3 experiments.

Figure 5 shows mean calculated clearances with ranges for the resin and carbon.   Clearances remained consistently high for cation exchange resin perfusion but were lower and more variable with perfusion over activated carbon.

An important feature of the use of the cation exchange resin Z225/21 is the pretreatment procedure necessary to minimise the removal of sodium, potassium, calcium and magnesium ions from the blood.   This pretreatment (Maini et al, 1976) consists of a rough equilibration of the resin with a con-centrated electrolyte solution of predetermined concentration in order to rapidly load the resin with cations, followed by fine equilibration with a solution having the same cationic composition as normal plasma.

In cases of paraquat poisoning, it is our view that plasma paraquat con-centrations should be reduced rapidly.   In this respect, haemoperfusion over Zerolit 225 SRC21 cation exchange resin, when used in combination with forced diuresis and the repeated oral administration of a material such as Fuller's earth, should prove advantageous.

ACKNOWLEDGMENTS

We wish to acknowledge the guidance of Professor R. M. Kenedi, Director of the Bioengineering Unit.   We are grateful to Miss J. Bowen for the preparation of illustrations and Mrs. M. Lynch for typing the manuscript.

REFERENCES

Abouna, G.M., Gilchrist, T., Pettit, J.E., Boyd, N.D., Todd, J.K., Courtney, J.M. and Maini, R. (1975) in "Artificial Liver Support", ed. Williams and Murray-Lyon, Pitman Medical, London, p. 180

Bailey, A., Maggs, F.A.P. and Williams, J.H.(1973) British Patent 1, 310, 011

Cameron, A., Courtney, J.M., Gilchrist, T., MacDowall, J. and Walker, J.M. (1974) Proc.Soc. Chem. Ind. 4th London Int.Carbon and Graphite Conf., Pennard Press, London, p. 227

Chang, T.M.S.(1972) "Artificial Cells", Charles C. Thomas, Springfield, Ill.

Charnley, J.(1970) "Acrylic Cement in Orthopaedic Surgery", Livingstone, Edinburgh and London

Courtney, J.M. (1969) Ph.D. Thesis, University of Strathclyde

Courtney, J.M., Gilchrist, T., Hood, R.G. and Townsend, W.B. (1976a)
Proc. ESAO 2, 210

Courtney, J.M., Gilchrist, T. and Dunlop, E.H. (1976b) U.S. Patent 3,983,053

Courtney, J.M., Gilchrist, T., Venn, R.F. and Lindsay, R.M. (1976c) in
"Biocompatibility of Implant Materials", ed. Williams, Pitman Medical,
London p. 183

Courtney, J.M., Fairweather, I.A., Gilchrist, T., Hood, R.G., Park, G.B.
and Smith, E.M. (1977a) in "Artificial Organs", ed. Kenedi et al, Macmillan
Press, London, p. 133

Courtney, J.M., Park, G.B., Smith, E.M., Gerard, S.M. and Winchester,
J.F. (1977b) Polymer surface modification and blood compatibility. Presented
at Polymer Surfaces Symposium, Durham.

Edwards, R.O. (1975) Ph.D. Thesis, University of Strathclyde

Falb, R.D., Grode, G.A., Luttinger, M., Epstein, M.M., Drake, B. and
Leininger, R.I. (1966) U.S. Nat. Tech. Inform. Serv., P.B. Report No. 173,053

Gander, R.J. (1967) U.S. Patent 3, 305, 513

Gaylor, J.D.S., Maggs, F.A.P., Park, G.B. and Smith, E.M. (1976)
Activated carbon cloth – a novel material for haemoperfusion 29th ACEMB 18,171

Gilchrist, T., Jonsson, E., Martin, A.M., Naucler, L., Cameron, A. and
Courtney, J.M. (1975) in "Artificial Liver Support", ed. Williams and Murray-
Lyon, Pitman Medical, London, p. 319

Gusman, S. (1960) U.S. Patent 2, 940, 950

Hood, R.G., Courtney, J.M., Gaylor, J.D.S. and Gilchrist, T. (1975)
Brit. Patent Appln. No. 44502/75

Idezuki, J., Watanabe, H., Hagiwara, M., Kanasugi, K., Mori, Y.,
Nagooka, S., Hagio, M., Yamamoto, K. and Tanzawa, H. (1975) Trans.
Amer. Soc. Artif. Int. Organs 21, 436

Lindsay, R.M., Rourke, J., Reid, B., Friesen, M., Linton, A.L., Courtney
J.M. and Gilchrist, T. (1976) Trans. Amer. Soc. Artif. Int. Organs 22, 292

Maini, R. (1975) Ph.D. Thesis, University of Strathclyde

Maini, R. and Winchester, J.F. (1975) Brit. Med. J. $\underline{3}$, 281

Maini, R., Courtney, J.M., Gilchrist, T., Winchester, J.F. and McKay, J.M. (1976) Proc. ESAO $\underline{2}$, 222

Maini, R., Baillie, H. and Stark, M. (1977) in "Artificial Organs" ed. Kenedi et al, Macmillan Press, London, p. 395

Muir, W.M., Courtney, J.M., Gray, R.A. and Ritchie, P.D. (1971) J. Biomed. Mater. Res. $\underline{5}$, 415

Muir, W.M., Gray, R.A., Courtney, J.M. and Ritchie, P.D. (1973) J. Biomed. Mater. Res. $\underline{7}$, 37

Park, G.B., Apiliga, M.T. and Fairweather, I.A. (1977) IRCS Med. Sci. $\underline{5}$, 140

Tuji, J. (1969) U.S. Patent 3, 477, 864

Utsumi, I., Ida, T., Kishi, S., and Hashimoto, T. (1963) U.S. Patent 3, 073, 748

Volker, T. and Wenzel, F. (1962) U.S. Patent 3, 070, 509

Walker, J.M. (1974) Ph.D. Thesis, University of Strathclyde

Winchester, J.F. (1977) in "Artificial Organs", ed. Kenedi et al, Macmillan Press, London, p. 280

COMMUNICATIONS

ASSESSMENTS OF TWO RAT MODELS OF FULMINANT HEPATIC FAILURE

FOR TESTING ARTIFICIAL LIVER DEVICES

E. Chirito, B. Reiter, C. Lister and T.M.S. Chang

Artificial Organs Research Unit
McIntyre Medical Sciences Building
McGill University
Montreal, Quebec, Canada

INTRODUCTION

Research in the treatment of fulminant hepatic failure is hampered by the lack of a suitable experimental animal model. We have looked into two animal models which can be conveniently used in large numbers for statistical analysis of effects of hemoperfusion on survival. One is carbon tetrachloride induced fulminant hepatic failure (1); another is the galactosamine induced fulminant hepatic failure rat model (2,3,4). These models seem to fulfill many of the requirements such as severe fulminant hepatic failure, reversibility and safety for research personnel. However, these animal models have not yet been used for the assessment of the effectiveness of treatment regimes for fulminant hepatic failure. Hemoperfusion has been used for patients with hepatic coma (5-13). The original finding (5,6) of hemoperfusion resulting in improvements of consciousness in grade 4 hepatic coma patients have now been supported by all centers. However, the effects on hemoperfusion in the improvements of long-term survival is not yet conclusive. For this, studies of a large series including rigid control studies is required. This is not too feasible in acute fulminant hepatic failure because of relatively small numbers of patients and the variations due to etiology, age, grade of coma and other factors. The present report is a feasibility study of assessing the use of these two fulminant hepatic failure rat models - carbon tetrachloride and galactosamine-as possible animal models for assessing the effects of hemoperfusion.

239

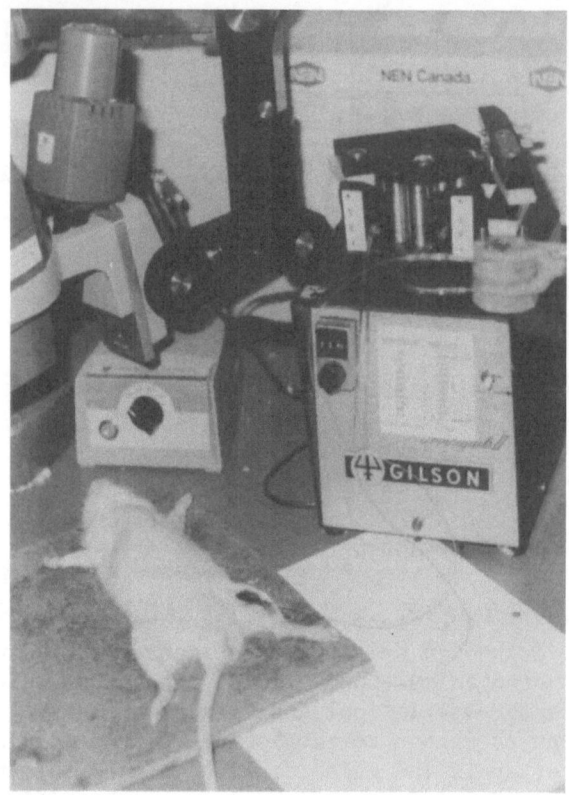

Figure 1
Equipments used in hemoperfusion studies in rat – including stereo
microscope for dissection and cannulation; Gilson Minipuls pump as
blood pump; and hemoperfusion chamber. 0.011 inch internal diameter
polyethylene tubings (Intramedics, #7410, Clay-Adams) were used for
cannulating femoral artery and vein. Each is joined to a 0.023 inch
internal diameter polyethylene tubings (Intramedic, #7410, Clay-
Adams); then to the 0.035 inch internal diameter Technicon auto-
analyser pump tubing in the Gilson Minipuls pump.

MATERIALS AND METHODS

Protocol for Hemoperfusion

In order to establish a suitable protocol for hemoperfusion,
studies were first carried out to establish suitable carbon tetrachloride and galactosamine dosages and techniques of hemoperfusion.
After the suitable treatment model system was established, study
was carried out to assess the use of ACAC hemoperfusion.

Hemoperfusion chamber was constructed as a miniaturized version of that previously described (14,15,16). The chamber was filled with 2 g of albumin cellulose nitrate microencapsulated activated charcoal (ACAC) prepared as previously described (14,15, 16).

Galactosamine Model

In the studies using galactosamine, male Wistar rats weighing from 266 to 302 gm were used. Each animal received an intraperitoneal injection of galactosamine (100 mg/100 gm body weight). Each treatment was carried out 48 hours following the administration of galactosamine. At this time, each rat was anesthetized with subcutaneous pentobarbital (40 mg/Kg body weight). The femoral artery and vein of each rat was cannulated under a stereo-microscope. The reason for choosing 48 hours is that in 3 hours, 20% of injected galactosamine was removed by the liver (4), so that by 48 hours, no galactosamine would be left in the circulation. Furthermore, 48 hours after injection, severe histological changes resembling acute liver necrosis are present (4). Death of the animal usually occurs about 4 days after injection. The rats were divided in 2 groups. 1 group received treatment with ACAC hemoperfusion for 1 hour at a blood flow rate of 1 ml/min. The control group received the same volume of priming solution through the femoral vein but no hemoperfusion was carried out. The priming solution is made up of glucose (10 gm/100 ml), albumin (12.5 gm/100 ml), and heparin (500 unit/100 ml). The total heparin dosage was 120 unit/Kg body weight. At the completion of hemoperfusion, 1.5 mg/Kg body weight of protamine-sulphate was infused. The animals were allowed food and 10% glucose ad. lib. throughout the study.

Carbon Tetrachloride Model

Similar studies were carried out using carbon tetrachloride administered into the duodenum.

RESULTS AND DISCUSSIONS

Carbon Tetrachloride Model

This rat model was found to be unsuitable for assessing the effects of hemoperfusion. The response of the animal to carbon tetrachloride was variable. Furthermore, the effects of carbon tetrachloride were not confined to the liver; varying degrees of pulmonary and renal damage makes it very difficult to accurately assess the effects of hemoperfusion.

Galactosamine

It was found that of the various dosages of galactosamine used, 110 mg/100 gm body weight produced severe fulminant hepatitis with a survival rate of 33%. The age and weight of the animal was found to be extremely important in reproducibility of results. The range of 266 to 302 gm was found to be a suitable range for adequate hepatic regeneration. The heparin dosage used was the minimum which allowed for adequate anticoagulation for hemoperfusion. It was found that these animals have severe clotting deficiencies and unless very low heparin dosages were used there were severe bleeding in the cannulation site, despite the administration of protamine sulphate after hemoperfusion. With proper heparin dosage, studies were successfully carried out. In the control group only 7 out of the total 23 rats recovered (30.4%). In the treated group 15 out of the total 21 rats recovered (71.4%). Death occurred in both cases at 3.0 ± 0.6 days. Those which recovered survived when followed for more than 1 month. The effects on survival of ACAC hemoperfusion as compared to the control was statistically significant to $p < 0.01$. Histological studies showed that the liver damage resembled severe acute liver necrosis. In those rats which survived, the liver regenerated to almost normal in 4 to 6 weeks. More detailed results of this study can be found elsewhere (16).

The present study has shown that the animal model of galactosamine induced fulminant hepatic failure in rats is useful in the experimental assessment of artificial support systems, important factors to be taken into consideration include the age, weight, heparin dosage, galactosamine dosage, blood flow rate, and time of treatment. The advantage of the galactosamine induced fulminant hepatic failure animal model is the severity of the fulminant hepatic failure which can be reversible. Furthermore, a large number of control and test animals can be used for statistical analysis.

REFERENCES

1. Paquet, K.J. and Kamphansen, V. (1975) Acta Hepato-Gastro-buterol, 22, 84-88.
2. Keppler, D., Lesch, R., Reuter, W., Decker, K. (1968) Pathology, 9, 279-290.
3. Decker, K., Keppler, D. (1974) Rev. Physiol. Biochem. Pharmacol., 71, 77-106.
4. Decker, K., Keppler, D. (1974) Progress in Liver Diseases, 4, 183-199.
5. Chang, T.M.S. (1972) Lancet, 2, 1371-1372.
6. Chang, T.M.S., Migchelsen, M. (1973) Trans. Amer. Soc. Artif. Intern. Organs, 19, 314-319.
7. Gazzard, B.G., Weston, M.J., Murray-Lyon, I.M., Flax, H., Record, CO., Portman, B., Langley, P.G., Dunlop, E.H., Mellon,

P.J., Ward, M.D., Williams, R. (1974) Lancet, $\underline{1}$(7870), 1301–1305.

8. Chang, T.M.S. (1976) Kidney Int., $\underline{10}$, S305–S311.
9. Gelfand, M. In this volume.
10. Amano, I., Kano, H., Takahira, H., Yamamoto, Y., Itoh, K., Iwatsuki, S., Maeda, K. and Ohta, K. In this volume.
11. Odaka, M. In this volume.
12. Silk, D.B.A. and William, R. In this volume.
13. Chang, T.M.S. (1969) Can. J. Physiol. Pharmacol., $\underline{47}$, 1043–1045.
14. Chang, T.M.S. (1972) Artificial Cells. Charles C. Thomas, Publisher, Springfield, Illinois, U.S.A.
15. Chang, T.M.S. (1976) Kidney Int., $\underline{10}$, S218–S224.
16. Chirito, E., Reiter, B., Lister, C. and Chang, T.M.S. (1977) Artificial Organs J., $\underline{1}$, 76–83.

USE OF ALBUMIN-CELLULOSE NITRATE MICROENCAPSULATED CHARCOAL

HEMOPERFUSION: IN ACUTE DIGOXIN TOXICITY IN DOGS

S. Prichard**, E. Chirito*, A. Sniderman**, and
T.M.S. Chang*

Artificial Organs Research Unit* and Cardiovascular
Research Unit**
McGill University and Royal Victoria Hospital
687 Pine Avenue, Montreal, Quebec, Canada

The incidence of digoxin toxicity remains high (1). The
recognition of the role of the kidneys in digoxin excretion and
consequently the need for reduced dosage in patients with
impaired renal function has diminished, but not eliminated the
risk of toxicity (2). Attempts to remove substantial quantities
of digoxin by either peritoneal or hemodialysis have been
unsuccessful due to their low clearance rates (3). Since the
vast majority of digoxin is tissue bound, any dialysis method
requires a high clearance rate from serum and rapid equilibration
from the tissue to plasma compartments. Albumin-cellulose nitrate
microencapsulated charcoal (ACAC) hemoperfusion has been shown to
be successful in the treatment of certain drug intoxications (4)
in addition to its use in renal failure (5,6). More recently,
this approach has been used for digoxin intoxication (7,8,9). The
present study examined the use of the ACAC microcapsule artificial
kidney prepared as described earlier (10,11,12), in dogs made
acutely toxic with intravenous digoxin.

The clearance of digoxin by ACAC hemoperfusion was estimated
at different serum concentrations at different times during
hemoperfusion. Digoxin was given in a loading dose of 0.05 mg/lb.
Samples were obtained in duplicate from the afferent and efferent
limbs at 1, 2, and 3 hours during the hemoperfusion. Digoxin was
measured by radioimmunoassay, and clearance was calculated.

The results for the first hour of hemoperfusion show that the
AV difference is linear and related to the afferent digoxin
concentration. The results during the second hour again show a

linear relationship between the AV difference and the afferent
digoxin level. The decrease in slope from the first hour
indicates a decreasing extraction efficiency for digoxin. By the
end of hour 3, no arterial/venous difference was noted, indicating
that the charcoal was saturated with digoxin. The clearance of
digoxin during hour 1 was 55.5 ± 5.0 ml/min, while during hour 2
the clearance decreased slightly to 48.4 ± 4.0 ml/min. The mean
clearance rate during the first 2 hours was 52.4 ± 4.0 ml/min.

If the removal from serum of digoxin exceeds that of tissue
release, the potential for a rebound increase in serum digoxin
after completion of hemoperfusion exists. To explore this
possibility, serial venous samples were collected for 3 hours
in two groups of dogs after completion of dialysis. There is no
evidence of a systematic rise in serum level following hemoperfusion. In each case, had digoxin not been released from
peripheral tissues, the digoxin content of the serum pool would
have rapidly been exhausted during hemoperfusion. Since this did
not occur and since there was no evidence of a rebound rise in
serum levels, it appeared that the rate of release of digoxin
from peripheral tissues is at least as rapid as the removal from
the serum pool by hemoperfusion.

We next determined whether there was an improvement in
digoxin induced arrhythmias following charcoal hemoperfusion.
All dogs had been anesthetized with sodium nembutol and received
the total dose of digoxin of 0.05 mg/lb in 3 increments over 1
hour. All developed ventricular tachycardias within 35 minutes
after the last dose of digoxin. Thirty minutes after the onset
of arrhythmias, 4 underwent ACAC hemoperfusion while 4 served as
controls. All were sacrificed 5 hours after the onset of the
experiment and the time during which ventricular tachycardias
persisted was noted. The mean duration of toxicity in the 4
control dogs was 204 minutes with 3/4 still remaining in a toxic
arrhythmia at the time of the sacrifice. The 4 dogs undergoing
ACAC hemoperfusion were all in sinus rhythm before sacrifice.
Since the experiment was terminated before the non-treated dogs
returned to sinus rhythm, the results express only a minimum
difference possible between the two groups. Even so, the
duration of the toxicity in the 4 treated dogs was significantly
less than in the treated dogs - 137 minutes vs. 204 minutes
($p < 0.05$).

Finally, we determined whether following ACAC hemoperfusion,
there was a change in the myocardial to plasma ratio of digoxin.
The myocardial to serum ratios were measured in 4 dogs sacrificed
8 hours after the administration of the digoxin. The myocardial
to serum ratio in the control animals is 51.3. However, in the
treated animals sacrificed 3 hours after hemoperfusion, at which

time any re-equilibration should have occurred, the myocardial to serum ratio was only 33.4. The difference between these two is significant at $p < 0.03$.

The results of these experiments therefore, indicate the following points.

1. ACAC hemoperfusion removes digoxin at a rate of at least 5 times that of peritoneal or hemodialysis, giving a mean clearance of 52 ml/min during a two hour hemoperfusion. It should be noted that if applied in the human situation, there are several manoeuvres which could be employed to increase this rate even further.

2. The removal of digoxin at this rate in the dog, appeared to have a beneficial effect on digoxin-induced toxic arrhythmias. This is perhaps related to a decrease in the myocardial to serum ratio of digoxin which was determined directly. Alternatively, the apparent beneficial effect on the arrhythmias might be due to another effect of the charcoal hemoperfusion unrelated to digoxin removal.

Acknowledgements

The support of the Medical Research Council of Canada (MRC-SP-4) is gratefully acknowledged. The technical assistance of Mr. C. Lister is gratefully acknowledged.

References

1. Ogilvie, R.I., Ruedy, J.: Can. Med. Assoc. J., 97:1450, 1967.
2. Evered, D.C., Chapman, C.: Br. Heart J., 33:540, 1971.
3. Ackerman, G.L., Doherty, J.E., Flannigan, W.J.: Ann. Int. Med., 67:718, 1967.
4. Chang, T.M.S., Coffey, J.F., Lister, C., Taroy, E., Stark, A.: Trans. Amer. Soc. Artif. Intern. Organs, 19:87, 1973.
5. Chang, T.M.S., Gonda, A., Dirks, J., Malave, N.: Trans. Amer. Soc. Artif. Intern. Organs, 17:246, 1971.
6. Chang, T.M.S.: Kidney Int., 10:S305, 1976.
7. Prichard, S., Chirito, E., Chang, T., Sniderman, A.D.: J. Clin. Invest. 409A, April, 1976.
8. Carvallo, A., Ramirez, B., Honig, H., Knepshield, J., Schreiner, G.E., Gelfand, M.C.: Trans. Amer. Soc. Artif. Organs, 22: 718, 1976.
9. Prichard, S., Chirito, E., Chang, T.M.S., Sniderman, A.D.: J. of Dialysis, 1:367, 1977.
10. Chang, T.M.S.: Can. J. Physiol. Pharmacol., 47:1043, 1969.
11. Chang, T.M.S.: "Artificial Cells", Charles C. Thomas, Publisher, Springfield, Illinois, 1972.
12. Chang, T.M.S.: Kidney Int., 10:S218, 1976.

CONVERSION OF UREA AND AMMONIA TO AMINO ACID USING SEQUENTIAL

ENZYMATIC REACTION WITH MICROENCAPSULATED MULTI-ENZYME SYSTEMS

J. Cousineau and T.M.S. Chang

Artificial Organs Research Unit
Departments of Physiology and Medicine
McGill University
Montreal, Quebec, Canada

Introduction

Adsorbents have been used in the artificial kidney and artificial liver in various forms. In chronic renal failure, adsorbents have been used effectively as a miniaturized hemoperfusion system in series with a hemodialyser or an ultrafiltrator (1,2,3). Adsorbents have also been used as a dialysate regeneration system to decrease the volume of dialysate for hemodialysers (4,5). In the artificial liver, charcoal hemoperfusion has been used as hepatic support (6,7). However, in these approaches using adsorbents, the removal of urea in chronic renal failure and the removal of ammonia in liver failure has yet to be optimized.

Since urea is a very unreactive compound which is not easily bound directly to sorbent, a method for the removal of urea has been developed to convert urea enzymatically to ammonia using microencapsulated urease (8-13). Ammonium could be bound to Dowex 50W-X12 or zirconium phosphate although these ammonia adsorbents have low capacity and also remove essential electrolytes. Another approach is the use of oxystarch for the removal of ammonia and urea (14-16).

This paper discusses the use of a microencapsulated multi-enzyme system for the conversion of urea and ammonia into an amino acid. This approach can be realized by using urease to convert urea into ammonia and appropriate enzymes which utilize ammonia as a substrate to form amino acids.

Microencapsulated Multi-Enzyme System

The approach for the enzymatic removal of urea and ammonia is schematized in Figure 1. Urease, glutamate dehydrogenase, and glucose-6-P dehydrogenase are enclosed inside semipermeable micro-capsules which are impermeable to enzymes but permeable to small molecules such as substrates, products, and cofactors. Urease converts urea into ammonia. The enzyme glutamate dehydrogenase incorporates ammonia to α-ketoglutarate to form an amino acid glutamate. Since the glutamate dehydrogenase requires the cofactor NADPH for its enzymatic reaction, the third enzyme, glucose-6-P dehydrogenase is used to recycle $NADP^+$ to NADPH as it converts glucose-6-P to 6-phosphogluconate.

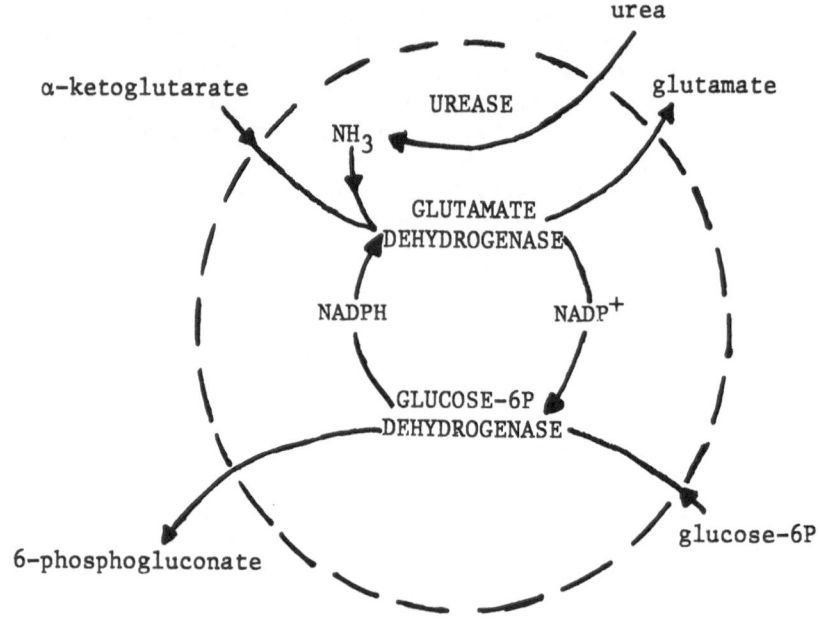

Figure 1

Schematic representation of the sequential enzyme reactions in the microcapsules.

Results

In absence of glucose-6-P, the production of glutamate from
urea (10mM) or ammonium acetate (40mM) depends on the initial
concentration of NADPH (0.21mM) and stops within 30 minutes.
However, in the presence of glucose-6-P, the oxidized form $NADP^+$
is continuously recycled to NADPH by glucose-6-P dehydrogenase,
and the initial concentration of cofactor can be lowered to 0.042mM.
Furthermore, the conversion of urea into glutamate achieved by the
three enzymes, urease, glutamate dehydrogenase, and glucose-6-P
dehydrogenase acting in sequence inside the microcapsules, is linear
when followed for 120 minutes (Figure 2). The rate of reaction
equals to the formation of 1.3 μmole glutamate per min per ml of
microcapsules. Similarly, the production of glutamate from
ammonium acetate achieved by glutamate dehydrogenase and glucose-
6-P dehydrogenase is also linear during 120 minutes (Figure 2).

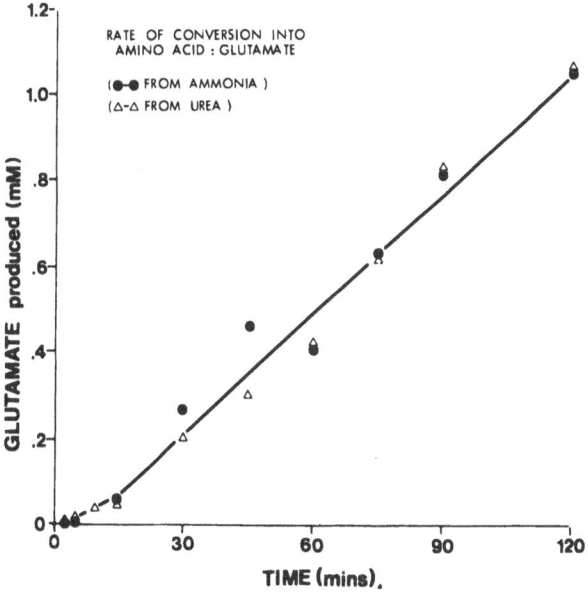

Figure 2

The formation of glutamate at a rate of 1.3 μmole per min per ml of microcapsules whether the microcapsules are supplied with urea or exogenous ammonium acetate corresponds to the removal of 0.65 μmole urea per min per ml of microcapsules or 2 mg urea per hr per ml of microcapsules.

Discussion

Since the first report in 1956 on artificial cells in the form of semipermeable microcapsules (17), the technique has been used to microencapsulate enzymes (8,18,19,20) or adsorbents like activated charcoal. Microencapsulated charcoal is now being clinically used for acute intoxication, uremia, and liver failure (1). With the demonstration of the possible use of microencapsulated multi-enzyme systems to recycle cofactors like ATP:ADP (21) and NAD^+:NADH (22), the future perspectives are much greater. Using this basic finding, we have now demonstrated the feasibility of self-sufficient artificial cells containing urease, glutamate dehydrogenase, and glucose-6-P dehydrogenase for the conversion of urea and ammonia into an amino acid. The advantage of this system is the non-toxicity of substrates and products of the reaction. The ammonia is converted into a non-essential amino acid which can be used for protein synthesis. The incorporation of glucose-6-P dehydrogenase within the microcapsules to regenerate the NADPH is also pertinent since glucose-6-P is a natural substrate present in the blood. With the cyclic regeneration of $NADP^+$:NADPH inside the microcapsules, the system can function with a low concentration of cofactor. The microcapsules containing the appropriate cycling enzymes appear to be a useful tool when free or immobilized cofactors must be regenerated, and the possibility of other multi-enzyme systems for the conversion of urea, ammonia, or other toxic metabolites could also be demonstrated.

Acknowledgements

The support of the Medical Research Council of Canada (MRC-SP-2) is gratefully acknowledged.

References

1.   Chang, T.M.S., Chirito, E., Barre, P., Cole, C., and Hewish, M.: Clinical performance characteristics of a new combined system for simultaneous hemoperfusion-hemodialysis-ultrafiltration in series. Trans. Amer. Soc. Artif. Intern. Organs 21:502, 1975.
2.   Chang, T.M.S.: Hemoperfusion alone and in series with ultrafiltration or dialysis for uremia, poisoning, and liver failure. Kidney Int. 10:S305, 1976.

3. Winchester, J.F., Apiliga, M.T., MacKay, J.M., and Kennedy,
    A.C.: Combined hemodialysis-charcoal hemoperfusion in the
    dialysis patient. Kidney Int. 10:S315, 1976.
4. Gordon, A., Lewin, A., Marantz, L.B., and Maxwell, M.H.:
    Sorbent regeneration of dialysate. Kidney Int. 10:S277, 1976.
5. Kolff, W.J., Jacobsen, S., Stephen, R.L., and Rose, D.:
    Towards a wearable artificial kidney. Kidney Int. 10:S300,
    1976.
6. Chang, T.M.S.: Hemoperfusions over microencapsulated adsorbent
    in a patient with hepatic coma. Lancet 2:1371, 1972.
7. Gazzard, B.G., Weston, M.J., Murray-Lyon, I.M., Flax, H.,
    Record, C.O., Portman, B., Langley, P.G., Dunlop, E.H.,
    Mellon, P.J., Ward, M.D., and Williams, R.: Charcoal hemo-
    perfusion in the treatment of fulminant hepatic failure.
    Lancet 2:1301, 1974.
8. Chang, T.M.S.: Semipermeable microcapsules. Science 146:
    524, 1964.
9. Chang, T.M.S.: Semipermeable aqueous microcapsules (artificial
    cells) with emphasis on experiments in an extracorporeal shunt
    system. Trans. Amer. Soc. Artif. Intern. Organs 12:13, 1966.
10. Chang, T.M.S. and Loa, S.K.: Urea removal by urea and ammonia
    adsorbent in the intestine. Physiologist 13:70, 1970.
11. Asher, W.J., Bovee, K.C., Frankenfeld, J.W., Hamilton, R.W.,
    Henderson, L.W., Holtzapple, P.G., and Li, N.N.: Liquid
    membrane system directed toward chronic uremia. Kidney Int.
    7:S409, 1975.
12. Sparks, R.E., Mason, N.S., Meier, P.M., Litt, M.H., and
    Lindan, O.: Removal of uremic waste metabolites from the
    intestinal tract. Kidney Int. 7:S393, 1975.
13. Gardner, D.L., Emmerling, D.C., Williamson, D.W., Baytos, W.C.,
    and Hassler, C.R.: Encapsulated adsorbent for removal of
    nitrogenous metabolites via oral ingestion. Kidney Int. 7:
    S393, 1975.
14. Giordano, C., Esposito, R., and Pluvio, M.: Oxycellulose and
    ammonia-treated oxystarch as insoluble polyaldehydes in uremia.
    Kidney Int. 7:S380, 1975.
15. Friedman, E.A., Fastook, J., Beyer, M.M., Rattazzi, T., and
    Josephson, A.S.: Potassium and nitrogen binding in the human
    gut by ingested oxidized starch. Trans. Amer. Soc. Artif.
    Intern. Organs 20:161, 1974.
16. Man, N.K., Drueke, T., Becker, A., Zingraff, J., Jungers, P.,
    and Funck-Brentano, J.C.: Clinical use of oxystarch. Kidney
    Int. 10:S269, 1976.
17. Chang, T.M.S.: Report of research project for B.Sc. Honours,
    Physiology, McGill University, Montreal, 1957.
18. Chang, T.M.S., MacIntosh, F.C., and Mason, S.G.: Semipermeable
    aqueous microcapsules. Can. J. Physiol. Pharmacol. 44:115,
    1966.

19.   Chang, T.M.S.: "Artificial Cells". Charles C. Thomas,
      Publisher, Springfield, Illinois, U.S.A., 1972.
20.   Chang, T.M.S. (editor): "Biomedical Applications of
      Immobilized Enzymes and Proteins", Volumes 1 and 2, Plenum
      Press, New York, U.S.A., 1977.
21.   Campbell, J. and Chang, T.M.S.: Enzymatic recycling of
      coenzymes by a multi-enzyme system immobilized within
      semipermeable collodion microcapsules. Biochim. Biophys.
      Acta 397:101, 1975.
22.   Campbell, J. and Chang, T.M.S.: The recycling of NAD^+ within
      semipermeable microcapsules containing a multi-enzyme system.
      Biochem. Biophys. Res. Commun. 69:562, 1976.

MICROENCAPSULATED CHARCOAL HEMOPERFUSION

FOR GALACTOSEMIA

P. Nasielski and T.M.S. Chang

Artificial Organs Research Unit
Departments of Physiology and Medicine
McGill University
Montreal, Quebec, Canada

In galactosemia, the elevation of galactose and subsequent metabolic products result in a variety of symptoms (1, 2) generally terminating in death. If this autosomal recessive enzyme deficiency is detected at birth diet restriction will alleviate the problem. However, for infants who have gone for weeks without a galactose-free diet, implementation of a restricted galactose diet has been of questionable benefit (3).

It has been well established that activated charcoal was extremely efficient in removing waste metabolites and toxins (4). However, until the application of microencapsulation (5, 6, 7, 8, 9), charcoal hemoperfusion was not used clinically because of its severe adverse effects of particulate embolism and platelet depletion. In the microencapsulated form charcoal hemoperfusion has been successfully used in chronic renal failure, acute drug intoxication and liver failure (9). Studies utilizing Union Carbide type activated charcoal microencapsulated with a ultra-thin semipermeable cellulose nitrate membrane were carried out. These investigations include in vivo and in vitro clearance studies for galactose.

METHODS

Encapsulation of the activated charcoal was performed as described by Chang (7, 8, 10) except the step for albumin-coating was omitted. The charcoal was Union Carbide's petroleum-base activated charcoal, 12-20 mesh, Columbis LCK. This type of charcoal, unlike coconut charcoal, was found to be effective in removing galactose.

A miniaturized version of the high density polypropylene extracorporeal shunt chamber was used (6, 7, 8).

The preparation of the solutions and the procedures used are described in detail elsewhere (11).

RESULTS AND DISCUSSION

Detailed studies were first carried out in aqueous solution and in plasma to assess the removal of galactose. With 1 gm of microencapsulated charcoal in 10 ml of galactose solution (80 mg/dl), the concentration decreased in 60 minutes to 43.7% (aqueous solution) and 46.8% (plasma) respectively.

Clearance studies were performed in vitro and in vivo. Using a flow rate of 1 ml/min/gm activated charcoal table 1 shows the extrapolated clearance values (ml/min) for different amounts of coated activated adsorbent. The values represent means and standard deviations. It was thought that these extrapolated values would be more indicative of the clearance obtained for humans. Values obtained from rat experiments were at glow rates of .7 ml/min and then extrapolated (11).

Preliminary in vitro work with microencapsulated enzymes galactose-oxidase and catalase may be another possible approach (11).

TABLE I

Extrapolated Clearance (ml/min)

In-Vitro (80mg/dl galactose)

Time	100 gm	200 gm	300 gm
5	46·1 ± 4·0	92·2 ± 8·0	138·4 ± 12
15	23·1 ± 2·7	46·2 ± 5·3	69·4 ± 7·9
30	15·9 ± 4·6	31·8 ± 9·1	47·8 ± 13·6

In-Vivo (1mg/ml gal/gm rat weight)

	100 gm	200 gm	300 gm
5	97 ± 2	194 ± 4	291 ± 6
15	78 ± 6	156 ± 12	234 ± 18
30	52 ± 12	104 ± 24	156 ± 36

ACKNOWLEDGEMENTS

The support of the Medical Research Council of Canada (MRC-SP-4) is gratefully acknowledged.

REFERENCES

1. Woolf, L.I.: Inherited metabolic disorders: Galactosemia. Adv. Clin. Chem. 5:1, 1962, Academic Press, New York, N.Y.

2. Hsia, D.-Y-Y.: Galactosemia. Charles C. Thomas, Publisher, Springfield, Illinois, 1969.

3. Shih, E.V., Levy, H.L., Karolkewiez, V., Houghton, S., Eflon, M.L., Isselbacher, K.J., Beutler, E., MacCready, R.A.: Galactose screening of newborns in Massachusetts. New Eng. J. Med. 284, #14:753, 1971.

4. Yatzidis, H.: A convenient hemoperfusion micro-apparatus over charcoal for the treatment of endogenous intoxications. Proc. Europ. Dialysis Transplant. Assoc. 1:83, 1964.

5. Chang, T.M.S.: Semipermeable microcapsules. Science 146: 524, 1964.

6. Chang, T.M.S.: Semipermeable aqueous microcapsules (artificial cells) with emphasis on experiments in an extracorporeal shunt system. Trans. Amer. Soc. Artif. Intern. Organs 12:13, 1966.

7. Chang, T.M.S.: "Artificial Cells", Charles C. Thomas, Publisher, Springfield, Illinois, 1972.

8. Chang, T.M.S.: Removal of endogenous and exogenous toxins by a microencapsulated adsorbent. Canad. J. Physiol. Pharmacol. 47:1043, 1969.

9. Chang, T.M.S.: Microencap. adsorbent hemoperfusion for uremia intoxication and hepatic failure. Kidney International 7:S387, 1975.

10. Chang, T.M.S.: Microcapsule artificial kidney: including updated preparative procedures and properties. Kidney Int. 10:S218, 1976.

11. Nasielski, P.: Galactose removal by microencapsulated adsorbent, M.Sc. Thesis, Physiology, McGill University, Montreal.

THE FILTRATION OF PLASMA FROM WHOLE BLOOD: A NOVEL APPROACH TO CLINICAL DETOXIFICATION

Franco Castino, Leonard I. Friedman, Barry A. Solomon*
Clark K. Colton**, and Michael J. Lysaght*

Blood Research Laboratory, The American National Red
Cross, 9312 Old Georgetown Road, Bethesda, Maryland 20014

A variety of techniques have been examined for the removal of toxins from the bloodstream. The most common of these, hemodialysis, has been available as a clinical detoxification procedure, and its utilization for the treatment of renal diseases is now widespread. In recent years, the limitations of hemodialysis have become apparent, particularly for the removal of high molecular weight toxins(1). Consequently, alternative approaches have been investigated. For example, polymeric membranes highly permeable to molecules with molecular weight up to 5,000 have been incorporated into devices that rely primarily upon convection, rather than diffusion, for the removal of toxins (2). These devices may offer some advantages over hemodialysis (3) and are currently under clinical study. However, both of these techniques are inadequate if the toxins are proteins or are protein bound.

Chemical sorbents in direct contact with blood may be useful for the removal of toxins, but their application has been hampered because of damage to blood components and risks of sorbent emboliza- tion (4). Encapsulation of sorbents with a biocompatible polymer is effective in reducing blood damage, but the resistance to the per- meation of large molecules is greatly increased (5). Attempts to perfuse uncoated sorbents with plasma obtained by continuous centri- fugation of whole blood have been frustrated by platelet losses (6).

Publication # 395 from the Blood Research Laboratory, The American
National Red Cross.
* Amicon Corporation, Lexington, Ma 02173.
** Department of Chemical Engineering, Massachusetts Institute of
Technology, Cambridge, Ma 02139.

Plasma exchange has not been widely used in the past because of the extreme difficulty and hazards of manual procedures (7). The introduction of continuous flow pheresis devices utilizing centrifugation has eased the problem, and a variety of immunological diseases have been successfully treated (8,9). The major obstacle to a widespread application of plasma exchange is the cost, complexity, and risk of the exchange procedure.

The objective of the studies reported herein was to develop a safe, efficient, reliable, and inexpensive continuous flow plasmapheresis system based on recent advances in microporous membrane technology (10). The removal of toxins from plasma obtained by filtration of whole blood could then be achieved by plasma exchange or by perfusion of sorbents, as suggested in previous reports (11). Since plasma would be completely free of cellular components, a biocompatible coating on sorbent particles would not be needed, and resistance to the permeation of large molecules or protein bound toxins would be eliminated. The present studies were limited to in vitro experiments utilizing whole human blood.

MATERIALS AND METHODS

The separation of plasma from whole blood was carried out using

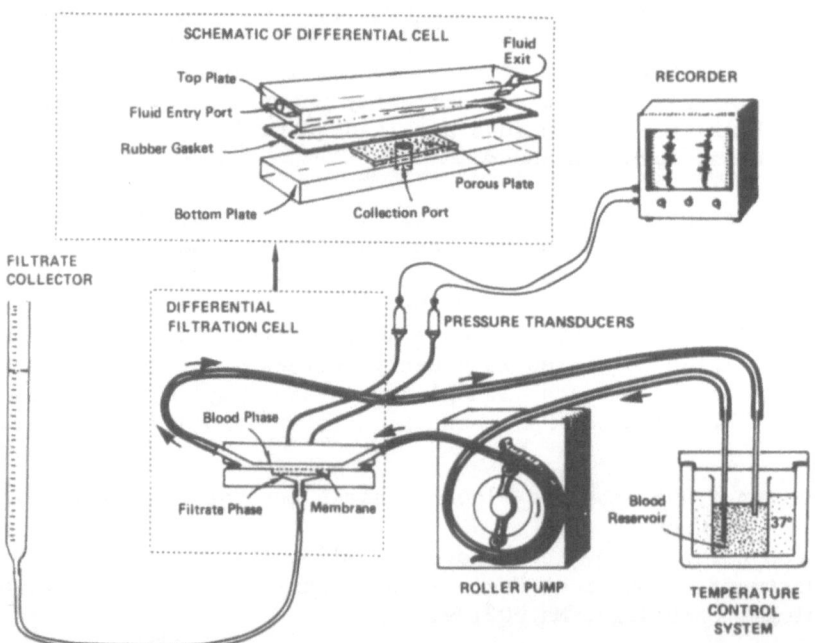

Figure 1: Diagram of the perfusion circuit and schematic of the differential filtration cell.

the perfusion circuit shown in Figure 1.   Standard hemodialysis lines
(Extracorporeal TS-110) and a roller pump (Sarns 5500) were utilized.
The filtration cell (Figure 1, insert) contained a straight channel
of rectangular geometry.   A single microporous membrane was mounted
in the cell between the rubber gasket and the bottom plate and was
supported on a sheet of porous sintered polyethylene foam which had
been machined flush with the surface of the bottom plate.   Polycarbonate membranes (Nuclepore Co., Pleasanton, Ca.), 0.6 μm pore diameter and 10 μm thick were selected on the basis of results reported
in previous studies (10,12).   The area available for filtration was
6.25 cm^2 (length 5 cm,   width 1.25 cm).   The height of the channel
was determined by six shims (plastic discs) placed within the gas-
kets.   Dye visualization studies indicated .that velocity was uniform
across the cell.   The flow was laminar under all conditions investigated.   Pressures at the beginning and end of the filtration area
were continuously monitored through ports drilled in the top plate
by means of strain-gauge transducers (Statham, P 23 ID) and recorded.   Mean transmembrane pressure (TMP) was calculated as the average
of these two values which differed by no more than 12 mmHg at the
highest shear rates.   Whole human blood containing citrate-phosphate-
dextrose (CPD) as the anticoagulant was used as the perfusate.   The
blood was stored at 4°C and was utilized less than 24 hours following
collection in order to minimize the occurrence of cellular aggregates (13).   Sterile, pyrogen-free saline (Travenol Laboratories
Inc., Deerfield, Ill.) was used for priming the circuit.   Filtrate
was collected in a 10 ml pipette with 0.1 ml graduations.   The liquid level was maintained at the same height as the filtration cell.
An event switch, connected to the strip-chart recorder, was activated for each ml increment of the filtrate volume.   The filtrate
was left open to the atmosphere unless otherwise indicated.

     Hematocrit (Hct), mean corpuscular volume (MCV), red blood cell
count (RBC), platelet count and mean platelet volume (MPV) were
determined by means of a particle counter (Electrozone Celloscope,
Particle Data Inc., Elmhurst, Ill.).   Hematocrit was also determined
by standard centrifugation techniques.   Plasma hemoglobin (plasma Hb)
was determined either by the cyanmethemoglobin method (14) using the
initial plasma as a reference, or by a modification of the tetra-
methylbenzidine method (15).   The concentration of individual plasma
proteins was determined by electrophoresis on agarose and cellulose
acetate (16), by automated immuno-agglutination techniques (17), and
by bidimensional immunoelectrophoresis on agarose with rabbit anti-
serum to human serum (18,19).

                          ENGINEERING EVALUATION

     Plasma was readily separated from whole blood by filtration
through the polycarbonate 0.6 μm pore diameter membranes.   The plasma
flux and the degree of hemolysis were dependent upon the following
parameters:

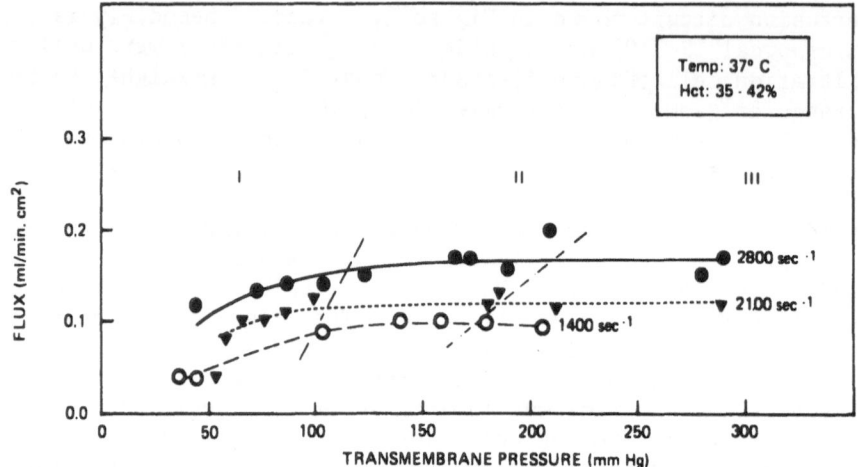

Figure 2: Plasma flux as a function of tranmembrane pressure at different shear rates.

Transmembrane pressure and shear rate. Figure 2 shows data obtained during experiments in which TMP was gradually increased by partial occlusion of the tubing distal to the blood exit port. The blood film thickness was 0.075 cm. Three different units of blood were used at flow rates of 100, 150 and 200 ml/min (shear rates 1,400, 2,100 and 2,800 sec^{-1} respectively). In each experiment, three separate regions were identified. At the lowest pressures (region I, TMP less than about 100 to 120 mmHg), plasma flux increased with increasing TMP. For intermediate values of TMP (region II), plasma flux was insensitive to TMP variations, and hemolysis did not occur. If the TMP was raised above about 180 to 210 mmHg

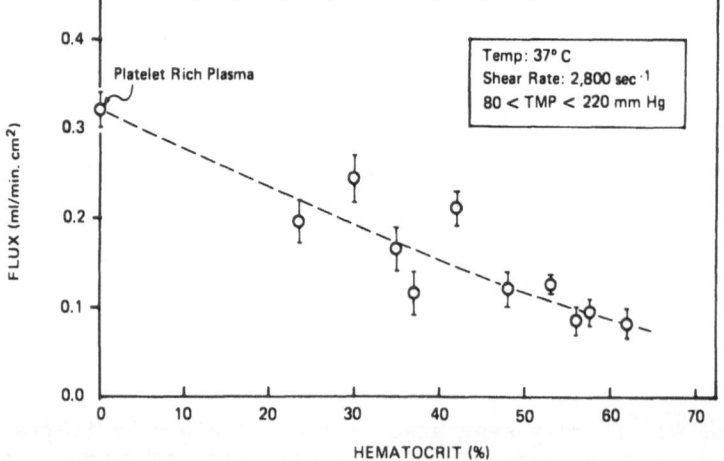

Figure 3: Plasma flux as a function of hematocrit at constant shear rate.

(region III), onset of hemolysis was observed, even though plasma
flux was the same as in region II. At any given value of TMP, plasma
flux increased as shear rate increased. The TMP threshold for the
transition from one region to another was also influenced by shear
rate.

Hematocrit and perfusion time. Ten units of blood of different
Hct were perfused through the filtration cell at constant shear rate
(2,800 sec^{-1}) and constant channel height (0.075 cm). TMP was maintained between 80 and 200 mmHg (region II of figure 2). Plasma
flux was repeatedly measured over a period of up to 60 minutes. The
values showed very little fluctuation from a time-averaged value that
decreased with increasing Hct, as shown in Figure 3. The value at
zero Hct was obtained with platelet rich plasma. The very small
variations of flux observed with time indicated that clogging of the
pores did not occur in these studies; this observation was supported
by scanning electron micrographs of the membranes at the end of
perfusion.

Plasma flux. In a separate series of experiments with channel
height at 0.033 cm and shear rate at 1,100 sec^{-1}, plasma flux was
predetermined by use of a tubing pump on the filtrate exit line.
The blood inlet pressure was held constant at 100 mm Hg, but the
pressure at the filtrate exit port decreased (and became negative
with respect to atmospheric pressure) as flux was increased. A re-
presentative experiment is illustrated in Figure 4, where plasma Hb
concentrations in the blood and in the filtrate phases are plotted
as a function of plasma flux. When flux was increased from 0.075
to 0.155 ml/(min.cm^2) Hb concentration in the filtrate increased
dramatically from about 50 to 700 mg%, whereas the Hb concentration

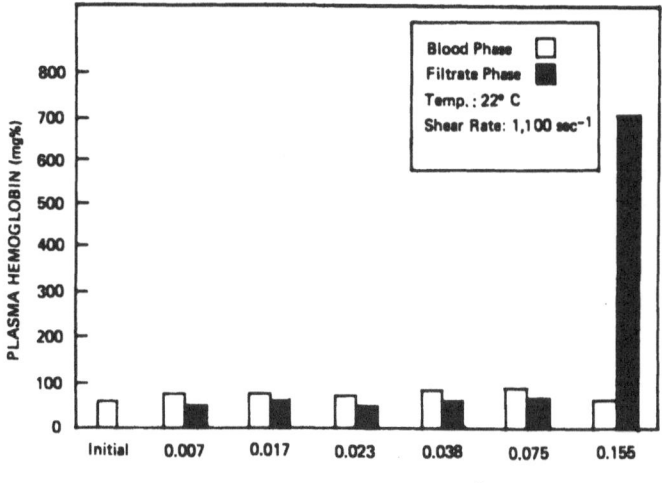

Figure 4: Hemolysis as a fuction of plasma flux.

in the blood remained constant. When plasma flux was decreased back
to 0.075 ml/(min.cm^2), Hb concentration in the filtrate promptly returned to its previous value. Although the existence of a threshold
in plasma flux above which massive hemolysis occurred was similar
to the transition from region II to region III in Figure 2, the relationship between the results from these different sets of experiments remains to be clarified. Existing theories for the deposition of cellular elements onto filtering walls (20) predict that
hemolysis occurs simultaneously with red blood cells deposition
when the so-called deposition parameter, a dimensionless group of
variables, exceeds a critical value. However, the values of the
deposition parameter calculated from the plasma flux data in the
absence of hemolysis (Figures 2 and 4) are up to one order of magnitude higher than that critical value. Hence, these results suggest
that the onset of hemolysis need not be coincident with the onset
of red blood cells deposition, but that an additional increment in
transmembrane pressure may be required in order to cause the red
blood cells to deform and enter into the membrane pores.

BIOLOGICAL EVALUATIONS

Cellular components. Unless hemolytic conditions were present
during the experiments, RBC, Hct and MCV remained constant throughout the perfusion. Platelet count and MPV were also constant, although a few platelets were observed in scanning electron micrographs of the membranes at the end of perfusion. Platelets were
never detected in the filtrate phase.

Plasma proteins. The protein distribution in the filtrate was
qualitatively and quantitatively identical to that of the perfusate
as determined by the techniques described in Materials and Methods.
An example of the results obtained with bidimensional immunoelectrophoresis is shown in Figure 5. This technique allows for the identification and quantitation of at least 30 protein species in plasma
(18,19). No difference between the concentration of any of these
species in the filtrate and blood phase was observed, even for the
biggest molecules (e.g., β -lipoprotein). These results are of particular interest in view of the reports that a variety of toxins
implicated in the etiology of several diseases are protein-bound(21).

DISCUSSION

Our initial results indicate that separation of plasma from
whole blood by filtration through microporous membranes is feasible.
Operational parameters have been identified which allow the process
to be carried out with minimal damage to blood components. The
plasma obtained by filtration is free of all blood cells. The proteins in the filtrate are qualitatively and quantitatively identical

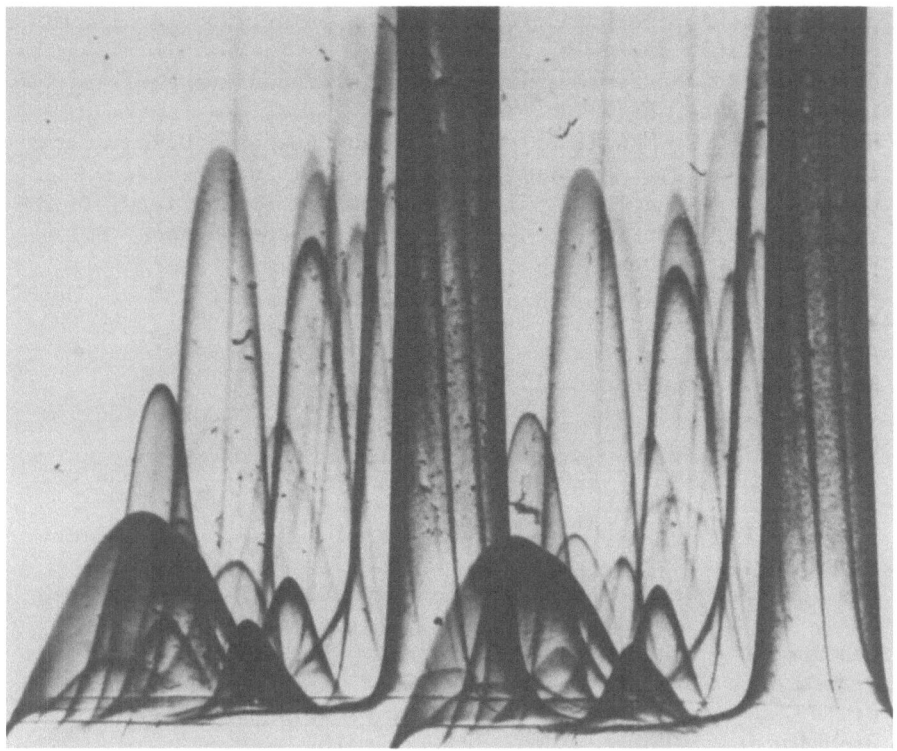

Figure 5: Bidimensional immunoelectrophoresis of plasma proteins
in the filtrate (left) and blood (right) phases.

to the plasma proteins in the original blood. Protein-bound toxins
could, in principle, be extracted continuously from the circulation
and removed by appropriate methods. Immunological disorders (hyper-
viscosity, Goodpasture's disease) could be treated by this process
much more efficiently than is currently possible. Further engineering studies are underway. Filtration modules have been designed and
built which operate at a blood flowrate of about 15 ml/min and which
yield a filtrate flowrate of 3 ml/min. We estimate that a prototype
device yielding 20 ml/min hemoglobin-free plasma from an inlet blood
flowrate of 70-80 ml/min will require less than 500 cm^2 filtration
surface area. The availability of such a simple, safe, economical,
and efficient filtration device could lead to completely new thera-
pies for a variety of conditions that are now relatively untreatable.

REFERENCES

1. Funck-Brentano, J.L., Man, N.K., Sausse, A., Zingraff, J., Boudet,

J., Becker, A.,and Cueille, G.F. Trans. Amer. Soc. Artif. Int.
Organs 22:163, 1976.

2. Colton, C.K., Henderson, L.W., Ford, C.A. and Lysaght, M.J.
    Lab. Clin. Med. 85:3:355, 1975.

3. Henderson, L.W. McGill Artifical Organs Research Unit Interna-
    tional Symposium. Montreal, Canada, April 20th, 1977.

4. Chang, T.M.S. Charles C. Thomas Publisher, Springfield, Il,1972.

5. Walker, J.M., Denti, E., van Wagenen, R., and Andrade, J.D.
    Kidney International, 10:S-320, 1976.

6. Weston, M.J., Mellon, P.J., Langley, R.D., Hughes, R.D., Dun-
    lop, E.H., Gazzard, B.G. and Williams, R. Clin. Sci. Mol. Med.
    48:187, 1975.

7. Keynes, W.M. The Lancet 1236, 1968.

8. Pineda, A.A., Taswell, H.F. and Brzica, S.M. Transfusion 15:
    510, 1975.

9. Lockwood, M. and Pearson, T. Haemonetics Pheresis Symposium,
    Boston, Ma., September 4, 1975.

10. Blatt, W.F., Agranat, E.A., and Rigopulos, P.N. U.S. Patent
    3,705,100, 1972.

11. Castino, F., Scheucher, K., Malchesky, P.S., Koshino, I., and
    Nose, Y. Trans. Amer. Soc. Artif. Int. Organs 22:637, 1976.

12. Castino, F., Scheucher, K., Malchesky, P.S., Nose, Y.
    Proceedings 29th ACEMB 18:292, 1976.

13. Bailey, D.N. and Bove, J.R. Transfusion 15:3:244, 1975.

14. Drabkin, D.L. Amer. J. Med. Sci. 217:710, 1949.

15. Holland, V.R., Saunders, B.C., Rose, F.L. and Walpole, A.L.
    Tetrahedron 30:3299, 1974.

16. Baux, M.D., Ackermann, P.G., and Gelson, T. The C.V. Mosby Co.
    Publisher, St. Louis, Mo, 1972.

17. Technical Publication # 1-UA4-01710-00. Technicon, Tarrytown,
    N.Y.

18. Weeke, B. Scand. J. Clin. Lab. 25:269, 1970.

19. Minchin-Clarke, H.G., and Freeman, T. Clin.Sci. 35:403, 1968.

20. Forstrom, R.J., Bartelt, K., Blackshear, P.L., Jr., and Wood,
    T. Trans. Amer. Soc. Artif. Int. Organs 21:132, 1975.

21. Zieve, F.J., Zieve, L., Doizaki, W.M. and Gilsdorf, R.B. J.
    Pharm. Exp. Ther. 191:1:10, 1974.

ACKNOWLEDGMENT

    This research was supported in part by NHLBI Contract NO 1 -
HB - 6 - 2928. The excellent technical assistance of Mr. Frank
Muolo and Mr. Allan Lovell is greatly appreciated. We are indebted
to the Center for Blood Research, Boston, Ma. for protein analysis.
We are grateful for the assistance received from the Biological
Ultrastructure Department, Blood Research Laboratory, for the elec-
tron microscope studies.

IONSIV F-80 AND IONSIV W-85: MOLECULAR SIEVE ZEOLITE

NH$_4^+$ ION EXCHANGERS FOR REMOVAL OF UREA NITROGEN

John D. Sherman

Molecular Sieve Department, Linde Division
Union Carbide Corp., Tarrytown Technical Center
Tarrytown, New York 10591

SUMMARY

New molecular sieve zeolite ion exchangers with high NH$_4^+$ exchange selectivities and capacities have been discovered and developed for use in a variety of applications. Preliminary tests show the LINDE IONSIV F-80 and IONSIV W-85 ion exchangers provide high NH$_4^+$ capacities in synthetic solutions similar in composition to blood serum or dialysate solutions.

The use of these new IONSIV NH$_4^+$ exchangers in conjunction with urease enzyme hydrolysis promises to provide significant improvements in urea removal for use in treatment of chronic renal disease.

INTRODUCTION

Improved urea-binding sorbents have been sought for many years for use in treatment of renal disease. Such sorbents could be employed in hemodialysis or peritoneal dialysis for dialysate regeneration, thus reducing the quantities of dialysate required and thereby reducing the size and weight of such systems. Alternatively, improved sorbents may be employed to remove urea in hemoperfusion or as an intestinal sorbent to bind urea and thereby augment the gastrointestinal excretion of nitrogenous waste products.

Unfortunately, although activated carbon is an effective sorbent for many waste metabolites and drugs, it does not possess sufficient capacity to remove urea effectively from dilute solutions. Other sorbents (organic resin ion exchangers, oxystarch, etc.) have also been studied, but a non-soluble, selective urea binding sorbent with high urea sorption capacity at physiological pH levels has not been found.

267

An alternative method of urea removal offers greater promise and has already achieved some success. In this approach urea is hydrolyzed (using urease enzyme) to form ammonium ions which are then removed by ion exchange.

Portable dialysis systems employing such a process have been developed ($\underline{1}$), and are sold by CCI Life Systems, Inc. Their REDY Universal Recirculating Dialysate System employs an immobilized urease enzyme catalyst to hydrolyze urea to NH_4^+, followed by an inorganic ion exchanger (zirconium phosphate) to remove the NH_4^+ cation, and a hydrous zirconium oxide anion exchanger to remove phosphate and fluoride anions. Ca^{++} and Mg^{++}, which are also removed by zirconium phosphate ion exchanger, must be added back in the desired concentrations to the regenerated dialysate.

We have recently reported ($\underline{2},\underline{6}$) the development of new molecular sieve zeolite NH_4^+ ion exchangers (LINDE IONSIV F-80 and IONSIV W-85 ion exchangers) which provide unique selectivities for NH_4^+ in the presence of other common alkali and alkaline earth cations. Such zeolites should, therefore, provide improved performance over zirconium phosphate in selectively binding ammonium ions to remove urea nitrogen.

BACKGROUND

Molecular sieve zeolites are crystalline, hydrated aluminosilicates of (most commonly) Na, K, Mg, Ca, Sr, or Ba cations. The aluminosilicate portion of the structure is a three-dimensional open framework consisting of a network of AlO_4 and SiO_4 tetrahedra linked to each other by sharing all of the oxygens. Zeolites may be represented by the empirical formula:

$$R_{2/n}^{n+}O \quad . \quad Al_2O_3 \quad . \quad X\ SiO_2 \quad . \quad Y\ H_2O$$

In this oxide formula X is generally equal to or greater than 2.0 since AlO_4 tetrahedra are joined only to SiO_4 tetrahedra; n is the cation valence. The framework contains channels and interconnected voids which are occupied by the cations and water molecules. The cations are quite mobile and they can usually be exchanged, to varying degrees, with other cations.

Although zeolites have attractive ion exchange properties, they did not find significant use commercially as ion exchangers until the early 1960's. This was largely due to lack of availability and lack of knowledge of their properties. The discovery by R. M. Milton and co-workers at Union Carbide that zeolites could be synthesized at convenient conditions (low temperatures and pressures) from reactive raw materials (e.g., freshly prepared aluminosilicate gels) led to the discovery of dozens of new zeolite structures. The fact that they could be synthesized by man assured their availability in commercial quantities in high purity, with reproducible properties.

The first commercial ion exchange uses were developed in the
early 1960's by Ames et al. for the processing of wastes from spent
nuclear fuel, and in the late 1960's and early 1970's for the removal
of NH_4^+ from municipal waste water. A number of other applications
of zeolite ion exchangers are in various stages of development.

The structure, chemistry, and use of zeolite molecular sieves
has been broadly reviewed in a recent monograph by Breck (3) which
includes a 64-page chapter extensively reviewing the theory, equili-
bria, and kinetics of ion exchange in zeolites. Applications of zeolites in ion exchange are described by Sherman (2).

Ion Exchange Properties of Molecular Sieve Zeolites

The ion exchange capacity of zeolite ion exchangers is a function of their SiO_2/Al_2O_3 mole ratio, since each AlO_4 tetrahedron in
the zeolite framework provides a single cation exchange site. Because some ion exchange sites are accessible only through small pore
openings in the porous framework, not all the exchange capacity of
some zeolites is available to large cations. The majority of the
total ion exchange capacity is available to the most common ions,
including NH_4^+. In special cases, however, separations based upon
ion size are possible.

In addition to some ion sieving effects, zeolites commonly exhibit high selectivities for ion exchange among ions which will easily
enter the zeolite pores. For example, LINDE IONSIV A-50 zeolite provides a striking selectivity for Ca^{++} over Na^+, compared with common
organic resin cation exchangers.

The ion exchange selectivity series for each of the most common
zeolites are reviewed in (2). Common organic resin cation exchangers
and some zeolites prefer ions of higher charge. However, some zeolites show marked selectivity for some monovalent cations over common divalent cations. For example, LINDE IONSIV W-85 exchanges NH_4^+
in marked preference to Ca^{++} and prefers Na^+ over Ca^{++}.

The observed ion exchange selectivities and loadings on zeolites
are dependent upon the pH (H^+ is a competing cation), temperature and
aqueous solution chemistry. The competing cations, choice of solvent,
presence of complexing agents, solution strength, and types of anions
present can each alter the quality of the ion exchange separation
which can be achieved (via the effects of these variables upon the
activities of the cations in solution, as is also true in the case
of the organic resin ion exchangers).

The molecular sieve zeolites have rigid, strong frameworks stable to high temperatures, oxidation/reduction, ionizing radiation,
and not subject (as are many organic resin ion exchangers) to physical attrition due to osmotic shock. For the same reasons, the ion

exchange properties of the zeolites are relatively more constant and
predictable over wide ranges of temperature, ionic strength, etc.,
than is often the case with other ion exchangers. Similarly, zeolite
ion exchangers should not tend to adsorb organic molecules or ions
and become "fouled" as readily as other ion exchangers.

Zeolites are also stable at elevated pH levels (e.g., pH 7-12)
at which other inorganic ion exchangers (e.g., zirconium phosphates,
etc.) tend to lose functional groups due to slow hydrolysis. Zeolites
are synthesized at elevated pH levels (e.g., pH 12-13) and temperatures (e.g., 100-300°C) and are quite stable at conditions only
slightly less severe than employed during their synthesis.

The chief restriction in the use of zeolite ion exchangers is due
to their limited acid resistance. Although some zeolites are stable
at lower pH levels ($\sim$pH 2), most zeolite ion exchangers should not
be employed below about pH 4-5 except for very brief exposures.
Operation at pH > 6 is preferred.

Ammonium Ion Removal from Waste Water

Ion exchange processes employing the zeolite clinoptilolite are
in various stages of use, construction, or planning in several loca-
tions in the United States for removal of ammonium ions from municipal wastewater (2). Although clinoptilolite performs quite well in
this service, exchangers with higher capacity should provide significantly improved overall process performance in this and related
applications.

Improved NH_4^+ Exchangers

Studies begun in 1968 at Union Carbide Corporation led to the
discovery that the LINDE IONSIV F-80 synthetic zeolite is more effective than clinoptilolite in removing NH_4^+ from wastewater (3,4).

During the same time period, exploratory tests were made of other
zeolites. It was discovered (5) that zeolites of the LINDE IONSIV
W-85-phillipsite-gismondine group provide superior NH_4^+ exchange
characteristics, even though these zeolites have lower theoretical
maximum cation exchange capacities compared to the LINDE IONSIV F-80
zeolite.

Initial column exchange studies compared phillipsite with clinoptilolite and LINDE IONSIV F-80 zeolites. These studies were later
extended to include the zeolites phillipsite, LINDE B, and LINDE
IONSIV W-85, which have three different (related) framework structures.
In order to examine the NH_4^+ exchange capacities and selectivities
of these zeolites, each was equilibrated with a mixed cation solution,
and the resulting zeolite solid samples were analyzed, providing the
results shown in Figure 1.

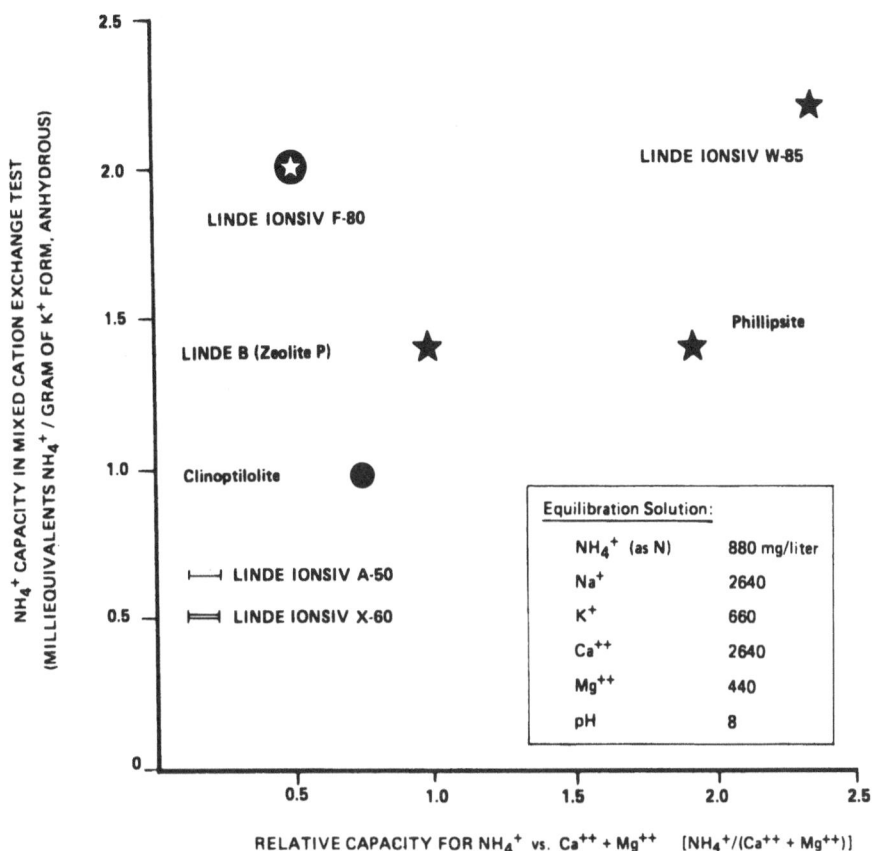

Figure 1: Performance in mixed cation exchange tests-
NH_4^+ capacity vs. selectivity.

As may be seen, the phillipsite-gismondine type zeolites (phillipsite, LINDE B and LINDE IONSIV W-85) provide higher NH_4^+ capacities
and selectivities compared to clinoptilolite. LINDE IONSIV W-85 zeolite provides the best performance of all, and it is superior to both
clinoptilolite and LINDE IONSIV F-80 zeolites in both capacity and
selectivity for NH_4^+ ion exchange.

Cyclic column ion exchange tests were made to compare the performance of LINDE IONSIV W zeolite with that of clinoptilolite for
NH_4^+ removal from municipal wastewater. The results ($\underline{2}$) revealed
that the LINDE W zeolite provides about 2.5 times greater NH_4^+ exchange capacity compared to Hector clinoptilolite.

NH_4^+ Exchange for Urea Removal

The extension of the use of these new IONSIV NH_4^+ ion exchangers to remove urea nitrogen should be quite straightforward. The NH_4^+ generated by urea hydrolysis will be exchanged onto the IONSIV NH_4^+ exchanger. The CO_3^{--} simultaneously generated must be neutralized by acid addition (directly or via use of a suitable buffer) to control pH at suitable levels ($\sim$ pH 7-8) to maintain the urease enzyme activity. The system chemistry is shown below.

SYSTEM CHEMISTRY

Urea Hydrolysis

$$(NH_2)_2CO + 2\ H_2O \xrightarrow[\text{Enzyme}]{\text{Urease}} 2\ NH_4^+ + CO_3^{--}$$

Neutralization of Ammonium Carbonate

$$2\ NH_4^+ + CO_3^{--} + H^+ \rightleftharpoons 2\ NH_4^+ + HCO_3^-$$

NH_4^+ Ion Exchange

$$(R_{2/n}^{n+})\ \text{Zeolite} + 2\ NH_4^+ \rightleftharpoons (NH_4^+)_2\ \text{Zeolite} + \frac{2}{n}\ R^{n+}$$

Overall Reaction

$$(NH_2)_2CO + 2\ H_2O + H^+ + (R_{2/n}^{n+})\ \text{Zeolite} \longrightarrow$$

$$(NH_4^+)_2\ \text{Zeolite} + R_{2/n}^{n+} + HCO_3^-$$

Preliminary tests of the NH_4^+ binding capacity of IONSIV F-80 and IONSIV W-85 NH_4^+ ion exchangers have been made in synthetic solutions approximating the cation composition of blood serum and in solutions containing only Na^+ as the competing cation.

In stirred-slurry contacting of the zeolite NH_4^+ exchangers in powder form with the mixed cation solutions, greater than 95% approach to equilibrium NH_4^+ exchange was achieved in approximately one minute even at room temperature. The ion exchange rates are even faster at normal body temperatures. In similar tests, zirconium phosphate provided much slower rates of NH_4^+ exchange.

The IONSIV NH_4^+ exchangers are much more selective and provide much lower Ca^{++} and Mg^{++} removal than does zirconium phosphate. However, some removal of Ca^{++} will occur, particularly on the IONSIV F-80 exchanger. This may be reduced by pre-equilibration of the zeolite with a solution of similar composition sans NH_4^+. The same is true for K^+ and other cations.

Based upon studies made on synthetic solutions of similar composition, the effective NH_4^+ binding capacities of the IONSIV F-80 and IONSIV W-85 in contact with blood or dialysate solutions have been estimated, as shown below.

Expected NH_4^+ Capacities at NH_4^+ Concentrations
Corresponding to 20-50 $^{mg}N/100cc$ (UN)

Zeolite	mEq NH_4^+ / Gram	gms urea equivalent / 100 gms zeolite
IONSIV F-80		
In Na^+ Solution	1.5-2.0	4.5-6.0
In Dialysate*	0.8-1.3	2.4-4.0
IONSIV W-85		
In Na^+ Solution	1.1-1.7	3.3-5.1
In Dialysate*	0.9-1.5	2.7-4.5

* Containing Ca^{++}, Mg^{++} and K^+ as well as Na^+ and NH_4^+

As may be seen, the equivalent urea binding capacities of these new IONSIV NH_4^+ exchangers are quite high, even in the presence of competing K^+, Ca^{++}, and Mg^{++} cations. For example, at a loading of 1.0 mEq NH_4^+/gram zeolite (or 3.0 gms urea equivalent/100 grams zeolite), the desired removal of 12-30 gms urea/day for treatment of chronic renal disease would require only 0.9-2.2 lbs/day of IONSIV NH_4^+ exchanger.

Typical properties of the LINDE IONSIV F-80 and IONSIV W-85 NH_4^+ ion exchangers in powder form are given on the following page.

Typical Properties of LINDE IONSIV NH_4^+ EXCHANGERS (6)

Property	IONSIV F-80	IONSIV W-85
Particle Size	Powder (1-20μm)	Powder (1-20μm)
Pore Openings	3.7Å	4.2Å
Bulk Density	0.59 gms/cc	0.63 gms/cc
Crystal Density	2.3 gms/cc	2.2 gms/cc
H_2O Content	12-17 wt%	15-20 wt%
Chemical Formula	$(Na_2O, K_2O)Al_2O_3$ $\cdot2\ SiO_2\cdot3\ H_2O$	$(Na_2O, K_2O)Al_2O_3$ $\cdot3.6\ SiO_2\cdot5\ H_2O$
Maximum Cation Exchange Capacity (mEq/gm, anhydrous)	6.0-6.7	4.8-5.3

ACKNOWLEDGEMENTS

The author wishes to thank S. R. Ash, M.D., for his invitation to discuss these new developments at the ASAIO meeting in Montreal in April, 1977, and Dr. T.M.S. Chang for his kind invitation of this chapter. Special credit is due to D. W. Breck and R. J. Ross, who shared in the discovery and development of these new NH_4^+ exchangers.

REFERENCES

(1) Maxwell, M.H., A. Lewin, and A. Gordon, "Sorbents in the Treatment of Chronic Renal Disease", Kidney International 7, S-383-S-386 (1975).

(2) Sherman, J.D., "Ion Exchange Separations with Molecular Sieve Zeolites", Paper presented at the 83rd National Meeting, American Institute of Chemical Engineers, Houston, Texas (March 20-24, 1977).

(3) Breck, D.W., "Zeolite Molecular Sieves: Structure, Chemistry, and Use", Wiley-Interscience, New York (1974).

(4) Breck, D.W., "Process for Removal of Ammonia from Waste Water Streams", U.S. Patent 3,723,308 (March 27, 1973).

(5) Sherman, J.D., and R.J. Ross, "Separations of Ammonium Ions from Aqueous Solutions", Ger. Offen. 2,531,338 (Feb. 12, 1976).

(6) Union Carbide Corp., Linde Div., "LINDE IONSIV F-80 Ion Exchanger", Ion Exchange Bulletin F-4092, and "LINDE IONSIV W-85 Ion Exchanger", Ion Exchange Bulletin F-4093 (1977).

PANEL AND GENERAL DISCUSSION

CHRONIC RENAL FAILURE AND FUTURE APPROACHES

Benjamin T. Burton

Artificial Kidney-Chronic Uremia Program, National
Institute of Arthritis, Metabolism, and Digestive
Diseases, National Institutes of Health, Bethesda, Md.

Historically the conservative treatment of chronic renal failure has been carried out with the aid of special diets which limit
the intake of dietary precursors of what I shall call, for lack of
a better word, "uremic substances" including cations such as potassium. In addition dietary management includes the restriction of
fluids in excess of insensible and residual urinary losses. This
type of management is primarily preventive. Other preventive
therapeutic steps include the use of gastrointestinal sorbents like
aluminum hydroxide, potassium-sequestering resins, and others such
as oxystarch to bind specific undesirable uremic substances (phosphate, potassium, urea) and to carry them out via the feces. All
of these preventive concepts of management of uremia must be looked
upon as adjunctive modes of therapy since in patients with a residual glomerular filtration rate below 3 milliliters per minute,
they alone cannot sustain life. As useful as the preventive concepts of uremic management continue to be, the mainstay of today's
therapeutic approaches to end-stage renal failure is based on the
removal of undesirable uremic substances from or with body fluids --
in brief, hemodialysis or peritoneal dialysis, and, more recently,
hemofiltration.

During the last few years we have seen signal advances in the
process of hemodialysis including the development of dialyzers with
large internal membrane surfaces which may permit us to decrease
treatment time considerably. Future approaches in hemodialysis no
doubt must include further sophistication of the apparatus with
emphasis on the use of a low volume of dialysate which is being
effectively regenerated at relatively low cost during the dialytic
process. This is essential to avoid the demineralization and purification of large volumes of dialysis water prior to use (and the

cost of the solutes contained in voluminous dialysates) and is a
prerequisite for further development of non-stationary hemodialysis
apparatus. A prototype of such apparatus already exists in the form
of the REDY system. The development of a light-weight, inexpensive
system of mixed sorbents to regenerate constantly a dialysate of
small volume is highly desirable for the design of new <u>portable</u>
artificial kidneys and it is absolutely indispensable should truly
wearable dialyzers ever come into routine use. Pivotal in this
development is the need for an effective sorbent for urea because
charcoal alone will not bind urea adequately at room or body temperature nor will it bind electrolytes which means that a potassium
sequestrant, among others, will also have to become a component of
the ideal sorbent mix for wearable dialyzers.

      Currently used methods of blood access continue to be the
Achilles heel of hemodialysis. For that and other reasons too
numerous to mention during such a brief presentation we must continue
to plan further optimization of peritoneal dialysis. The recent
renaissance of peritoneal dialysis, including the development of
closed-cycle, automated treatment and daily short-term self-dialysis,
continues with current work focused on enhancement of mass transfer
with the aid of specific vasoactive or diuretic drugs or sodium infused with the dialysate. In addition we look toward the further
development of improved peritoneal access methods and to novel methods
of peritoneal lavage such as "reciprocating peritoneal dialysis" in
a stationary mode of application and "low-volume, continuous, ambulatory peritoneal dialysis" for additional expansion of the horizon of
peritoneal lavage. The former would be characterized by the use of
a relatively small volume of peritoneal dialysate which is constantly
being regenerated and infused in and out of the abdominal cavity at
an optimal stroke volume. The latter would be based on the constant
retention in the peritoneal cavity of a small volume of dialysate
which equilibrates optimally with the patient's blood and which is
periodically "voided" by the patient as he replaces it, four to five
times per 24-hour cycle.

      One of the most fascinating future aspects of artificial kidney
development involves hemofiltration. Recent rapid developments in
Europe have shown it to be both a feasible and clinically effective
treatment method for the uremic patient. Since, however, <u>convective</u>
transport on which this imitation of the action of the natural glomerulus is based does not result in an optimal clearance of small
molecules, it is foreseeable that in artificial kidneys of the future
an element of <u>diffusive</u> transport involving a modicum of dialysis may
also be included. Reference here is to future development of stationary equipment and it is highly premature to even consider at the
moment anything but stationary equipment in this new area of hemofiltration.

One can foresee future developments in hemofiltration which would pit the principle of pre-dilution of blood prior to hemofiltration against that of ultrafiltration of undiluted whole blood combined with downstream replenishment of the blood volume with a man-made sterile nonpyrogenic solution. Several years may elapse before the clinical advantages and disadvantages of these respective approaches are fully elucidated. Moreover, future experimentation may well emphasize the desirability of the partial use of diffusive transport through membranes with the use of dialysate concomitant with or following hemofiltration, and there is no reason why this should not become a component of the stationary artificial kidney of the future.

The most important development of the future, however, revolves around the selective processing of the filtrate obtained by hemofiltration. In current usage in Europe, for instance, approximately 20 liters of ultrafiltrate are being removed from the patient during a 5-hour treatment. Approximately 18 liters of a lactated Ringer's solution are being replaced simultaneously. The refinement of the future which must be sought here encompasses sophisticated means of removing undesirable uremic substances from the constantly elaborated hemofiltrate, followed by the simultaneous reinfusion of the purified filtrate into the patient. Such a development indeed would, for the first time, enable us to speak truly of an artificial kidney because the hemofiltration process would imitate the action of the natural glomerulus and the subsequent selective processing of the ultrafiltrate and reinfusion of the remaining fluid would constitute artificial renal tubular action and would complete our imitation of the divine prototype. It would also return to the patient some, if not all, of the desirable solutes in the ultrafiltrate. Moreover, pragmatically speaking, this would also avoid the high cost of 18 liters of a sterile, nonpyrogenic replacement electrolyte solution, and would solve the present technical impasse created by a regulation of the U.S. Food and Drug Administration that sterile fluids for intravenous infusion may not be marketed in containers holding more than 2 liters each.

In theory such selective processing could be carried out with the aid of an optimal mixture of sorbents, both specific ones (for the binding of urea, potassium and other electrolytes) and nonspecific ones, like charcoal (until our knowledge improves concerning the true nature of the most important "uremic factors").

The knowledge gained in past experiments with hemoperfusion will have to play a particularly important role in this selective purification process, except that many technical difficulties which now bedevil perfusive processing of whole blood will present less of a problem when the medium to be perfused is an aqueous filtrate, and this will, no doubt, simplify future experimental approaches.

For the foreseeable future such an overall system of purification for semi-uremic blood, composed of hemofiltration (with or
without simultaneous or subsequent hemodialysis) followed by selective purification of the filtrate and subsequent reinfusion of the
latter, will require a formidable and complex apparatus and thus
we should look upon it for the time being as a _stationary_ means of
treatment. Moreover, even this "artificial kidney" will continue
to be subject to the many drawbacks -- led by the continued problems
of blood access -- which beset the manipulation of blood. On the
other hand, it is quite possible to foresee successful additional
optimizations with relation to peritoneal dialysis, possibly even
constant ambulatory peritoneal lavage, with or without auxiliary
dialysate-regenerating wearable sorbent cartridges.

Which brings us to the last and most important point to be
emphasized while outlining future approaches to treatment of uremia:
that there is a need for a _multiplicity_ of experimental directions
which must be followed in the future in contrast to a structured
approach toward a pre-conceived (and possibly prematurely conceived)
concept of a single "ideal artificial kidney" of the future. Based
on our fairly dismal biochemical and metabolic state of knowledge
in the realm of uremia, it is scientifically inconceivable to do
otherwise since at best what we have engaged in heretofore, however
successful to date, is still largely empirical.

STATUS OF ARTIFICIAL LIVER SUPPORT: 1977

Paul D. Berk, M.D., F.A.C.P.

Section on Diseases of the Liver, National Institute
of Arthritis, Metabolism and Digestive Diseases
National Institutes of Health, Bethesda, Maryland 20014

From the title of this symposium and the distribution of papers, one might mistakenly conclude that artificial liver and artificial kidney development were proceeding in parallel. In fact, progress in these two areas is decades apart. Artificial kidney devices are a standard form of therapy which is currently sustaining the lives of more than 20,000 people in the United States alone (1). In contrast, the sum total of all patients in hepatic failure ever treated with any experimental hepatic support device appears to be approximately 200. Moreover, analysis of the available data on the minority of survivors leaves uncertain the extent to which the devices employed contributed to their recovery.

The motivation for the interest in artificial hepatic support systems is obvious. Whereas the availability of artificial kidney devices has substantially improved survival of patients with renal disease over the past two decades (2,3), conventional management has yielded no corresponding improvement in the survival of patients with liver disease. In particular, the death rate from fulminant hepatic failure is generally believed to be approximately 85% in adult patients (4). It is obviously hoped that an artificial hepatic support system could improve this unsatisfactory situation.

Because of the widely accepted analogy between the physiologic roles of the liver and kidney (5), many of the techniques currently being tested in artificial liver devices are borrowed directly from the field of nephrology. However, the liver/kidney analogy cannot be carried too far. In particular, while the synthetic functions of the kidney - such as the production of erythropoietin - improve the quality of life, long experience with anephric patients demonstrates that these functions are not essential for survival.

In contrast, the liver's role in such areas as glucose homeostasis and clotting factor synthesis is such that the prolonged survival of an anhepatic patient is currently inconceivable. Hence, in contrast to chronic renal dialysis, artificial hepatic support systems must be looked on as temporary measures for use in the patient with acute, but reversible hepatic failure. In this setting, the critical factor for survival is the ability of the liver to regenerate and render the artificial device unnecessary.

Within the setting of acute but reversible hepatic failure, what should be asked of an artificial hepatic support system? A fundamental goal ought to be the restoration of consciousness in the comatose patient, since coma itself is a major contributing factor to the secondary complications which are so often the cause of death (6). At this point, one quickly comes up against the overwhelming ignorance of basic pathophysiology which characterizes our knowledge of this area. Is coma in acute hepatic failure due to the accumulation of toxic compounds, i.e. is it due principally to hepatic excretory failure, or is it due to brain deprivation of a critical substance produced by the liver? There has been evidence on both sides of this question for 25 years (7-9), but the question remains essentially unanswered.

Assuming - and it is an assumption - that accumulation of toxins is the major problem to be dealt with, what is the nature of the compounds to be removed from the body, either because they contribute to coma or inhibit hepatic regeneration? Table I lists many of the currently recognized biochemical abnormalities which are demonstrable in patients with hepatic failure (10-12). None of these abnormalities is pathognomonic, and none shows an absolute correlation with either the state of consciousness or the prognosis. Hence, it remains uncertain whether hepatic coma is due to one of these recognized metabolic abnormalities, the synergistic effects of several (13,14), or to factors as yet entirely unrecognized.

Against this lack of essential information, a number of strategies for the design of an artificial hepatic support system have been employed (Table II). Three basic principles have been invoked in these approaches: hemodialysis of potential toxins through a membrane, removal of potential toxins by direct contact with sorbents, or the use of living liver tissue to achieve the same ends. The last approach has the added potential advantage of supplying the hypothetical liver-derived factors necessary for normal cerebral activity. Details concerning several of these approaches are presented elsewhere in this monograph. While the list appears exciting and innovative, the basic concepts behind all of these approaches were available by 1960 (5), and work since then has largely consisted of technical or engineering, rather than conceptual advances. Hemodialysis with conventional (15) and polyacrylonitrile (16,17) membranes, charcoal hemoperfusion (18,19),

TABLE I

KNOWN METABOLIC ABNORMALITIES IN HEPATIC COMA
(NONE PATHOGNOMONIC)*

1) Amino acids increased in blood, brain, spinal fluid, urine,
   with disproportionate increase in aromatic, relative to
   branched chain compounds

2) Mercaptans increased in breath, blood, urine

3) Fatty acids increased in blood

4) Neurotransmitters decreased in brain and muscle

5) False neurotransmitters increased in brain, muscle, blood,
   urine

6) Neurotransmitter metabolites increased in spinal fluid

7) Ammonia increased in blood, muscle, brain, spinal fluid

8) Glutamine increased in muscle, brain, spinal fluid

9) α-Ketoglutaramate increased in spinal fluid

10) Pyruvate, Lactate, Citrate, α-Ketoglutarate increased in blood
    and muscle

11) α-Ketoglutarate, Fumarate, Malate, Oxaloacetate decreased in
    brain

12) Brain O_2 and glucose utilization decreased

13) Ketone production decreased

14) Affinity of Hb for oxygen reduced

---

*Modified from reference 10.

---

and perfusion through both cation (20) and anion (21) exchange
resins have undergone clinical trials in patients with hepatic
failure. Neutral resins have been employed in drug intoxicated
patients (22) and in animal models of fulminant hepatic failure
(23), whereas affinity chromatography (24,25) and perfusion through
isolated hepatic microsomes (26) and enzymes (27), or through
liver cells grown in tissue culture on hollow fiber capillaries

TABLE II

APPROACHES TO THE DEVELOPMENT OF AN

ARTIFICIAL HEPATIC SUPPORT SYSTEM

I.   Hemodialysis

A) Convenional

B) "Second-generation" - hollow fiber, etc.

II. Hemoperfusion Through Sorbents

A) Charcoal

B) Resins

1) neutral (XAD-2, XAD-4)

2) cation exchange

3) anion exchange

C) Affinity Chromatography (Albumin-agarose gel)

D) Biologically Active Adsorbents

1) gel-entrapped hepatic microsomes

2) solubilized, carrier-bound hepatic enzymes

III. Hemoperfusion Through Living Liver Tissue

A) Liver slices, "chunks", cell suspensions

B) Liver cells in tissue culture

---

(28), have been employed thus far exclusively in animal systems.
There is, of course, additional human experience, principally
from Japan and the United States, with devices which employ liver
slices, chunks or isolated cells, often in combination with
dialysis and resin perfusion, but it is impossible to determine
the role of any one component of these more complex systems (5).

It will be obvious from the proceedings of this symposium that the two variables receiving the greatest attention are patient survival and "biocompatibility". In the absence of detailed understanding of the favorable biochemical changes to be produced by an artificial hepatic support device, improved patient survival, at best a crude endpoint (vide infra), remains virtually the only available parameter of device efficacy. With regard to "biocompatibility", a great deal of effort has gone into developing devices with bland surfaces which do not induce hemolysis, or platelet or white cell aggregation (29), but the effects of these various coatings on the adsorption of toxins appear inevitably to be unfavorable to a greater or lesser degree (30). Recently, calcium chelation with citrate anion has been shown to virtually eliminate platelet losses over a variety of sorbents including uncoated charcoal (31). Hence, the use of "regional" citrate anticoagulation during hemoperfusion may have useful clinical applications under certain circumstances. An alternate approach would be the perfusion of the artificial hepatic support system with cell free plasma, produced by a continuous flow blood separation device. Attempts to use the IBM/NCI celltrifuge for this purpose were unsuccessful because the intrinsic efficiency of that device was inadequate to produce sufficient volumes of plasma with sufficiently low platelet counts (32). Recently a new type of continuous flow centrifuge has been developed with the capacity to generate high flow rates of cell and platelet free plasma (33). Alternatively, ultrafiltration of whole blood through a cellulose acetate hollow fiber capillary device has been used as a simple and inexpensive method of generating platelet free plasma for subsequent sorbent perfusion (34). If either of these devices proves to be successful and can be incorporated as an integral part of an artificial hepatic support system, then much of the current concern with "biocompatibility" and considerations of the properties of various coating materials may be rendered irrelevant.

One of the major problems in the field of artificial hepatic support systems is evaluating where we are. Of all the devices tested, the oldest - conventional hemodialysis - has the best published survival statistics: 3 of six patients with fulminant hepatic failure treated by this approach survived (5,16). That the patients were on three continents, and that 25 years were required to accumulate the small series emphasizes the lack of enthusiasm for this approach among hepatologists (35). Perhaps there is a substantial negative experience which is unpublished. It is of interest to note that the call for a multicenter controlled trial of this therapy, made some 20 years ago (15), has never been answered.

In 1972, Benhamou and colleagues undertook a detailed review of all the published data on the therapy of fulminant hepatic failure (36). Three of their conclusions bear careful scrutiny.

At that time, they concluded that:

(1) The death rate in severe acute hepatic failure (SAHF)
averages 80-90% but is subject to considerable variation as a
function of age, sex, etiology, and unknown variables. Even for
viral hepatitis with coma, well documented survival rates with conservative therapy have varied from 15-50%. Therefore, therapeutic
success in an isolated case (or even in a small uncontrolled series)
is of no significance.

(2) Published case reports do not accurately reflect the
effects of therapy. Thus, 91.7% of all subjects of isolated case
reports survived, compared to only 36.8% of patients in series of
2 or more. Survival correlated inversely with the size of the
series.

(3) Authors tend to publish isolated cases with a favorable
outcome attributed to a given therapy but not to publish cases in
which therapy has failed. In fact, it might be argued that the
best future one can wish for a sufferer from SAHF is to undergo a
new treatment and have his case published - "be published or
perish".

Have we progressed since that 1972 review? After carefully
reviewing the more recent data, the only unequivocal statement
that can be made is that we are not sure. As illustrated in
Table III, charcoal hemoperfusion appeared at one point to offer
a substantial improvement in survival. Subsequently, following a
switch from hand-made to mass produced columns, results were less
good [(37) and M. Davis, personal communication], and the series
was terminated after a run of 18 consecutive deaths (R. Williams,
presented at the N.I.H. Conference on Fulminant Hepatic Failure,
Bethesda, Maryland, February 9, 1977). This study, which was not
a randomized controlled trial, serves to emphasize the critical
need for such trials in assessing all progress. Is charcoal hemoperfusion ineffective for the treatment of acute hepatic failure,
or has the art of making and coating the right kind of charcoal
merely been temporarily lost? At this time, we simply do not know.
While one must have great sympathy with the need for short uncontrolled phase I trials of new devices, it seems a pity that the
role of charcoal cannot be assessed with certainty despite its use
on more than 100 patients. It should be emphasized that non-
contemporaneous, non-randomized controls simply will not do.
Differences in patient material or in subtle aspects of supportive
care may greatly influence the outcome. This is clearly illustrated
by the results obtained with the new RP-6 polyacrylonitrile
dialysis device, which has resulted in 33% survivors in London (8
of 24 patients) but 21% survivors (5 of 24) in Paris (16,17). The
former, but not the latter, was believed to represent an improvement
over results obtained in the same unit with conventional therapy.

TABLE III

CHARCOAL HEMOPERFUSION IN ACUTE HEPATIC FAILURE WITH GRADE IV

ENCEPHALOPATHY: EXPERIENCE AT KINGS COLLEGE HOSPITAL, LONDON

Patients	Survivors	% Survivors	Date
1–22	10	45	May, 1974
1–37	14	38	September, 1974
1–65	21	32	September, 1975
23–37 (n = 15)	4	27	
38–65 (n = 28)	7	25	

It seems apparent that more information about basic pathophysiology is essential to the rational design and utilization of
artificial hepatic support devices. In this regard, recent
theoretical studies have shown that the hemoperfusion schedule
employed in fulminant hepatic failure may be almost as important
as the device itself in depleting slowly exchanging extravascular
metabolic pools of toxic metabolites (38). Optimization of the
treatment regimen will be dependent on identification of the
metabolites to be removed, and intimate knowledge of the kinetics
of their internal transfer between blood and critical extravascular
compartments such as brain and/or cerebrospinal fluid. An animal
model of acute hepatic failure which closely approximates the
human situation would be of enormous value for many relevant lines
of investigation. It also seems evident that more attention to
controlled trials and to basic statistical principles will be
essential if we are to know where we are now, let alone where to
go next.

The view presented above is clearly somewhat pessimistic.
This pessimism is, in part, related to the nature of the problem
itself. Hepatologists, after all, are accustomed to viewing the
world with a jaundiced eye.

REFERENCES

1. Burton, B. T.: Overview and state of the art. In <u>Proceedings</u>
    <u>of the 9th Annual Contractors Conference of the Artificial</u>
    <u>Kidney Program of the National Institute of Arthritis,</u>
    <u>Metabolism and Digestive Diseases</u>, DHEW Publication No. (NIH)
    77-1167, U. S. Department of Health, Education and Welfare,
    Washington, 1967, pp. 188-192.

2. Klebba, A. J., Maurer, J. D., Glass, E. J.: Mortality trends
    for leading causes of death: United States, 1950-1969.
    National Center for Health Statistics: Data from the National
    Vital Statistics System, Series 20, No. 16, U. S. Department
    of Health, Education and Welfare Publication No. (HRA) 74-1853,
    U. S. Government Printing Office, Washington, 1974.

3. Maher, J. F., Nolph, K. D., Bryan, C. W.: Prognosis of
    advanced chronic renal failure. <u>Ann. Intern. Med</u>. <u>81</u>:43-47,
    1974.

4. Trey, C.: The fulminant hepatic failure surveillance study.
    Brief review of the effects of presumed etiology and age on
    survival. <u>Can. Med. Assoc. J</u>. <u>106</u>:525-527, 1972.

5. Berk, P. D., Martin, J. F., Scharschmidt, B. F., Plotz, P. H.:
    Current status of artificial hepatic support systems. In
    <u>Progress in Liver Diseases</u>, Volume V, Chapter 24, H. Popper
    and F. Schaffner (Editors), Grune and Stratton, New York,
    1976, pp. 398-417.

6. Gazzard, B. G., Portmann, B., Murray-Lyon, I. M., Williams, R.:
    Causes of death in fulminant hepatic failure and relationship
    to quantitative histological assessment of parenchymal damage.
    <u>Quart. J. Med</u>. <u>44</u>:615-626, 1975.

7. Geiger, A.: Correlation of brain metabolism and function by
    the use of a brain perfusion method <u>in situ</u>. <u>Physiol. Rev</u>.
    <u>38</u>:1-20, 1958.

8. Opolon, P., Huguet, C., Granger, A., Gallot, D., Bloch, P.,
    Bidallier, M.: Comparison of single and cross hemodialysis
    with a donor through cuprophan and a new polymer membrane.
    In <u>Artificial Hepatic Support</u>, R. Williams and I. M. Murray-
    Lyon (Editors), Pitman, London, 1975, pp. 186-201.

9. Roche-Sicot, J., Sicot, C., Peignoux, M., Bourdiau, D.,
    Degos, F., Degos J-D., Prondi, D., Rueff, B., Benhamou, J-P.:
    Acute hepatic encephalopathy in the rat: The effect of cross
    circulation. <u>Clin. Sci. Mol. Med</u>. <u>47</u>:609-615, 1974.

10. Zieve, L.: Metabolic abnormalities in hepatic coma and poten-
     tial toxins to be removed. In Artificial Hepatic Support, R.
     Williams and I. M. Murray-Lyon (Editors), Pitman, London,
     1975, pp. 11-26.

11. Schenker, S., Breen, K. J., Hoyumpa, A. M. Jr.: Hepatic
     encephalopathy: Current status. Gastroenterology 66:121-154,
     1974.

12. Zieve, L., Nicoloff, D. M.: Pathogenesis of hepatic coma.
     Ann. Rev. Med. 26:143-157, 1975.

13. Zieve, L., Doizaki, W., Zieve, F. J.. Synergism between
     mercaptans and ammonia or fatty acids in the production of coma:
     A possible role for mercaptans in the pathogenesis of hepatic
     coma. J. Lab. Clin. Med. 83:16-28, 1974.

14. Zieve, F. J., Zieve, L., Doizaki, W. M., Gilsdorf, R. B.:
     Synergism between ammonia and fatty acids in the production of
     coma: Implications for hepatic coma. J. Pharmacol. Exp. Ther.
     191:10-16, 1974.

15. Kiley, J. E., Pender, J. C., Welch, H. F., Welch, C. S.:
     Ammonia intoxication treated by hemodialysis. N. Engl. J. Med.
     259:1156-1161, 1958.

16. Opolon, P., Rapin, J-R., Huguet, C., Granger, A., Delorme,
     M-L., Boschat, M., Sausse, A.: Hepatic failure coma treated
     by polyacrylonitrile membrane hemodialysis. Trans. Amer.
     Soc. Artif. Int. Organs 22:701-710, 1976.

17. Silk, D. B. A., Chase, R. A., Hanid, M. A., Davies, M., Trewby,
     P. N., Williams, R.: Haemodialysis using the RP6 membrane
     in fulminant hepatic failure and its effects on amino acid
     levels. Abstracts of the 23rd Annual Meeting, Amer. Soc.
     Artif. Int. Organs 6:80, 1977.

18. Chang, T. M. S., Migchelsen, M.: Characterization of possible
     "toxic" metabolites in uremia and hepatic coma based on the
     clearance spectrum for larger molecules by the ACAC micro-
     capsule artificial kidney. Trans. Amer. Soc. Artif. Int.
     Organs 17:246-252, 1973.

19. Gazzard, B. G., Weston, M. J., Murray-Lyon, I. M., Flax, H.,
     Record, C. O., Portman, B., Langley, P. G., Dunlop, E. H.,
     Mellon, P. J., Ward, M. B., Williams, R.: Charcoal hemo-
     perfusion in the treatment of fulminant hepatic failure.
     Lancet 1:1301-1307, 1974.

20. Juggi, J. S.: Extracorporeal cation exchange circuits in
     the treatment of hyperammonia of liver failure. Med. J. Aust.
     1:926-930, 1973.

21. Lopukhin, U. M., Shurkalin, B. K., Leykin, U. A., Evseev, N. G.,
     Molodenkov, M. N., Kuznetzov, V. N., Gorchakov, V. D.,
     Blagosklonov, A. S.: Bilirubin removal by anion exchange
     resin (Letter). Lancet 2:461, 1975.

22. Rosenbaum, J. L., Kramer, M. S., Raja, R., Boreyko, C.: Resin
     hemoperfusion: A new treatment for acute drug intoxication.
     N. Engl. J. Med. 284:874-877, 1971.

23. Gazzard, B. G., Buxton, B. H., Winch, J., Machado, A. L.,
     Flax, H., Williams, R.: Effects of haemoperfusion through
     charcoal or XAD-2 resin on an animal model of fulminant
     hepatic failure. Gut 15:482-486, 1974.

24. Scharschmidt, B. F., Plotz, P. H., Berk, P. D., Waggoner, J.
     G., Vergalla, J.: Removing substances from blood by affinity
     chromatography. II. Removing bilirubin from the blood of
     jaundiced rats by hemoperfusion over albumin-conjugated
     agarose beads. J. Clin. Invest. 53:786-795, 1974.

25. Scharschmidt, B. F., Martin, J. F., Shapiro, L. J., Plotz,
     P. H., Berk, P. D.: Hemoperfusion through albumin-agarose
     gel for the treatment of neonatal jaundice in premature
     Rhesus monkeys. J. Lab. Clin. Med. 89:101-109, 977.

26. Denti, E., Luboz, M. P.: Preparation and properties of gel-
     entrapped liver cell microsomes. In Artificial Liver Support,
     R. Williams and I. M. Murray-Lyon (Editors), Pitman, London,
     1975, pp. 148-152.

27. Brunner, G., Jaworek, D.: A new approach towards an extra-
     corporeal management of liver failure: The use of detoxifying
     enzymes bound to artificial membranes. Abstracts of the VI
     Meeting of the International Association for the Study of the
     Liver, Acapulco, October 20-24, 1974.

28. Wolf, C. F. W., Munkelt, B. F.: Bilirubin conjugation by an
     artificial liver composed of cultured cells and synthetic
     capillaries. Trans. Amer. Soc. Artif. Int. Organs 28:16-27,
     1975.

29. Bruck, S. D.: Blood compatible materials for extracorporeal
     assist and related devices. In Artificial Hepatic Support,
     R. Williams and I. M. Murray-Lyon (Editors), Pitman, London,
     1975, pp. 68-82.

30. Walker, J. M., Denti, E., Van Wagenen, R., Andrade, J. D.: Evaluation and selection of activated carbon for hemoperfusion. Kidney International 10:S320-S327, 1976.

31. Scharschmidt, B. F., Martin, J. F., Shapiro, L. J., Plotz, P. H., Berk, P. D.: The use of calcium chelating agents and prostaglandin E_1 to eliminate platelet and white blood cell losses resulting from hemoperfusion through uncoated charcoal, agarose gel, and neutral and cation exchange resins. J. Lab. Clin. Med. 89:110-119, 1977.

32. Weston, M. J., Mellon, P. J., Langley, P. G., Hughes, R. D., Dunlop, E., H., Gazzard, B. G., Williams, R.: Resin column perfusion with whole blood or plasma separated by the continuous flow celltrifuge. Clin. Sci. Molec. Med. 48:187-192, 1975.

33. Ito, Y., Suaudeau, J., Bowman, R. L.: A new flow-through centrifuge without rotating seals applied to plasmapheresis. Science 189:999-1000, 1975.

34. Yamazaki, Z., Fujimori, Y., Sanjo, K., Sigiura, M., Wada, T., Inoue, N., Oda, T., Kominami, N., Fujisaki, U., Hayang, F.: New artificial liver support systems for hepatic coma. Abstracts of the 23rd Annual Meeting, Amer. Soc. Artif. Int. Organs 6:99, 1977.

35. Keynes, W. M.: Hemodialysis in the treatment of liver failure. Lancet 2:1236-1238, 1968.

36. Benhamou, J-P., Rueff, B., Sicot, C.: Severe hepatic failure: A critical study of current therapy. In Liver and Drugs, F. Orlandi and A. M. Jezequel (Editors), Academic Press, New York, 1972, pp. 213-228.

37. Gazzard, B. G., Weston, M. J., Murray-Lyon, I. M., Record, C. O., Williams, R.: Experience at King's College Hospital with charcoal hemoperfusion: Overall results in 37 patients. In Artificial Hepatic Support, R. Williasm and I. M. Murray-Lyon (Editors), Pitman, London, 1975, pp/ 234-241.

38. Berk, P. D.: A computer simulation study relating to the treatment of fulminant hepatic failure by hemoperfusion. Proc. Soc. Exp. Biol. Med., 1977 (in press).

TREATMENT OF ACUTE INTOXICATION

George Schreiner, M.D.

Nephrology Division,
Georgetown University Hospital
Washington, D.C., U.S.A.

My interest in detoxification began after my high school prom.
Seriously, it began as a medical student when Dr. Theodore Koppanyi,
who was then Professor of Pharmacology at Georgetown, carried out a
very interesting but rather basic experiment, and that is, he took
a group of dogs, poisoned them with barbital and phenobarbital in an
amount that killed all of them and then took another group of dogs
and gave then the same doses, and infused very, very rapidly a huge
amount of saline into the dogs to dilute their circulating plasma
concentration, and some of these dogs lived and did not go into
congestive heart failure, but more importantly, they woke up. Immediately, this suggested to many of us that there was, at least in
the case of these particular drugs, a relationship which we have
subsequently defined, and which I think is a very important concept:
i.e. - there are a group of drugs and substances which have a time-
dose cycotoxic relationship, that is, there is a relationship between the exposure of the cells to a critical concentration of the
molecule, and to a period of time, and that removal or lowering of
the dose by any technique, whether it be drug removal, dilution, or
what have you, can lessen the clinical toxicity of that particular
compound. There are obviously poisons which don't have a time-dose
cycotoxic relationship, but in the case of sedatives and particularly
those drugs which do have a time-dose cycotoxic relationship, it
seems a simple basic truth that the same blood stream which acted
as a railroad to carry the molecules in from a vein or from the
stomach, can also act as a railroad to carry the molecules in the
reverse direction - that is, all railroad tracks go potentially in
two directions; and if so, one needs only to have a removal technique
which will lower the plasma concentration sufficiently to begin to
move the transport in the opposite direction. Now this is an

imperfect analogy because substances highly soluble in fat, obviously may be captured in the fat depots or in particular membranes and
there may not be a reversible situation. By and large however,
molecules which are carried, particularly by albumin as a transport
protein, are reversible by a decrease in concentration.

    Now the other thing is that the sooner you get the patient with
the highest possible blood level, the more dramatic your results
will be in terms of the amount removable, and the more dramatic will
be your clinical change. This is because everything virtually
known, has a maximum binding capacity and therefore, you will bind
up to whatever that maximum may be for the bigger compounds and
what is in excess of that is then freely soluble in plasma water
and is extractable either by tissues, by intrabody renal mechanisms,
but also is much more freely extractable by excorporeal methods
such as dialysis and hemoperfusion, peritoneal dialysis, dilutions,
etc. So therefore, the earlier you get the patient up on the curve,
the more drug you can remove. The other variables, obviously, as
you've heard talked about today, have to do with the interval of
time between the moment that the person takes his dose and has it
adsorbed, to a point where he enters the medical care system, and
what is the length of time between the moment he hits the medical
care system such as a emergency room to get to a detoxification unit
for example, whether it be hemoperfusion or hemodialysis. This is
very important because if you read the literature literally everyone
says that I'm getting the tough patients, but everyone else is selecting the easy patients. This is not true if you look over epi-
demeologic situations. In fact, one of the things accounting for
the variations in statistics, is that in lot of jurisdictions its
the bad cases who die before they get into the entry system, and
therefore, leave the investigators with the selective better cases.
You really have to know the demography of the poison situation.
Our first phenobarbital case, for example, had a higher blood level
than an single patient in London in which the blood level taken by
the medical examiner post-mortum - that is, these were all the dead
cases - and we had living patients with higher blood levels than the
highest level in the dead patients in London. So this has a lot to
do with which cases are selected, sometimes they are easy ones, and
sometimes they are the dead ones; and this will affect your percentage of response.

    In 1950 we got our first artificial kidney actually on the NIH
grant to study the removal of poisons, and as Dr. Kolff remembers,
it was one of the first artificial kidney units in the U.S. Shortly
thereafter we decided that maybe resins would be better, and in
1951-52 with Dr. Arthur Pallotta we did a series with a Dowex lactate
ion-exchang resin - this is an experiment from 1952 showing the
actual changes in plasma drug level before and after our resin columns. We also have done this with charcoal. One of the problems

that we ran into was platelet removal and it was apparent early on
that platelet removal from columns did not just depend on the column
and the contents, but also on the platelets, because successive
removal Slopes were quite different using the same resins, hemo-
dynamics, and geometric configurations. This suggests that perhaps
there is a population of platelets which is more susceptible to
aggregation and removal, and damage by the column. This particular
point is still being approached experimentally, and I think that we
need to pay some attention to what's going on with the platelets
and not just what is going on with the column. This indicates by a
study by De Myttenaere et al. that Glutethimide can be removed very
easily and quickly by a 100 gm charcoal column and that charcoal may
also do this in a repeated and very abrupt fashion. The important
point I want to make is that the dynamics of detoxification have to
take into account, not only the technical removal rate and side
effects of the treatment, but the dynamics of each particular drug,
to know whether or not we can accomplish something in a given population of patients. Part of the things we need to know are such
things as clearance and half-life. Dr. John Maher, a lifetime
colleague of ours will now present this.

INTERRELATION OF HEMOPERFUSION, PLASMA CLEARANCE AND HALF LIFE

John F. Maher, M.D.

Division of Nephrology, Department of Medicine
University of Connecticut Health Center, Farmington,
Connecticut

One goal of therapy of acute poisoning is to achieve a maximal rate of elimination. In the past two decades, forced diuresis and hemodialysis have been used for this purpose most successfully in the management of water soluble intoxicants (1). Lipid soluble poisons are removed only minimally, in part because of low clearances and large distribution spaces (2). Hemoperfusion, however, achieves higher clearances, even of lipid soluble toxins (3,4,5).

Clearance by these techniques is from plasma that is repleted by solute diffusion from extravascular spaces. Water soluble solutes which are rapidly cleared by diuresis or dialysis, also diffuse rapidly from extravascular water into and from plasma and may be considered distributed in a single compartment. Larger solutes and those with a high lipid affinity often diffuse so slowly that not only is clearance by dialysis slow, but also, with more rapid elimination, e.g. by hemoperfusion, a disequilibrium results between body pools. Such solutes should be considered distributed into two compartments (Figure 1). If the second compartment is much larger than the more exchangeable pool or if diffusion is much slower into the exchangeable compartment than out of it, the following will occur. Plasma concentrations will decrease more rapidly than anticipated, the calculated distribution space will be inappropriately small and there will be a secondary rise in plasma concentrations after the procedure terminates.

The rate of decline in plasma concentration, the plasma half life relates to the volume of distribution (V) and the plasma clearance (C) by the formula, $T 1/2 = .693 V/C$. Knowing half life and clearance, the volume of distribution can be calculated (Figure 2). Solutes with high clearances and long plasma half lives must have

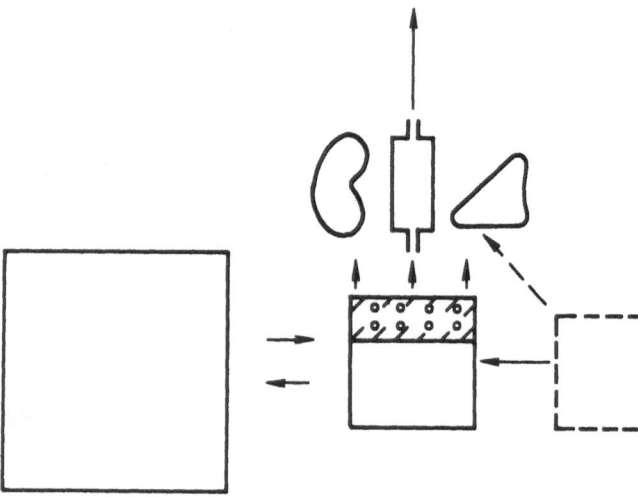

Figure 1. Arrows indicate intercompartmental solute kinetics.

large distribution spaces. Conversely, solutes with short half
lives must have very high clearances or small distribution spaces.
Under conditions where the plasma concentration has previously been
stable, influx equals endogenous plasma clearance and net removal
can be considered equal to extracorporeal clearance. If extracorporeal clearance is high relative to the endogenous clearances, the
half life should decrease considerably. When the calculated distribution space is smaller than the normal value, because the half life
is very short relative to the clearance, however, it is consistent
with delayed intercompartmental transfer. The magnitude of this delay may be a major factor limiting therapy of poisoning by techniques that increase elimination of toxins. Because most poorly
dialyzable toxins have distribution spaces exceeding 100 l and many
have high metabolic clearance rates, a rapid decrease in plasma concentration should not be explained only by extracorporeal clearance
of solute from the total distribution space. It should also be
noted that the plasma extraction ratio factored by the extracorporeal blood flow rather than plasma flow gives spuriously high clearance values unless the solutes are equally distributed in erythrocytes and cleared during the extracorporeal circuit which does not
happen with hemodialysis (6).

Assuming negligible intake in the postabsorptive state, the
plasma concentration may be stable or even decreasing slightly as a
procedure such as dialysis or hemoperfusion begins. If equilibra-

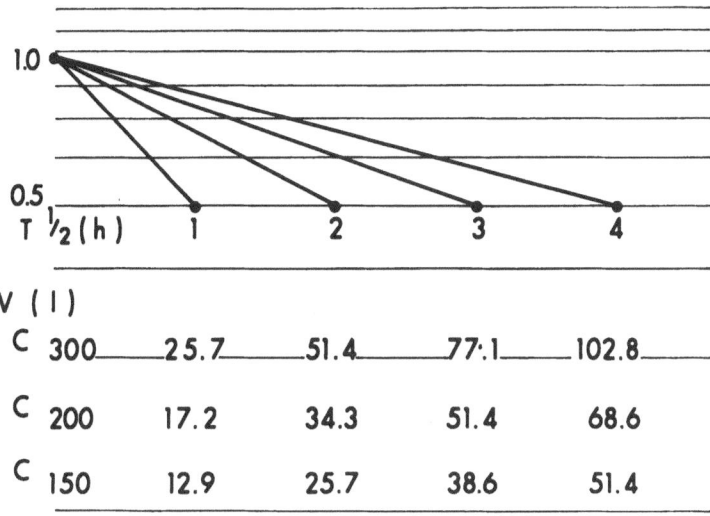

Figure 2. Based on apparent plasma half lives and clearances, distribution spaces can be calculated.

tion is rapid throughout the distribution space during the period of increased elimination, there should be a negligible rebound increment in plasma concentrations after the procedure terminates (Figure 3). The extent of the rebound can be inversely proportional to the fraction of the pool actually affected by the procedure.

Clinical improvement with hemoperfusion suggests that toxins stored in some pools are relatively innocuous. Thiopental exemplifies this behavior (7). Moreover, the elimination rate of toxins by metabolism, the usual dominant mechanism for lipid soluble toxins, may decrease with higher concentrations. This may be explained in part by a rate limited degredation process, i.e. concentration dependent kinetics, and in part by the clinical effects of toxicity such as shock (8). Thus, after treatment, the elimination rate may be increased because of clinical improvement and a decrease in plasma concentration to a level where elimination kinetics are first order.

Pharmacokinetic principles must be considered when interpreting the data from hemoperfusion therapy. Moreover, careful observations should provide new insights about the disposition of poisons by intoxicated patients. Finally, if the elimination rate greatly exceeds intercompartmental transfer, it argues for earlier and repetitive use of hemoperfusion and should stimulate investigation of methods to modify the rate of intercompartmental equilibration.

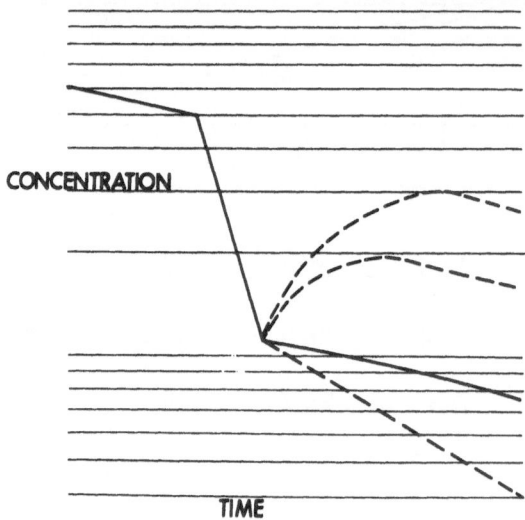

Figure 3. Hypothetical plasma concentrations plotted against time
illustrate possible courses after hemoperfusion.

REFERENCES

1. Schreiner GE, Teehan BP: Dialysis of poisons and drugs. Trans Am
Soc Artif Int Organs 18:563, 1972
2. Maher JF, Schreiner GE: An evaluation of the effectiveness of
dialysis for sedative and analgesic poisoning. Proc Eur Dial Transpl
Assoc 5:246, 1968
3. DeMyttenaere MH, Maher JF, Schreiner GE: Hemoperfusion through a
charcoal column for glutethimide poisoning. Trans Am Soc Artif Int
Organs 13:190, 1967
4. Chang TMS, Coffey JF, Lister C, Stark R, Taroy E: The clearance
of the ACAC microcapsule artificial kidney for glutethimide, methyprylon and methaqualone: In vitro and in patients. Trans Am Soc
Artif Int Organs 19:87, 1973
5. Rosenbaum JL, Kramer MS, Raja R, Winsten S, Dalol F: Hemoperfusion for acute drug intoxication. Kidney Int 10:S341, 1976
6. Nolph KD, Bass OE, Maher JF: Acute effects of hemodialysis on removal of intracellular solutes. Trans Am Soc Artif Int Organs 20:
622, 1974
7. Brodie BB, Bernstein E, Mark LC: The role of body fat in limiting
the duration of action of thiopental. J Pharm Exp Ther 105:421, 1952
8. Maher JF: Determinants of serum half life of glutethimide in intoxicated patients. J Pharm Exp Ther 174:450, 1970

GENERAL DISCUSSION

Thomas Ming Swi Chang

Artificial Organs Research Unit
McIntyre Medical Sciences Building
McGill University
Montreal, Quebec, Canada

ARTIFICIAL KIDNEY

The different novel approaches discussed in this symposium
include dialysate regeneration, wearable artificial kidney, portable
artificial kidney, hemofiltration, encapsulated charcoal hemoperfusion, oral adsorbents and combinations of these approaches. Each
of these different approaches has certain advantages and disadvantages and a combined approach of the different principles appears
most promising. Except for hemoperfusion, the general comparative
perspectives of the different approaches have already been discussed in detail by Professor Kolff in the opening lecture and by
Dr. Burton in the panel discussion. In the case of encapsulated
charcoal hemoperfusion, extensive clinical trial for chronic renal
failure has just been initiated as commercial systems become more
widely available recently. Except for water, electrolytes and urea,
encapsulated charcoal hemoperfusion removes the same uremic metabolites as dialysate regeneration except that hemoperfusion can do
this much more efficiently. Adsorbent hemoperfusion in series with
hemodialysis tested here has now been used successfully by a number
of centers. This has resulted in a significant decrease in the time
required for treatment. It is also being tested here in series
with a small ultrafiltrator to form the most compact artificial
kidney that is presently available. However, this latter approach
will require the further development of more effective system to
remove urea. Further development of urea removal systems are also
required by most of the other novel approaches in artificial kidneys.
Approaches using oxystarch and other adsorbents to adsorb urea or
microencapsulated multi-enzyme systems to convert urea to amino

acids discussed in this symposium are further steps towards this
aim.

DETOXIFIER FOR ACUTE DRUG INTOXICATION

The effectiveness of encapsulated charcoal hemoperfusion and
resin hemoperfusion for acute drug intoxication in suitable cases
has been demonstrated by all centers which have carried out clinical trials. However, speakers and panelists also emphasized the
importance of taking into consideration: compartmental distribution,
time-dose cytotoxic relationships, plasma drug levels, affinity of
adsorbents for the drugs, and other factors. Panel discussion of
this area has already been described in detail by Professor Schreiner
and Professor Maher and therefore will not be discussed further here.

ARTIFICIAL LIVER SUPPORT

This aspect has already been summed up in some detail by Dr.
Berks. In the case of fulminant hepatic failure, our findings in
1972 that hemoperfusion with encapsulated charcoal temporarily
improved the consciousness of Grade 4 hepatic coma has now been
conclusively supported by other centers. Our suggestion that this
may be due to the removal of toxins in the "middle molecular weight
range" has been confirmed by studies elsewhere using dialysis membrane with high permeability to middle molecules. However, despite
a total of more than 100 cases carried out around the world in
different centers statistical demonstrations of the effects of
encapsulated charcoal hemoperfusion on long-term survival are still
not available. This is related to the problem of assessing the
long-term effectiveness of hemoperfusion due to the small number of
patients in any one center; variations of survival rate related to
age, etiology, and grades of coma; and different types of charcoal
hemoperfusion systems being used. It would appear that it might be
easier to obtain conclusive results using suitable animal model
systems for fulminant hepatic failure. The most popular animal
model which has been used for the assessment of hemoperfusion for
fulminant hepatic coma is the partially hepatectomized dog, followed
by devascularization. Unfortunately, this model can only be used to
demonstrate whether treated animals live a few hours longer, but
not for long-term survival. Another animal model is reported at
this symposium of the use here of the galactosamine induced fulminant hepatic failure rat for assessing the effectiveness of hemoperfusion for complete recovery and survival. Further studies
carried out here using this model have shown that early initiation
of hemoperfusion; the blood flow rates and other factors are important determining factors in the recovery of the treated animals.

   The complexity of the metabolic and synthetic functions of the
liver is such that a complete and successful artificial liver
support system will most likely have to be a combination of the
different principles and approaches described in this symposium.
In addition, other approaches using immobilized enzymes, cell
extract or cells are also potentially important. In the case of
terminal renal failure, one would not dream of testing the effect
of long-term survival of the patients by using encapsulated charcoal
hemoperfusion alone without looking after water, electrolytes and
urea. Liver has an even more complicated metabolic and synthetic
function, yet we are apparently testing individual systems each of
which may support only part of the numerous metabolic and synthetic
function of the liver. By doing this, we may commit the grave
error of prematurely misjudging the effectiveness of various liver
support systems. Much more basic and animal studies are required
to arrive at a complete liver support system to effectively change
the long-term survival of "end stage" grade 4 hepatic coma patients.
On the other hand, if further basic research in animals here continues to substantiate this, earlier initiation of treatment in
grade 2 coma using even a partial system like microencapsulated
charcoal hemoperfusion would increase the chance of recovery when
the liver still has partial function.

                        Adsorbent Hemoperfusion

   At this point of development, many attempts to modify and
extend the encapsulated charcoal hemoperfusion approach have been
made, resulting in the availability of different hemoperfusion
systems. This is an important and necessary step leading to final
optimal systems which can combine acceptable clinical performance
with ease of large scale industrial production. On the other hand,
it should be strongly emphasized that at this point of development
one should not attempt to make any generalizations related to
charcoal hemoperfusion on the basis of studies on one or two of the
different systems available at present. There are great variations
in membrane thickness, membrane permeability, adsorbent capacity
and clearance characteristics among the different systems. What is
more important is that the in-vivo blood compatibility of the different systems varies greatly. In those which are not as blood
compatible, the extra coating of fibrin and blood cells on the
surface will greatly decrease an apparent high in-vitro clearance.
Furthermore, the response of the critically ill patients may also
be different. Thus, it is advisable to specify the exact type of
charcoal hemoperfusion system when discussing clinical or experimental results.

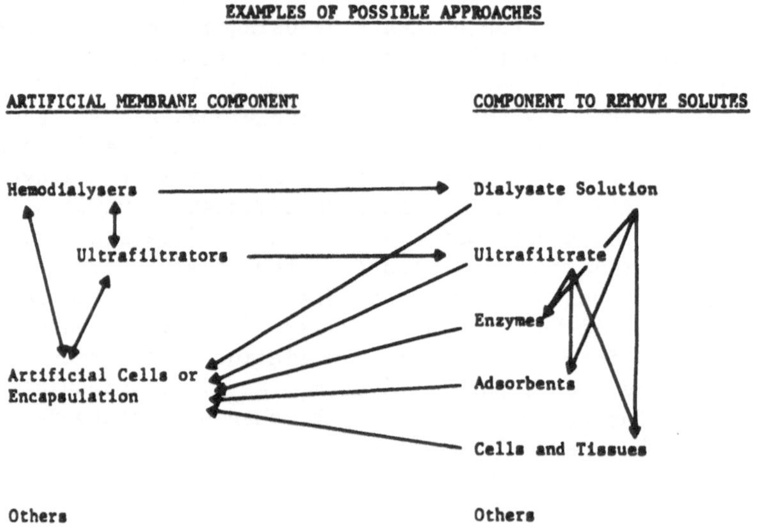

EXAMPLES OF POSSIBLE APPROACHES

Figure 1

GENERAL DISCUSSION

This symposium concentrates mainly on adsorbents and the artificial membrane components related to hemodialysis, hemodia-filtration and artificial cells (encapsulation). However, as can be seen in Figure 1 there is an unlimited number of components to remove solutes crossing those membrane components. Furthermore, there are possibilities in combining the 3 different membrane components in various ways (Fig. 1). Some of these combinations have already been tested clinically. Progress in artificial kidney, artificial liver and detoxification can be best made by keeping an open mind and combining the advantages of the different approaches.

INVITED SPEAKERS, SESSION CHAIRMEN* AND ORGANIZING COMMITTEE**

Dr. I. Amano   Chief, Department of Artificial Organs,
                                Biodynamics Research Institute, Nagoya,
                                Japan.

Professor K. Atsumi*   Director, Institute of Medical Electronics,
                                Faculty of Medicine, University of Tokyo,
                                Tokyo, Japan

Dr. B.H. Barbour   Chief, Nephrology Section, White Memorial
                                Medical Centre, Los Angeles, California,
                                U.S.A.

Dr. P. Berk   Chief, Liver Section, NIAMDD, NIH Clinical
                                Centre, National Institute of Health,
                                Bethesda, Maryland, U.S.A.

Dr. B.T. Burton   Chief, Artificial Kidney Program, Associate
                                Director, NIAMDD, National Institute of
                                Health, Bethesda, Maryland, U.S.A.

Professor S. Carriere*   Professor of Medicine, Hospital Maisonneuve-
                                Rosemont, Montreal, Quebec, Canada

Dr. L.A. Castro   Co-Director, Nephrology Division, Gross-
                                hadern University Hospital, University of
                                Munich, Munich, Germany

Professor T.M.S. Chang**   Professor of Physiology, Professor of Med-
                                icine, Director, Artificial Organs Research
                                Unit, McGill University, Montreal, Quebec,
                                Canada

Dr. A.S. Chawla**   Assistant Professor of Physiology, Head,
                                Biomaterials Research, Artificial Organs
                                Research Unit, McGill University, Montreal,
                                Quebec, Canada

305

Dr. E. Chirito   Lecturer in Physiology, Artificial Organs
                              Research Unit, McGill University, Montreal,
                              Quebec, Canada

Dr. J. Courtney   Bioengineering Unit, Strathclyde University,
                              Glasgow, Scotland, U.K.

Dr. J. Cousineau   Research Fellow, Artificial Organ Research
                              Unit, McGill University, Montreal, Quebec,
                              Canada

Dr. T.A. Davis   Senior Chemical Engineer, Southern Research
                              Institute, Birmingham, Alabama, U.S.A.

Dr. E. Denti   Head, Artificial Organs Division, Sorin
                              Biomedica, Saluggia, Italy

Professor E. Friedman   Professor of Medicine, Downstate Medical
                              Centre, State University of New York, New
                              York, N.Y., U.S.A.

Professor   Professor of Medicine, Department de
J.L. Funck-Brentano*   Nephrologie, Hopital Necker, Paris, France

Dr. M.C. Gelfand   Co-Director, Dialysis & Transplantation,
                              Assistant Professor of Clinical Medicine,
                              Georgetown University Hospital, Washington,
                              D.C., U.S.A.

Professor C. Giordano   Professor of Medicine, Director, Nephrology
                              Division, University of Naples, Naples,
                              Italy

Professor A. Gordon   Clinical Professor of Medicine, UCLA Medi-
                              cal Centre, Los Angeles, California, U.S.A.

Dr. R. Goulding   Director, Poison Unit, New Cross Hospital,
                              London, England, U.K.

Professor L. Henderson   Professor of Medicine, Associate Chief of
                              Staff (Research), VA Hospital, University
                              of California, San Diego, California, U.S.A.

Dr. J.B. Hill   Director, Hemodetoxifier Program, B.D. Re-
                              search Centre, Research Triangle Park,
                              North Carolina, U.S.A.

Professor M. Kaye*   Professor of Medicine, Director, Division
                              of Nephrology, Montreal General Hospital,
                              McGill University, Montreal, Quebec, Canada

Professor W.J. Kolff   <u>Honoured Guest Lecturer</u>
                             Professor of Surgery, Director, Artificial
                             Organs Division, Director, Institute of
                             Biomedical Engineering, University of Utah,
                             Salt Lake City, Utah, U.S.A.

Professor T. Lindholm*   Professor of Medicine, Njurkiliniken, Med.
                             Klin. B. Lasarettet, Lund, Sweden

Professor F.C. MacIntosh**   Joseph Morley Drake Professor, Department
                             of Physiology, McGill University, Montreal,
                             Quebec, Canada

Professor J.F. Maher   Professor of Medicine, Director, Nephrology
                             Division, University of Connecticut,
                             Farmington, CT, U.S.A.

Dr. A.M. Martin   Consultant Physician, Medical Renal Unit,
                             Department of Medicine, Royal Infirmary,
                             Sunderland, England, U.K.

Dr. Y. Nose   Head, Department of Artificial Organs,
                             Cleveland Clinic, Cleveland, Ohio, U.S.A.

Dr. M. Odaka   Associate Professor of Surgery, Chiba
                             University School of Medicine, Chiba, Japan

Dr. Robert P. Popovich   Associate Professor, Chemical & Biomedical
                             Engineering, The University of Texas at
                             Austin, Austin, Texas 78712, U.S.A.

Professor J. Price*   Professor of Medicine, University of
                             British Columbia, Vancouver, B.C., Canada

Dr. S. Prichard   Cardiovascular Unit, Royal Victoria Hos-
                             pital, Montreal, Quebec, Canada

Dr. R. Qules   Dialysis Unit, St. Erika Hospital, Stock-
                             holm, Sweden.

Professor J.L. Rosenbaum   Professor of Medicine, Head, Renal Section,
                             Albert Einstein Medical Centre, Phila-
                             delphia, PA, U.S.A.

Professor G. Schreiner   Professor of Medicine, Director, Nephrology
                             Division, Georgetown University Hospital,
                             Washington, D.C., U.S.A.

Dr. J. Seely*   Associate Professor of Medicine, Director,
                           Division of Nephrology, Royal Victoria
                           Hospital, McGill University, Montreal,
                           Quebec, Canada

Professor S. Sideman   Professor and Chairman, Wolfson Dept. of
                           Chemical Engineering, Technion-Israel
                           Institute of Technology, Haifa, Israel

Dr. D. Silk   Consultant Physician, Liver Unit, Senior
                           Lecturer in Medicine, King's College Hos-
                           pital & Medical School, London, England,
                           U.K.

Professor R. Sparks   Professor of Chemical Engineering, Director,
                           Biological Transport Laboratory, Washington
                           University, St. Louis, Mo., U.S.A.

Dr. D.S. Terman   Associate Professor of Immunology, Baylor
                           College of Medicine, Houston, Texas, U.S.A.

Miss J. Toms**   Secretary, Artificial Organs Research Unit,
                           McGill University, Montreal, Quebec, Canada

Dr. J. Winchester   Nephrology Division, Dept. of Medicine,
                           Georgetown School of Medicine, Washington,
                           D.C., U.S.A.

Professor L. Yaffe   Vice Principal, Administration, McGill
                           University, Montreal, Quebec, Canada

INDEX